PHILIP DARMSTAEDTER

Jones And The Watchers Way

Jones T. Harver And The Watchers Way

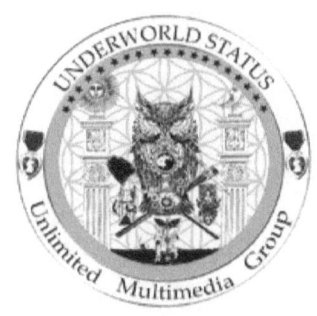

First published by Underworld Status Multimedia Group LLC 2021

Copyright © 2021 by Philip Darmstaedter

All rights reserved. No part of this publication may be reproduced, stored or transmitted in any form or by any means, electronic, mechanical, photocopying, recording, scanning, or otherwise without written permission from the publisher. It is illegal to copy this book, post it to a website, or distribute it by any other means without permission.

First edition

Editing by Kufanya Gentry
Illustration by Andres Rodriguez

This book was professionally typeset on Reedsy.
Find out more at reedsy.com

This novel is dedicated to anyone who has struggled with mental illness and the families who support their loved ones in their times of need. This book is dedicated to the task forces that exist to understand the mentally ill coming up with new methods to help them rather than treating them the same as criminals during their confusions and delusions. A novel, loosely inspired by real experiences, all names have been altered.

Contents

Acknowledgement   iii
Jones T. Harver And The Watchers Way   1
Prologue – Cold Walls and a Journal   2
Chapter Two – The Great Plan   10
Chapter Three – The Interview   29
Chapter Four - Arrival   45
Chapter Five – Splitting Journey   59
Chapter Six – A Day's Job   88
Chapter Seven - Static Beach   103
Chapter Eight - Fall   120
Chapter Nine – Depression Trip   129
Chapter Ten – District Nothing   147
Chapter Eleven - Unclear Discovery   164
Chapter Twelve – Scattered Infiltration   185
Chapter Thirteen – Therapeutic Judgment   211
Chapter Fourteen – Drowning Trap   229
Chapter Fifteen – Grand Escapist   237
Chapter Sixteen – Musical Heart   251
Chapter Seventeen – Imagination Reincarnation   268
Chapter Eighteen – Chase   275
Chapter Nineteen – Mind Chess   304
Chapter Twenty – Warrior Radio   342
Chapter Twenty-One – Split Soul   361
Chapter Twenty-Two – Cleaning After Nepharius   382
Chapter Twenty-Three – Archonic Disaster   407
Chapter Twenty-Four – Celebration Collision   441

Chapter Twenty-Five - Mira's Reality	453
Chapter Twenty-Six – Flash Back	465
Chapter Twenty-Seven – Mira's Appearance.	481
CHAPTER FINALE - THE LETTER	495

Acknowledgement

I want to take a short moment to thank the people involved in helping this book further come to life. Thank you to my editorial team Ivan Ornelas, my mother, my father and my friends for being avid readers. Special thanks to Kufanya Gentry for helping with this project work. I would also like to thank Bill H. for inspiring me to write, my wife for being supportive, Princess. Thank you to my friends who have helped me understand better how to navigate through the publishing industry such as Lora G, Dan Haight and other published authors. Thank you to you, the reader who I hope I've inspired to better the world with progressive ideas and understand mental health from everyone who needs it.

Jones T. Harver And The Watchers Way

Written by Philip A. Darmstaedter

Prologue – Cold Walls and a Journal

The truth is, the world is always cold — like these four psych ward walls. Do you understand what that means? As I sit here writing to you? Yes, people are fighting for their right to live among one another. Like babies that fight for their right to live when no one can understand them. Mothers that are kin to their young try to protect them with their warmth. However, no one talks about what goes on within the coldness, the low-paid among the rich bickering abounds about who their next best son will be. Most of all, you feel the cold in the darkness that surrounds us at night when we go to bed. Sometimes I write this as if it was my last thought, but I'll give you a damn story before it is. One strives for greatness, but we are only as awesome as how we are judged by others. From what I've seen, the people who don't care usually make it out on top; anywhere from the hardcore criminals to those who find the loopholes in the legal system.

Yes, this is the cold hard world we live in. Why should I waste my breath on you? You of all people as I stare at these psych ward walls slathered in white and bumpy asbestos. Honesty? Integrity? Hah! The truth is simple… this world will take from you what it wants; when it wants and where it wants if you don't beat it first. I am Sir Jones, of the Musical Warriors and this is my story. The last of my kind really, somehow a writer and a reader educated by the masses. Never really got called human, but never really cared. Just kind of up and accepted it wherever I went.

PROLOGUE – COLD WALLS AND A JOURNAL

Anyhow, my story starts here on earth in a brazen place among men. It begins when I was a young boy, mostly picked upon and attacked by the wolves of the lands. Do you know what it's like to stare at a wolf dead in the eyes as it flashes its teeth? The taller, fat boys would attack me as I sat there taking in their shitty comments upon the self-esteem that I'd built within myself. Ah yes, these crude words beg you to put yourself in my shoes, don't they? Well, growing up I wasn't much for gifting roses. Rather, I enjoyed the simplicities that followed. A mother who was too smart for my good, a brother who outplayed me, and a father who gave support from far away. All of them meant well, but none of them knew the simple demon lurking inside this story-telling fool. The man from an original rich family plays the guardian of the earth. Yet for it, I get tossed in a psych ward holding cell? Are these people even deserving of my right to earth's existence?

Regardless, today was harsh. I'd been told that even if I wrote these words, the days would go by without remembrance. What's one young buck to do anyway against a world of wolves, thieves, hidden magicians, and destroyers? So, I'll write my troubles and stories, the story of the Mars 42 man. Yes, that's apparently me in this earthly world. An arbiter from mars under the guidance of 42, whatever that means. An agent name was given to me by a distant planet. The oracle who was consistently captured, the ion man, and the dead among the living. I'll get to all that later on. However, in this real world of books and writings, fuck it! There are millions of writers, songs, and other things. After all, just look at all the books! Anyway, sit tight and hold onto your chair so it doesn't rock back and forth. It will be a long journey before this writing is over. Call it Jones' Secret Journal, I suppose. At last, it's a secret to this damned psych ward. But it is not a secret to you, clearly, to you who is reading this now.

"Ahem", Jones cleared his throat and picked up his journal as he looked at the table in front of him next to the empty chair in the room. He continued reading his journal.

It was the year 1983 when I started my passive journey to the outside lands. Lands on the far side of the mountain were woven in grassy fields with flowers wide as the eye could see. The sunset was vast as the rose bushes mixed with the yellow-flowered poppies. "Jonesy! Jonesy!" Niles yelled. His yellow hair extended, flowing in the wind over his shoulders. His voice was so deep the bass waves could be heard throughout the area. "Jonesy! God damn it, get over here!" Yes, the man of his time, the great one too. Grandfather Niles headed down to tell me I needed to get my ass off the mountain tops and run across to the wooden barn pasted in black; pure black burnt from the ashes of a long worn-out battle during his time. "Jonesy! Cut that wood will ya?" annoyed at my slowness he looked at me. My mind wandered back and forth; wondering what to do with the little strength I had in my arms. Moving towards the ax that lay behind the haystack, I swung. I deeply inhaled before making a landing strike, splitting the wood barely down the middle. A few more chops and maybe I'd have a way through the everlasting wooden block.

"Not like that!" Niles screamed out as he walked over wrinkles showing in the sunny day as the midafternoon came along. Grabbing the ax, he made a powerful swing cracking the wood in two." Jonesy, have I ever told you that the world is filled with precious secrets that are hidden away within the wheels of time itself?" he said, breathing heavily. Contemplating for a moment he stopped, reluctant to say whatever was on his mind. "Niles, what the fuck are you talking about?" I replied with a hasty sass. I was eager to get back to chopping wood to perfect form for the fire. My old man went over to the back of the barn pulling out a book, woven with vines, green-colored to the touch. A face is written into the text that just reads "Species" as the title. Glossing over the Species I reached out and Niles took it away. "Not until you finish chopping. However, should you choose to open this book you must be careful. The Species book shows the darkest ends of humanity's greatest kept secrets. Some places you may even end up in if you go running your mouth." He then turned after pointing a stern fist towards the sky.

PROLOGUE – COLD WALLS AND A JOURNAL

"There are ways out there, ways to get out there with your mind. People say you can't break the speed of light, but no one ever thought that thought travels faster than the speed of light." My grandfather broke his statement and continued chopping. Jones continued to write in his journal as a psychiatrist walked through the psych ward hallway. "That's right, sir, madam, I will take you into my past as I finish writing in my journal here, I will read it to you. Whoever you may be, whoever reads this. Niles knew something I didn't...we'll get to that later along with how I am getting out of here. Looking back through the pages, he mumbled to himself. Yes, little me, little Jonesy didn't understand a word at the time, as every word sounded like a jumbled puzzle. Little old me didn't realize that song names were the way that the secret societies were communicating; that through the music itself the universe would react. Or that within the mind, life forms of another world existed, disguised as humans living among people using music to show who they truly were. For example, take that insane person that you saw walking down the street in their world acting strange –they are the Watchers, such intense creatures.

My grandfather went back towards the house as if a gigantic weight was lifted off his shoulders, always a bit of an oddball, but I never knew why until he told me about the book's existence. Little farm boy me. Who knew I'd be telling you this story from a psych ward, a Mars 42 agent forced against his will to obey the laws of earth society?

"Jones, it's almost time for dinner," the psychiatrist yelled from down the psych ward hallway. "Okay! I will be there soon!" Jones replied as he continued to read from his written journal. His roommate stared at him with curiosity from the psych ward as Jones recalled his past to himself, mumbling, staring at the journal. Jones's disheveled face with his beard spiking out from under his chin due to the pills that affected his growth. His fingernails beyond repair continued to write. His hair was brown and wavy almost down to his shoulders. Jones had gained weight much more than his fit figure in the past. His blue eyes traveled back to the journal slowly as he recalled his journey starting in Hawaii, finishing up his last statements. Writing them down in hopes his roommate would gain interest.

A few years have passed as I waltz through the urban areas. I am older now and apparently still sane. Niles had gotten old and wiser beyond his years. He could no longer house me on the farm. After a long debate and discussion of who would take me on, I ended up in my mother's house with my Species book. While zoning out in my computer chair, I started downloading applications and instantly transmitting data, quantum computing was after all a reliable commercialized source. I hadn't much to do among these big walls of the castle that we called home. While looking out my window I felt as if my hair was growing gray, watching the people go by. The Species book was staring me in the face. I couldn't help but start reading. "Sleep very little, speed up your thoughts, and don't stop. Never stop, but never speak, creep to creep your mind will leak; realities will be created among other things, but don't break the chain or else ring…ring…ring."

"Ring, ring, ring?", I said quietly to myself. "What the hell does that mean?" I had heard of a man lacking in sleep who had gone a whole two weeks without it. Many claimed he was going into the future, stating times that would happen; maybe this was a way to connect with the stardust of our subconscious self within the universe.

Letting out a big sigh I decided it would be intense but may be worthwhile just to see what it was like; after all, I had no work and nothing to focus on. The worst that could happen was a possible failure to sleep and an auto knockout, right? If by chance I could get into this future world, the realities of life might not be so boring. Oh, how I was so wrong! I went onto the internet searching out a guy on my phone that I didn't even remember meeting. An old war veteran by the name of Nepharius. There wasn't much to him but his ability to create, or so I believed. As a former high-grade military enlistee, I wanted to ask him what high-profile military places were like, bases, and other historical items. I had a thirst to learn about ancient times, way back, made by humanity for humanity. "Jones," Nepharius started typing. "Simply see everything for what it is, not what it says it is and other worlds will open up to you. There are places seen that people out there will tell you if you seek it." he wrote.

Within those two sentences, I received a few links. Videos started formulating under his words. I received documentaries of ancient Egyptian rulers, CSI and CIA documentaries, and the movie Men in Black. Whatever questions tempted my curiosity, Nepharius seemed to have an answer. "What about the Green Species book?" I asked curiously. Nepharius took a long time to write back to that, contemplating about something he's never heard of. "Come see me in Hawaii," he wrote. "Hawaii? How the fuck am I going to get there?! I'm miles away and have no place to stay?" stating the obvious facts. More importantly, I had no way home. I wasn't making money anytime soon with only volunteer PR work for Animal Beats, a music label company.

Nepharius kept mentioning crazy things and ideas, like the third eye. He wanted to escape from Hawaii; it was like a prison to this man. He was scathed in scars from the past. "Bring the book, I'll pay," he wrote, snapping me out of my reverie from his rapid train of thought. What was there to lose? I mean, I already fuckin' lost everything anyway and there was no place left to go, I already was living a boring mundane life that was worth escaping from. "Okay, I'll fly to Hawaii if you help me decipher what's in these pages. As a front, we'll claim we're working together. Maybe I can stay for a whole week." I replied. In agreement, Nepharius signed off of Facebook.

"If a spiritual type of man wanted to show me the archives of humanity and ways of the world, why shouldn't I go?", I thought quietly to myself. But I was beginning to question my sanity and began thinking about the complications I would end up having to go through as I traveled. I began looking around the room at old stuff made from different cultures. Fine glass vases from China, two in brilliant blue with flowers in red, above those, in contrast, the one with golden lines running up and down with a brass top. I got up to get a drink from the fridge, "This world is so boring, I wish I could create." All within a few seconds, thoughts flooded in. I hit the pipe to try to calm the anxiety; after all, traveling was never my strong point. I decided to journal my thoughts. "A spiritual journey and a front for work, music, and magazines — Truth on we'll call it!" Jones muttered to himself in the psych ward thinking about how he had carried it with him all of this time.

I started turning back towards my room from the kitchen, calmer now. I gallantly waltzed into my room with coffee in hand. I heard the front door open; my brother had come home from work. "Did anything interesting happen today?" Reber spoke in a semi-mundane voice. A man with a couple of cats, he's smart, tech-like, but extremely skeptical. A tall lanky man who could eat his fill and wouldn't be fatter than a string bean. This man could eat three burgers and still look like a twig. I smiled, "Not much! I'm about to take a short vacation; maybe a weeklong one." Reber turned to him, surprised, "Who's paying?" I smirked, "Doesn't matter, does it?" I headed towards the front door without a care in the world, deciding to go on a stroll.

Another psychiatrist walked through the psych ward, "Jones, it's time for your daily meal." she said walking towards the room where he was journaling. Looking up, Jones replied, "Be right there! I'm proofreading and finishing writing today!"

"Can I read that journal when you go to eat?" Jones' roommate asked. "I've just eaten." "Yes, why yes! Read it out loud and read it with form. Others should know of my journey. It would be boring if I read the whole thing out loud to you, wouldn't it?" Jones smiled as he walked out the door. Jone's roommate picked up the journal and continued to read "I, Sir Jones viewed the trees, yes, Sir Jones I will read your story as if I am you". His roommate mumbled. Jones viewed the trees, green and simplistic. It was soon fall; the leaves still hadn't turned to that deep summer red that Jones knew all too well. The walk seemed long, little cars on a small two-way road, close to an unused military base, a train that ran over a bridge with a sign that said, "Do Not Enter", referring to people who took the walk towards the pathways. After a good 20 minutes, Jones came upon the Veterans Center Hall.

There, Jones could pay his respects to those who simply wanted him around. He passed it every day after walking past the dam near the reservoir. Reaching the center of town in a little known place called Lafayette, there's a single bar, your too-good-for-simple Safeway and Whole Foods grocery store battling it out to see which corporation would come out on top, a candy shop and a gym that seems to be barely used within the town limits. "Royce Candy," the building says, copying the Willy Wonka style sign from the movie people used to watch more than three times in a row as a kid. The rest of the town consists of car shops and fancy restaurants; not much to screw about with here.

Jones realized he had gone pretty far in a short time, after all the trip to Hawaii would take place in a day or two and he had to prepare. Turning back through the trees he noticed his phone battery was getting low, not that it mattered much in this day and age with chargers everywhere and a Starbucks down the street. Jones's life wasn't much to follow on social media. Furthermore, the sun was setting, and he had to get back home. The green cover Species Book seemed open to interpretation. Jones had finally reached his decision. He decided he would do what the book said. He would not sleep and see where it took him.

Chapter Two – The Great Plan

The next day started bright and early as Jones's alarm rang loudly, almost knocking him out of bed, startling his peaceful slumber. "Shit, I'm late!" Jones rushed over grabbing the closest items that he left out among the brown bag. He threw his toothbrush and phone charger in after having packed fully last night. "Hawaii, here I come!" shouting to himself. Jones stayed up researching all last night for fun, heeding the woven green book's wording; peeking into randomized cults and societies that existed in the weirdest documentaries he had been given by Nepharius. "Reber!" Jones bellowed, "Reber, get up! I'm late!" His brother was to drive him as he didn't have enough money to head to the airport in a cab. Reber's cat ran by him, crashing into a door, knocking over a clock that broke on the ground. Jones didn't care or think much of it as Reber rubbed his eyes while disappointingly shaking his head.

"Okay, give me five, man," he quietly replied as he picked up the pieces from the clock, and then headed to the restroom to get ready. "Hurry up Reb! Flight leaves in an hour and you know those lines." anxiously waiting by the front door. Reber, dragging his head around with shadows under his eyes, looked into Jones' eyes, "You sleep last night?" "Yeah, yeah," Jones replied. Jones waved Reber away, "C'mon, we've got to head to the airport." Jones reached for the door. Reber commented under his breath, "Could 'a slept in, but insteadWe I have to carry your ass to the airport." Jones stared back, threw his hands up, and said nothing as the both of them went

CHAPTER TWO – THE GREAT PLAN

towards the car. Taking the green woven book with him, Jones got in his brother's car. "Music!" Jones said as the car turned on.

"How 'bout some Rock?" His brother flipped on the radio switch in his car, a 2006 BMW. "Alright, let's just listen". As the satellite radio surfed through the channels, SoundCloud lay dormant in Jones' phone. He hadn't started collecting music yet. Both brothers were completely silent on the way to San Francisco just waiting to arrive at the airport. "Today's weather is slightly overcast." Jones heard on the radio. "Another day, who cares?" he thought. Twenty minutes passed and they arrived at the airport. Reb pulled up curbside at the departures area. "Be safe, good flight yeah?" he said. Jones hopped out. "Off to the magical land of Hawaii," he stated sarcastically as he closed the car door and Reber drove off without looking back.

"Let's see, Gate 22B?" Jones rushed towards the TSA Security line. "ID and ticket please, Sir." requested the Agent. "Ma'am I only have 30 minutes to board. Anyway you can get me by all this?" The TSA Security Agent was unamused. "Sorry Sir, this line is only for premium passengers!" Jones started to go into his head again, "Mundane and boring. Money will always win, I guess." Jones handed his ticket, waiting in line. The sign read: "Expected Wait Time 20 minutes" Time was passing slowly. Jones scanned the crowd playing a game with himself trying to find the funniest costumes. He came across a crazy-looking guy dressed in a brown fedora hat, from the olden times. The color was washed out. He had new, green shoes with a black design. He was wearing a jacket that seemed different from the rest, and it had air conditioning cooling on it. "Man, bet that hat cost a lot," Jones said to the random man. He looked at Jones, "Well, $300 normally, but my friend makes these." replying as he went through the line. "Oh Sir, we'll upgrade you right away." said the TSA Security Agent.

The man showed his phone to the attendant, decorated and colorful, but sleek black in the right lighting. "Huh, never seen that before," Jones thought to himself as he finally passed through security not realizing that the man disappeared into the distance getting ahead of him. Jones headed towards the airplane. "Ah made it on time!" Ten minutes left until boarding." Jones said, looking quietly at his phone.

Pulling out his laptop and the Species Book he packed, Jones started writing music. He loaded up Fruity Loops; a digitized music writing program that many used before. A girl in the boarding area looked him up and down. She seemed to be working at a faster pace than normal. Catching her eye, he smiled. She was wearing a hat; similar to the other man's fedora hat, with dyed hair and contacts that made her eyes red as strawberries. It reminded Jones of the strawberries he used to buy in the supermarket. Feeling odd, Jones got up to stand in line while the woman continued to sit. Ten minutes passed and the plane started boarding. The woman got right up and went ahead of both lines to the left. "First class?" Jones asked the woman. She looked back, "Just a traveler going about my way."

There was nothing special that he could make out. Sleep-deprived, Jones simply believed he was flying to Hawaii. "Where're you from?" he asked, as she passed the doorway. "Monterey. Gotta keep it moving!" No one had ever really talked to Jones in this manner before. "Guess I'll check it out," he said as she disappeared into the distance of the hallways that were darkened with a yellow tint. As he boarded the plane, he wished for a faster, better way. Similar to the two people Jones had just seen. It was almost as if they were completely different people as if they weren't from around here. They seemed inhuman, or perhaps upgraded humans. Jones didn't sleep on the flight. He was too busy and preoccupied, focused on trying to stay awake and trying to write a song. "I'll call it 'Universal'," he said, smirking to himself, preparing to upload it to SoundCloud later.

Already two days had passed since Jones had slept. By this time, he was going through social media as fast as possible trying to gather data for

CHAPTER TWO – THE GREAT PLAN

Nepharius' magazine and the music meetup. Nepharius had paid for the flight and a taxi ride to the top of Kauai Hills where his big house resided. Turns out, he had made a lot of money from one of his books that focused on a conspicuous consumption crowd that believed in the book's teachings. It wasn't any of Jones' business though, and little did he care. As the plane landed, Jones headed towards baggage claim where a man, who was dressed in black, waited. "Apparently, I'm important enough for a formal greeting by my very own taxi driver, huh?" cracking a small joke. They headed for the car. The man in black didn't say a word, just smiled and reached for the Global Positioning System. "Where are you headed?" he asked, waiting patiently for a response. "Kauai Hills, to see Nepharius." The man's eyes went wide briefly, "Right away, Sir." Jones asked, "What do you think about our new phones?" trying to make small talk. "We're bound by them sometimes" he replied, working the GPS.

A simple press on the dot and off the car went faster than usual. The taxi shot up the street, out of the airport. Jones sat there quietly, freaking out in his head about what to do next. The man signaled for Jones to relax; it was as if he knew exactly what the actions taken against his driving were going to be. Maybe it was just Jones' sleep deprivation. Maybe it was being in a new place that stressed him out. Odd things were happening around him which he could not deny, and this was only his second day without sleep. "You are special. We'd like to cordially invite you to the CJX Music Show. Tap to accept our invite and that's all." Best regards, J Cougie." Jones opened up his email as he arrived at Nepharius' doorstep. The two had never met before. Nepharius opened a bit, trying to be cautious not to worry his guest, following the pattern that the other man in black had so courteously done before. Nepharius was bulked up, muscles wide, well built, skin black, and tanned. "Ethiopian," he said as if to read Jones' thoughts on the matter. "Ah, never would have guessed." Jones was smiling like an idiot, trying to hide his nerves from the previous encounter. "That was Buji. Don't mind him., said Nepharius, cutting right to the point. Come, there's work to do."

Truth on Magazine wasn't exactly all that great of a name, but it did have an interesting ring to it," said Jones. The two sat down and started discussing the details of the magazine. "I've met a musician who's a type of church fanatic. He'd be a great man to start with. His story holds with the rest of the crowds. Ask him simple questions and get back to me on the matter." Dumbfounded, Jones stared into the distance, contemplating what he would write. "Why a fanatic?" Jones asked hesitantly. Nepharius's deep green eyes peered into Jones' eyes. He leaned in close as if to make a point. Skeptical that he was being watched, but stern and straightforward in his voice, "Because, there's nothing better than making a magazine that will report on everything in the universe, wouldn't you say?" Jones peeked over Nepharius's shoulder and out the window to see if this was a joke. Was this all in his head? Reality seemed to be intermixing and slipping away as ideas poured into his mind. Was he going insane? "Who am I?" he asked Nepharius with great concern.

It was as if there was something hidden away in this Universal World, something Nepharius knew but wouldn't say. In their silence, Nepharius reached over and patted Jones on the back. "Within time, Jones. For now, we need an artist! I have a few in mind, but if you have anyone better, we can get started sooner." Jones agreed, nodding slightly and then mumbling to himself. He was so sleep-deprived that he thought he was communicating when all he was saying was gibberish. Yet somehow Nepharius understood him. "You've got a long way to go kid. Go get some rest."

Jones passed out. He could see the details in his mind of this brand-new place, floating in the universe. He was seeing the galaxies and the stars. There was a table of five people staring back at him. All of them were cheering at Jones for starting up this magazine with Nepharius. Seems that Nepharius was quite possibly a very famous person who had been gone for a long, long time. "How do you know Neph?" A woman came up from behind Jones as he floated there. Jones twitched. "How uncomfortable".

CHAPTER TWO – THE GREAT PLAN

he thought. "I heard that," she said. "My name's Mira."

Mira was dressed in black and blue. She had pearls around her neck that were multicolored. Her skin tone lightly browned as she leaned in infringing upon his space. On top, Mira wore a golden overcoat with a black hood. Her eyes glowed blue."You can hear my thoughts?" Jones asked with dismay. "Yes, I can," she replied sharply. Then laughing, "Keep your thoughts clean, will you? In this universe, everyone can hear what you're saying. You're a wild kid."

She leaned further in, "Kid if you know him, expect trouble. The man's sort of a universal pirate." she said with dismay. "A very popular universal pirate, with the talents of music and writing." Jones sat there listening intently while he sat on the chair near the bar. He spun lightly to the left catching himself from falling backward.

"Yes,6:00 pm, from the stream of consciousness connected throughout the planets of the galaxy. Trapped from Nepharius's captivity to attempt to keep us all here, like himself. Nepharius is physically stuck but moves freely throughout this stream that you're currently in. As do some of the watchers out there." "Watchers?" Jones replied with a confused look on his face.

He froze as the bar he sat at with her felt all too real. Jones was stunned by Mira's clothing and communication flowing directly towards him. He could see the sound float through the space in the air as she spoke, each color of frequency becoming clearer to him. "Yes, watchers. Normal people like you and I are walking the earth. Nepharius with his two artifacts in hand trapped them in their own ideas, their own imaginations. Now they roam the streets mumbling to themselves, attempting to get here." Jones put down his plastic cup that turned multi-colored as the drink reversed up into his mouth without him lifting a finger. "Why here?" He said slowly, afraid to move. Mira paused for a moment, "Because Jones, here is where we can shape our future. Only the watchers who have been enlightened know this. No other human, no other person walking close to you will ever know this unless." Mira paused, not wanting to reveal the rest to Jones. "Unless what?" Jones said cautiously not knowing what would happen next. "Unless they are like you" Mira got up and snapped her fingers. "That is enough Jones, we'll be speaking sooner than you expect."

She started to fade in the distance in the back of Jones's mind as he drifted further in towards the stars. Jones woke up. Looking around him, he was lying on the tile floor of his guest house. It was almost 6:00 pm. An old lady was standing over him asking if he was okay. Jones looked at her. He was now reoriented back to reality. Jones got up off the floor and backed up. "What's your name?" Jones asked. "Mira, my boy. Don't be alarmed. I just saw you starting to pass out by your door. You seemed in need of trouble. Is everything alright?" This woman was older, wrinkled beyond her age. With pure white skin, long white hair, and a face marked with a brown mole, she had spaces in between her teeth as if she had been chewing on ice. None of this made any sense to Jones. She was not beautiful like the Mira in his dreams. Not even close. Jones started to freak out. "Please leave right this instant!" Then stammering, "T-T- Thank you for waking me. I have to go!"

Opening his phone and now understanding that there was some form of connection with the mysteries from the green-covered book, he started to believe in a new level of communication. Jones looked at his email. "Club CJX is going on. Where are you at?" the message beeped on his phone. Somehow the contact information was showing up directly on his phone. Notes started writing themselves. Jones blinked again and it was gone. He went quickly to his spam email to check the events going on. There was no such thing as a Club CJX. He checked the area on Google and found another club called Rusty's Tech Show. Booking a ticket for five dollars, Jones decided to chase after his mind. Maybe somewhere deep down, he believed he could change the world with his ideas. Somehow,

CHAPTER TWO – THE GREAT PLAN

Jones wanted to figure out how to solve the mysteries and rules that he was self-creating. On the brink of insanity, there was no turning back.

Two weeks after this incident, Jones took a flight out from Hawaii back to his home base in California. The trip to Hawaii had confused Jones, leaving him troubled. Jones realized that he needed to earn some money to live. After his mother picked Jones up from the airport, the two of them got into it before opening the front door. Jones realized that he needed to earn some money to live. "Jones, there's a Juice Shack in town that I hear is hiring. Go already and apply!" she briefly mentioned.

Jones retorted as he headed for the shower, "Okay mom, I hear you. Thanks for telling me about the Juice Shack." Rolling his eyes, Jones closed the shower door to end the conversation, turning on the water full blast. After a long shower, Jones hopped into bed to review his notes and prepare for the next day. He was very tired from the flight home. Trexor had sent a text. "Hey, dude! Welcome home from Hawaii! Want to come over?" Jones replied texting back, "Sure man. I'll be right over."

After a few short minutes, Jones unpacked his clothing and headed over to Trexor's house. As the two of them met, Jones fell asleep right away near Trexor's couch while watching T.V. Jones had trouble sleeping as many ideas passed through his head. His dream world started to feel realistic. There were many faces of people that he felt he knew, dressed up as their best selves. The women and men looked as if they were at the Oscars, dancing vibrantly around the galaxy floor. A car flashed by with three strange old men wearing brown top hats. They were war veterans, with white skin that was covered with blue and red veins. These three men turned slowly towards Jones surrounding him. Without any words, their fingers pointed at him and he woke up.

"FUCK!" he said out loud. Jones' friend looked right at him. "Dude you okay?" Trexor stared at Jones, confused by his actions. "I just had the weirdest dream." Jones shook his head. "I don't know. Do you think different worlds can be connected?"

Trexor laughed, "Bro, smoke some weed. I think you need this more than I do."

Jones took the joint and gave it a puff. "What time is it?" he asked, questioning Trexor. He felt it as if it was a brand-new day. Trexor looked at his phone, "It's beer o'clock. You've been asleep for almost ten hours." "Fuck! Fuck! Ten hours?" Jones swore again. "The show! Shit! We need to go!" Trexor sat Jones back down. "Chill out bro. What type of music is it?" "Electronic Dance Music," Jones replied excitedly.

"Not my scene, bro." Trexor coughed as the smoke hit the ceiling. "I'll get us an Uber." Jones grabbed his phone and called on one. The name on his phone read "Goar".

Jones read his phone. His phone said that Goar will be there in 20 minutes. "Okay, I have time." As Jones got up, he threw whatever clothing he had back on, there was a knock on the door. "GOAR HERE!" the man said, slender with spiky hair, brazen but clean. And he smelled like a million bucks. "What?" exclaimed Jones. "I thought it said 20 minutes." Jones read his phone again. It said time zero until arrival.

Goar smiled, "You might have misread 20 minutes as 2 minutes."

Jones must have been so sleep-deprived that he was misreading the time. However, in his mind, this world was changing as he felt the presence of Goar at his doorway.

"This is too fucking crazy," Jones said to himself as he spoke under his breath. "Okay, this invite will solve everything." Goar silently waited for Jones to walk to the Uber car. Judging him, Goar wondered if the man was crazy, watching him talking to himself. "Oh, great. Another one to deal with." Goar thought.

As Jones got into the car, he leaned back in the rear seat, barely opening his eyes. "So, what do you do, Goar? Besides driving for Uber?" Jones

CHAPTER TWO – THE GREAT PLAN

inquired with his eyes closed. Goar laughed, "Well, I'm retired. But you know that garage near the mall? I own it." "You know people are always getting lost in there. You should put some lights up inside — like they do in Europe — to tell people where they are." Jones suggested.

Goar laughed again, his smile turning into a thinking man's pose.

"You know Jones, that's not a bad idea." Jones then furthered the conversation. "Also, those flying cars? Yeah, we need them in this day and age. I know there are a few out there, but not too many successful ones." Goar sat silently listening to what Jones had to say as Jones rambled on half asleep. Goar was trying to make sense of his words. "Would you like some music?" Goar asked.

Jones mumbled, "Sure…" barely making sense of what he was saying or where he was. Yet somehow Goar was able to understand him. Jones blinked, trying to will his eyes back open. Goar's hairstyle became clean-cut. His sweater now becoming a suit. Has Jones noticed? He couldn't open his eyes, nor did he care anymore as his head spun from exhaustion. The radio popped on, "Here on Galactica Brazur! We have Steph Scarso! One of the galaxy's pop star's new hits." Jones blinked. "Here on baseball today…"

Goar started closely tuning in, "It's going to be a great game." Goar said, trying to bring Jones back to the conversation. Jones mumbled at this point inaudibly. He blinked again. In his mind, the pop star was singing an unheard-of song. He grabbed his iPhone and went on SoundCloud to play from the EDM list. Somehow his phone had connected to the unreleased music. "Hey! I was listening to that ball game!" Goar sighed. "Well, you're the passenger." For the rest of the ride Jones silently sat with Goar. In his notes he put down Goar's name, not knowing why. Jones just felt that he and Goar had connected. Arriving at the club, Goar shook Jones awake, "Hey guy, get up." Jones tipped Goar and got out of the car. Seeing the bottled water, he asked if he could take that and a piece of gum. "Sure.

And thanks." Goar let Jones get slowly out of the Uber ride.

The sign read "Rusty's Tech Show." As Jones approached the building, it was completely run down by rain, rusted as if it hadn't been used in years. No lines of people waiting to get into the club. The security guard immediately lit up when he saw Jones. "Get in man! You're early!" stating it as if he knew who Jones was. "Early for what?" he asked, mumbling. The security guard shined a light on his face. Jones immediately woke up. "What did you say??" the guard questioned, feeling offended by the comment. "Early for what?" Jones asked again, now fully alert as a man dressed in all black with threatening intent.

The guard backed up realizing Jones hadn't said anything incriminating and smiled, "For the party!" he said. After a quick check to make sure Jones had no weaponry, he walked inside. There was a big projector with lights and people were already dancing.

   Yet the club still felt empty as if not many people were showing up. Jones hopped onto Facebook and hit "going" on the event page. As he sat down in one of the seats he was approached by a woman. "Where are you from?" Jones inquired. The woman replied, "Galaxy Mars." Jones laughed, "What are you supposed to be?"

Her partner showed up and they were both dressed with spikes and silver knuckles. They were white-skinned with dark makeup, one green and one black in costume. Both of the women had red hair covered in velvet crossings with sparkles under their eyelids. Jones simply smiled as one sassed at him, "Bulbonii's. C'mon. How could you not know that?" Jones laughed, "Yeah and I'm the man who's making the galactic magazine with the king musician pirate." saying it sarcastically without thought. Instantly the woman grabbed him, "Yo! You don't say things like that out loud." They pushed him on the dance floor. He hadn't noticed, but the speed at which everyone showed up was monumental. The projector that showed dull pictures was now flashing lights. The crowd was filled with creative people.

CHAPTER TWO – THE GREAT PLAN

Hats that weren't flashing before now flashed brightly with red words attached to them. Costumes ranged anywhere from an octopus to dresses of deep red, made out of rusted iron, to fit the theme of the night. It was almost as if people dressed like the universe they were from — making a statement. Jones couldn't believe it.

"OWW!! THIS IS CLUNNZIE FROM CLUB CJX! HOW ARE YOU ALL DOING RIGHT HERE?? WE HAVE A VERY SPECIAL GUY HERE TONIGHT!" pointing right at Jones. The stage crew followed J. Clougie's finger and invited Jones to come towards the front. Jones waddled his way over to the front as a couple of younger kids snickered, "That bro is way too drunk." Smoke blew in Jones's face from the machines. It seemed that the stage crew was attempting to put on their best show. JJones'spresence alone had changed the way people in the club interacted.

"THIS IS THE MAN WHO IS GOING TO CHANGE OUR UNIVERSE FOR EVEN MORE CREATIVITY! YOOOOW!" CLUNNZIE shouted again. "LET'S GET THIS SHOW STARTED! HANDS UP!" In reality, the dance floor was full. However, no one was shouting at Jones. Jones was swaying there as one of his friends showed up to the party. Massi shook Jones' shoulder, "Hey man, you called. Fuck man, we've been to so many shows together. It's been forever." Jones, more awake now, said, "Yeah; I need to get some water." "No man, you need a beer!" Massi held the beer up to Jones. "My man, take it." People started to question Jones's position in the world. He could feel the tension of the high-level energy starting to leave the room. A blonde woman came over wearing nothing more than panties and a bra, completely covered in colored jewels and rainbow stockings. "Jones. Water. It will keep you in this world." she whispered.

Jones saw Massi drunk off the beer in his hand. He felt the disapproval of his friend Massi's antics. Jones looked at the water case starting to rule out beer from his diet, "If water will keep me in this world then I better drink this instead of beer." He went around to the case to pick one up.

Many of the people on the dance floor saw the separation between the two wondering what this crazy man was going to do next.

Jones walked to the in-house bar. "Do you have any healthy beer that's like water? 'Cause apparently, water is an important thing tonight." requested Jones.

The bartender eyed Jones for a bit, deciding whether to accept the sass or not. Jones ended up closing his eyes, falling back into Club CJX mode. He noticed that the room had even more people now. The labels on the liquor bottles read — "red Kavs, blue Kavs, and gold Kavs". Jones sat down and looked around. The bar had green glowing lights, constantly moving. He read a sign, "Put your hands under the bar." As Jones scoffed at the stupidity of the idea, he did what it asked. "Why doesn't this bar just spray water? My hands are so damn dirty." Jones said aloud.

The bartender raised an eyebrow. "What?" Jones repeated himself, this time louder. "Yeah! Why doesn't this bar have a spray that just shoots out water if you press a button? You know, kinda like those grocery store vegetable aisle hose sprays." The bartender just laughed, "Here's a napkin with some water. The restroom over there."

As Jones got up to leave, water spritzed all over his hands. Jones quickly sat back down contemplating his next move. At that same moment, his friend Massi had come up and given him a pat on the back. Massi, wondering wherJones'ss had gone, was glad he had found him. Massi accidentally spilled some water on Jones's hands from behind. Seeing the wet napkin already on the bar, Massi said nothing, sat down, and watched. Jones didn't seem to notice Massi's presence as Jones was locked in conversation with the bartender.

Jones asked the bartender, "So what's with all these labels? These Kavs." The bartender said, "Well, gold is our premium. It's very healthy. Whereas the red and the blue aren't as tasty, in my opinion," knowing that Jones, from his perception, didn't seem to be in his right mind. Jones said, "I'll take

CHAPTER TWO – THE GREAT PLAN

that one." pointing to the premium label, "Pass it my way." The bartender took it down from the top shelf replying sarcastically. "One tasty, healthy drink coming right up." Massi caught on to what the bartender was doing. Jones finally noticed Massi but it was too late. Massi already made his move, belligerently starting a scene with Jones.

"Oi, that ain't healthy bro. He's taking advantage of you!", Massi warned Jones. Jones zoned out, dipping back into Club CJX mode. Massi's presence started to disappear as if his old world didn't matter. Jones was becoming addicted to the idea of thinking that the ideas in his head were becoming his new reality. Massi reached out and paid for the expensive drink scowling at the bartender. Jones waved at Massi to stop being so belligerent. "Alright, man. It's okay. He said it was healthy, so it is healthy!" as Jones took a sip. The expensive mixed drink filled him, imagining the taste of refreshing mint and feeling no effects on his mind. Jones smiled at Massi and the bartender. "See now, it's a great time. I have to get to reporting." Jones smiled.

Massi sighed not realizing yet that Jones had been in his own little world. "Stay here. I'm going off to the restroom," Massi said in a disapproving voice. As soon as Massi left, Jones got up from the bar. He went over to the stage to start talking to the crew from Rusty's Tech Show. "Hey, Brother!" the man said who was dressed in an army suit. He came up with a basic salute like he knew who Jones was. The two of them hugged as if they were old friends who hadn't met for a long time, yet the two souls had never met once. "How have you been?" Jones smiled back, "I've been fine, just traveling around for a while. You?" The man gave him another hug, "Same! It's so good to see you. The private bar is behind the stage." the man said.

An artist name that Jones hadn't heard of before got on stage. The music started flaring up. "Jones! Heard you were becoming a galaxy reporter? The big job you know!" the soldier said approvingly. Jones wondered how far the sound of those spoken words traveled — seeing the lights that were once stationary fall down from the roof. A woman dressed in an elephant inflatable costume walked by as another got on stage to dance. The soldier continued, "You know Jones, go mingle! Enjoy this celebration. It's all yours. You're going to be great. We're going to be so free with something to read." Jones laughed. What had he gotten into? Did he truly understand the scale of the sparks of a movement that he was becoming a part of? The soldier pushed Jones on stage and Jones went towards the woman who was dancing.

"Hiiii!," she waved. "Combat's kind of fun don't you think?" Fit beyond anyone Jones had seen, but still holding a beautiful physique, she started circling him as he circled back. Jones laughed, "What kind of combat are we talking about here?" She poked at him with a single finger, "This one." Jabbing towards his side, he avoided it. Jones jabbed back. Playfully the two were entranced in this motion, letting their worlds collide, not caring about the time nor setting. "Name's Shell and yes, I'm a combat expert. Do you want to learn sometime? You should come to my class." she stated invitingly. Jones found a lead for the magazine. "What type of music do you play there?" Jones winced as he lost focus. Shell had jabbed him right under the rib with her finger. Though it wasn't enough to damage him, it still dealt enough pain to stop the circling. "You've got to keep up. You should come home with me tonight." jumping straight to the point. "I'd love to, but I can't. Obligations," replied Jones. She frowned, giving a pout, "Oh, why does it matter?"

Jones's memory flashed back to what Nepharius had told him, "People will want to play, they won't want to work. Throw off your temptations. You're better than this." Jones frowned too, "Sorry beautiful. Obligation. I'm supposed to report on that guy over there." Jones didn't understand at the time that his statement "who he was reporting on" in his own words was creating his world, but somehow, he knew. When the next performer got up on that small, two-step stage, it all clicked. This was his work. She

CHAPTER TWO – THE GREAT PLAN

walked off and started flirting the same way with others. Jones had turned down his first expert's invite unknowingly. As the DJ got on stage, the crowd's reaction became crazier. Now the club was filled, almost as if people teleported there. The people were moving around at inhuman speeds in bursts of motion. When dancing, the people would slow down. A simple movement from place to place got the person there at a ridiculous speed. Jones joined in running around the giant warehouse dancing in a circle around everyone else while spinning and twisting whichever way he could. Jones couldn't comprehend why the place felt like this. He started to crumble. Everything started spinning. The alcohol started to kick in more than he had expected. "Are you all ready? Who's here from Mars?" the DJ shouted, getting a rapid response. The crowd yelled cheerfully in return as they went back to their dancing.

Massi went off looking for Jones again but couldn't find him. Dancing towards the front of the club, Massi spotted Jones on stage. He headed toward the stage to go and collect him. With this interaction, Jones's mind came back to reality. "Where have you been? I've been looking for you all night!" Massi yelled. "Jones, that's awesome! You were on stage!!! What in the world. Do you know these people?" Jones just smiled, "No idea."

Jones ran over to the corner and took a water bottle. Massi wondered what he was doing. He kept his distance. Like a clown would twist a balloon, Jones started making shapes with a closed water bottle. The plastic reformed within Jones's hands. "Hey, a pony!" he said to Massi. Massi gave him a pat on the back, "You've lost it, man." The water bottle seemed to melt in Jones' hands, into an orb that he could drink from. Massi looked at the water bottle on the floor, twisted into a small knot, unopened, "Come on Jones, let's go." Jones looked back at the DJ, "Hold on. I have to ask this guy some questions." Massi sighed, "I'm going back to the dance floor."

Massi turned and walked back towards a woman to dance with. Jones walked alongside him briefly. "You should dance with him!" Jones said to the woman. She laughed and smiled at Jones but appeared hesitant at the idea of dancing with Massi.

Jones wandered back to the V.I.P. section as Massi became sucked into the music — like a pack of animals, where time wasted was an afterthought. As the set was ending, the lights, the energy, and everything seemed to fade. "Hey! Nice set man! "Jones exclaimed. The DJ waved back, "Thanks, appreciate it."

Jones took out his phone with his notes, "So, what did you do before this?" The DJ frowned, "Not going to even ask my name?" Jones apologized right away, "Oh man, sorry! What's your name.? Mine's Jones." He reached out to shake his hand. The DJ looked at him, "What's up, name's Foue. I was an engineer beforehand, but there was so little progression in that area, I gave it up." Jones was starting his first report.

"So why engineering?" Jones continued. Foue answered, "Well simply put, because I can build upon what's already there. I can create even faster."

The interview lasted for twenty more minutes with harder questions as the conversation progressed. As it was ending, the crowd disappeared slowly. Massi was calling Jones to go outside as it had become late. Jones, feeling tired, had taken the notes on his phone. He thought to himself that it would be awesome if his words could be uploaded to the cloud. Words appeared on his phone screen briefly. "We'll work on it." The words disappeared as quickly as they came. At this point, nothing was phasing Jones. He felt a tug on his arm. It was Massi signaling it was time to go.

Massi was all smiles, "That was so fun, man. Oh my god, we have to do this again, man. This was great!" They hopped in Massi's car. Massi pulled out his bong and started lighting up the weed. Putting on some hard music from the UK grime, Massi started to cool down. Jones sat in silence collecting his thoughts. "Yeah, man. Let's just get home." Jones mumbled as he drifted off. Massi started to drive after blowing out a few

CHAPTER TWO – THE GREAT PLAN

puffs of smoke hitting the gas pedal at a rapid rate. He took off down the road away from Rusty's Tech Show.

The wind blew past on Jones' face as the lights and trees whisked by. Massi seemed to be in his zone as he was playing his darker grime music. Jones started to fantasize about a lady, blonde with curls. She was on the beach, smiling in his dreams, telling him slowly to come over to her and look across the ocean. The rocks were shimmering as she was walking towards him. Yet she never ended up getting to Jones. And he never reached her. It was as if his mind had a block. "Focus. You can drift later." a voice whispered. Jones woke up as the voice hit his ears. Massi was poking him for the last two minutes wondering when his friend would wake up.

"Yo, we're here," Massi said as he opened the car door.

"Thanks for the ride," Jones replied in short, as he closed the door to Massi's Porsche 911. Almost as if he was to be there rapidly in case of emergencies. Jones slowly waded into the guest house while staring at the ceiling. He thought to himself, "A universal car that could travel the galaxies would be amazing. The color yellow would be worthwhile." He flopped down on his bed. Jones thought, "Later. I have to focus." the words silently coming out of his mouth. Nepharius rang his phone waiting on the other end for Jones to pick up. Jones noticed it vibrating on the counter and hesitated. Right as he listened from his bed the phone voicemail went off on speaker.

"We will talk tomorrow when you wake up, but here you go!" Nepharius sent him a link to the ancient Egyptian documentary. "You wanted inspiration for stage productions and writings, right? Watch this. These places exist!"

Nepharius was very excited, but Jones couldn't muster the energy. "Okay, I will try to watch these links later," he mumbled before passing out. "I got our first interview. He was an engineer. It was tough to grab his attention and there was a woman who kept poking me the whole time." Nepharius laughed, "Okay, once I went down the red carpet to meet and talk to D'.

I didn't want to talk to anyone else. I told him what I was there for and what I needed. He started to talk to me then. Just approach it like that and you won't have any trouble. Stay well, my friend."

Running through what just happened Jones drifted off into a deep sleep. Now fully in the dream world, he could recall all of the people on the dance floor and the craziness he felt. He could see them clearly, having fun and laughing. The woman in particular that he had touched once on the dance floor came to him in his dream.

"You wouldn't come home with me, so I had to come to you tonight." she cooed. "What are you trying to do? Jones said, knowing full well what she wanted. "Shh! It's Shell. Just shut up." She stuck her hands down his pants. Jones, understanding the power that he had gained, felt it. Throughout the dream, the feeling connected him to her. Fully going into a deep slumber, Jones was able to finally rest.

Chapter Three – The Interview

The next day, Jones awoke to the sound of a light breeze hitting his window. Sun was illuminating through his window as a beam of small light went in on his leg. The world was becoming more interesting to him from a dull gray place to a colorful one filled with wonders. He looked down as his pants were wet from the night before. "No way," he stated, exasperated at the results he got in the morning. Looking towards the ceiling, he saw a magazine cutout of Einstein. Right next to that was a picture of a gray jeep. His attention to detail had kicked in. Barely getting out of bed, Jones rolled over. Nepharius called, "Hey, we're expecting a call from this artist soon. Are you ready?" Jones rubbed his head, putting on a new pair of underwear and pajamas, "Yeah" he yawned. "Let me grab a cup of coffee really fast." Nepharius spoke again, "Also, I was thinking that we need a logo. Can you get us one?"

Jones thought for a moment, "Well, I know an artist who's not bad. Maybe she can draw us one." Nepharius smirked on the other end, "Yeah, an eyeball would be great. It'd go right over a galaxy background." Jones started hitting ideas back and forth with Nepharius, "We can have two women— one winking with blonde hair and one brunette on the other end. You know, Yin and Yang style." Nepharius sounded surprised, "These are some great ideas. I know some great producers for the music that we'll be playing soon." Jones shrugged, "What do you mean music we'll be playing soon?" Nepharius seemed surprised again, "You don't know?

We start with the magazine to gain traction with others and then promote ourselves through it. Figured you'd understand that."

Nepharius sighed, "Well no problem." In short, he said, "Get me that artwork done!" The artist will call you around 2:00. You have lots of time until then. Get up and shower." "Uh…Thanks?" Jones said, scratching his head. Jones decided to sit down in the chair out back next to the pool, sipping his coffee and thinking about his next move. "It'd be cool if this coffee cup could just close itself electronically." The mug did not react, but in Jones's mind, he could picture it. "Why not just put a napkin over it?" Ms. P giggled from the background as she gardened. His mother had golden blonde hair and brown eyes. Although much older, she still had a young physique. "It's hot out, Jones. You should go back inside." Jones retorted, enjoying the sun, "Well, I'm not the one outside gardening."

The garden was filled with roses, daisies, and different apple trees. There hung a giant fig tree next to the pool. Tomatoes and plums had bloomed as they had been in season. Moss covered the ground in the crevices around the poolside that was paved with red bricks. The water, calm, as if staring right into the ocean, where little triangles were making patterns across the pool.

They both laughed as Jones sipped his coffee. He took the napkin and put it over the mug as it hit back down on the coaster. Looking at his phone for the time, he wondered if his notes could ever be uploaded automatically to the cloud again so he would never lose them. Jones thought he'd send out an idea to his friend at Google later. Why not after all? It'd make his life easier.

"Oh, look at the time. It's nearly time for the 2:00 phone call." Jones went back inside and sat at his computer chair. Turning on his home production system, where two yellow and black KRK speakers were, Jones picked up his iPhone 6. Hand-held and fully charged, Jones got to work. "Hi,

CHAPTER THREE – THE INTERVIEW

this is Jones from Nebulous Magazine! How are you today, Bhusty?" The man had a deep voice. He was calm and collected but proud of his work. "I'm good today, thanks for asking." Jones had never done a phone call interview before. This was his first time. Pulling up his notes on the computer screen, he tapped his fingers to release any nerves that were building in him.

"First, this is an interview. You are aware of this right?" Jones began. Bhusty took a moment. In the silence, Jones's nerves shot up thinking he would hang up. Instead, Bhusty politely replied, "Yes, thank you for taking the time. My management team told me." Jones let out a big sigh, "So, I hear you make Christian electronic dance music. So, it's the Christianity religion with a musical spin on your electronic work? Do I have this right? Can you tell me a little about how you got into this?" Jones asked. Bhusty sounding confident in his abilities started to talk and let loose. Jones could hear it through the phone. "Yeah, growing up I had no place to go but church. I was a broke kid with not much to spare. You see, the music is sort of the universal language and I figured…I figured I could communicate to so many people through this without having to worry about the feelings."

Jones replied ecstatically, "Absolutely. Music is a portrayal of a language everyone can understand." "Next question." Jones asked, chuckling as he read it, "If you had a pickle on stage instead of a microphone, or a pickle-shaped microphone, what would you do?" Bhusty sounding surprised, "Could you repeat that?" Jones repeated the question and Bhusty said it again aloud to himself. "You know kid, I like this interview. It's very different. I'd probably eat the pickle." Jones and Bhusty both laughed. After about thirty minutes, the two of them finished all of the interview questions. Feeling accomplished, Jones pulled up his Microsoft Word and looked at his work. As he was about to relax his phone rang. He answered without looking to see who was calling. "Hello, Jones here." "Nepharius here," he replied. "Good job on the interview. Send it over!" Jones wondered how Nepharius instantly knew that the call had been completed. Jones hadn't even reported back the full story. As requested, he emailed the documents at the man's request. Nebulous Magazine was truly becoming a reality in the stream of the galaxy.

Heading to the kitchen to grab some food, Jones didn't want to clean his plate that he saw sitting in the sink from the night before. "If only this plate would rinse and clean itself. The sides could come up and scrub this damn thing." he thought. "Maybe my next house will have a robot on the sink side that can hand scrub these things for me." Jones sighed looking at the dirty plate. Jones wasn't sure why he was so agitated. Opening up his phone after getting a message from SoundCloud, Jones turned his music on. "A new day of listening." Jones smiled to himself at his first accomplishment. On the SoundCloud application, Jones couldn't believe what he saw. It read, 'Bhusty's Secret Single'. As he shut his eyes and re-opened them, the single disappeared. Jones shut his eyes and re-opened them again attempting to will the single back. On the phone 'Bhusty's Secret Single' appeared again.

A little voice inside Jones's head started to speak, "Stop Jones! You mustn't will against others' wills." Jones thought back to himself, "What do you mean? Others' wills? It's there on my phone!" Feeling agitated, he put the dirty plate back in the sink. Half-finished, it sat there alone with Jones believing it was finished and clean. Jones hopped in his car. The feeling of irregularity was taking over his thoughts. He revved the engine and drove out towards the mall on the bright sunny day. "For a galaxy agent, being in a car powered by music would help. Maybe something joyful." In his mind, the voice came again, "Build this world, Jones. Why don't you?"

Jones looked out at the sky for a moment. He wasn't sure how to answer his question asked to himself. Locked in his mind, wanting to test out what he might be able to accomplish, had him driving around in circles within his head. While he was daydreaming, a car honked at him. Jones closed his eyes again. When he reopened them; the car was completely

CHAPTER THREE – THE INTERVIEW

gone. No sound, no car. Jones was convinced he made the car disappear with the use of his mind. He frowned at the thought. Driving into the same parking lot that the Uber driver, Goar, owned, Jones stopped for a moment, wondering if there would ever be any changes around the same old stomping grounds. Spiritually feeling the wind across his face, he decided that the wind was telling him where to head next.

"There!" Jones said to himself as his eyes turned towards a visualized parking spot. The space was empty before Jones had finished turning the corner. There were two red cars parked on either side, as if the world was guiding him where to go, to be more efficient with his time. Jones took a moment and shook his head, thinking that despite all the weird occurrences happening around him, most were coincidences. Yet he still wanted to believe that maybe this was a different world that he could pursue on his own. He opened the car door of his silver vehicle, shutting the loud music off. He walked happily towards the stairwell. People smiled back at him knowingly, as if they secretly understood what he was doing. Yet, the smiles were simply because Jones had run off to his world inside his head and was smiling himself. Walking down the stairs, Jones felt each step's vibration. The ideas swelling within his head made it ache. He needed to get away from his own devious thoughts. The flight of stairs was almost ending. 'Level

Three' was written on a green-colored leaf to symbolize the cosmic environmentalist grassy feel around him. Arriving at the bottom of the stairs, Jones took a deep breath. His thought was to walk around the mall to get some fresh air so that he could recuperate and gather his thoughts and ideas. While walking towards the shopping mall he observed lots of people, well dressed, flocking towards the various shops. At the main intersection, some people crossed diagonally. Others were walking across the street using the sidewalks in a normal fashion. Jones sat on the curb next to the pizza parlor right in between two short red poles. These red poles lead to the architecture of the whole mall with a sign outlining all the stores' locations and a category listing below. The bench he sat near had a name engraved on it, worn out by time. Jones didn't care much to read it.

Closing his eyes to absorb the sun's natural energy, he started to dream for a moment. "Not yet," the woman on the beach in his dream said. This woke him up. Jones looked around him. At the main intersection where people crossed, the lights had doubled on top of one another. "Huh? That wasn't there before!" Jones said to himself, scratching his head. "And neither was that! Now there were two crosswalk signs on top of one another. One showing the original crosswalk sign and one showing a much newer crosswalk sign on top of it. The sign above had a much newer look only as a trolley passed through. The trolley was different too. It was painted green and red, having gold on the side where people were to board.

Jones in his "off-self" state of mind had started to notice the world around him in ways he hadn't seen before. As he sat up, he felt he had to explore the layout of the mall. Remembering that his phone was becoming a necessity, he diagonally crossed the main intersection and then waltzed into the adjacent iPhone store. "Hi! My name's Alex. Heard you needed some assistance!" Jones was about to object, "No, I…I…"

Then Jones made the connection, "Of course those from the galaxy would be able to read his mind, right?" Jones pondered for a moment. "Here," Jones said, giving his phone to Alex. "Thanks! I'll have this updated for you right away, galaxy man!"

Other workers and people in the store were looking at what seemed to be a bumbling idiot and a man trying to help. Right then, a big burly man came through the door. He started attempting to rap right in front of everyone. Without hesitation, after a single note of rap, the I-team politely told him to leave. "MY CAREER!" "YOU'RE RUINING MY CAREER!" The burly man shouted, storming out in anger. Everyone was now alert in the store. "What's that guy's problem? My gosh, we're in public," various customers

CHAPTER THREE – THE INTERVIEW

said quietly, not wanting the other weird man to be overheard. Jones was amused that they were whispering about him. Finding the idea funny, he grabbed another phone, turned on the oldies, and started singing. Alex put his hand to his face in embarrassment at first, then laughed when a crowd gathered.

After one first practice note was sung, Jones attempted to mime a Frank Sinatra oldie. Then, slowly and surely, he started hitting the notes right on the key. An older lady stood there listening, mesmerized. Jones then asked to spin her around the store. She agreed to laugh. As Jones copied all of the notes and movements, a small crowd of twelve people gathered around. The crowd clapped along as they watched in wonderment. One customer frowned in dismay and yelled at him to stop signing.

Jones retorted, "What? You don't like music?"

As half of the crowd agreed with Jones, and the rest agreed with the complainer, as quickly as the crowd had gathered, it dispersed. One of the iPhone store managers told Jones to stop singing and dancing as he was disturbing the store. Then a clerk came out of the very back of the store to give back Jones's phone. "All updated. Have a case too." extended her hand giving him the free case.

Unpaid, Jones left the store as if the case was given to him without a second thought. Everyone went back to what they were doing. While walking across the street he briefly closed his eyes and then reopened them, willing the lights to change from red to green. He thought that if the world would stop for a moment, the crosswalks would be safe to cross. Jones crossed with the green light and everyone else started moving again. Lost in between his inner mind and reality, he wasn't sure what to do anymore, but knowing his "screw it" attitude, he just didn't care.

Jones imagined walking the streets, with colorful lights strung across, crosswalks flashing. and the sidewalk taking shape in front of him as if to guide him properly. Every rule that he set upon himself, he started to remember. He started to follow these new rules to that eternity of the rabbit hole that was being discovered in his mind. "Red is bad. Green is good. Yellow is happy." New rules started to come together, succeeding in what they meant. There was no gray, as the rules of black and white became absolute. Extremities were now becoming normal in Jones's mind as he swayed in between his lifestyle on earth and in the galaxy.

Jones started to run without care. Without reason, he began to feel like he was powerful in the mundane world that surrounded him. Running as fast as his body would allow; people seemed as if they were coming out of their bodies. People were blurred in doubles as if he took a computer mouse and gave them the photoshop effect. This gave him a whole new perception of how people were viewed through his own two eyes. Ideas rushed into his mind as he went towards the parking structure stairs. Voices became apparent from afar. Due to his consistent lack of sleep, as his body was put in a constant state of stress, his senses doubled. However, as Jones grew addicted to this feeling, he also grew addicted to the thought that he could heighten his senses by having his body in a frenzy. Jones did not want to go back to sleep.

Jones ran up the stairs. Hopping into the car, Jones floored his gas pedal and turned his electronic music up to full. People around him were cautious, wary of the way he recklessly drove. People started to disappear around him as he wished them to be gone. They were disappearing simply by his very thought. "I must be good," Jones said to himself. "I must be responsible with all this." trying to control his thoughts from being heard by the galaxy. "This will be my greatest battle to overcome." Driving home as fast as he possibly could, for the first time Jones felt freedom. Jones arrived through the front door, ran straight to his room. His mother, a bit confused, acknowledged him as if nothing different had happened.

She waved, "Hello. Welcome home! You seem chipper." He smiled, "Just

CHAPTER THREE – THE INTERVIEW

happy. I closed my first interview." Running to his computer, he hopped on and started to look at the link about patterns and theories. The links and ideas that Nepharius sent him were incredible but dangerous. Jones sat down and read. "So, if I follow these theories, I will start to unlock these secrets. Huh?" throwing on his headphones. He began watching the link. As a guy named Saaim came on screen, the video started.

"Imagine a world connected by memories. A world connected by patterns and geographical shapes. The triangle is exactly that. You see, the triangle is one of the perfect geometrical shapes. If one looks through each time, he or she may find the perfect alignment of where to go next. With this knowledge, you can tell who is looking at you, where your life is going, and what may even happen next." Jones repeated the last statement to himself, "What may even happen next?"

As the video ran in the background, he decided that he would test these theories. Walking outside towards the pool, he looked down inside. Seeing the triangles at the bottom of the pool he would catch the sun's rays beaming through each white triangle. Then Jones would look up and then back down at the pool again. He would match his fingers in a triangle directly aligning it with the wooden post from the overhang in the roofline. There was something mysterious about this, but Jones didn't know yet where this would head. The phone rang a second time breaking Jones' focus. He picked it up. "Nepharius here again. Saw you watched the link. What did you think?" Jones took a moment to himself before replying as he started to pace around the pool area. Despite his lack of sleep, he sounded cool and collected. Nepharius isn't picking up the signal that Jones was already too far gone.

"Well, the ideas are interesting. Who's our next expert?" he asked, wondering what Nepharius was after. Nepharius hesitated, "I don't think you're ready. Take the Iron Trail until you reach the Army Base. You will see tanks. Pass by them and head down to the school with the Knights

Emblem as their coat of arms. Ever heard of the Retragrammatron?" Jones, scratching his head, didn't understand. "The what?" he replied curiously. Nepharius sighed, "Do I have to tell you everything? The Retragrammatron. It stems from tetragrammaton. Just Google it.

Listen, I want you to start doing an exercise regime to get buff. All of our guys have to become buff for what we're about to do later in life. You will do 500 pushups, 700 squats, 100 pull-ups, 250 leg-ups. 350 dips, a 5 mile run twice a week, 1-day sprint for cardio, 100 breath practices, and deep sit-ups at least every day. Wear unique clothing, clean-cut and fitted." Thinking for a moment about what he just heard, he wondered how he would have time for anything else. Jones had already exhausted all of his own time and now, here Nepharius was asking for more.

Jones decided that he would Google it later. First, he needed to clear his head. Walking back inside, he scratched his head, then put on his White Sox cap. It appeared most successful men and women seemed to be wearing a brown fedora hat based on the magazine cutouts hung at the top of his wall. Saaim, the man in the video seemed to have one too, so he wondered. His mom shouted at him, "Jones! It's time to get your glasses renewed." He forgot that he had an appointment with the eye doctor that day. "Where are we going mom?" he said back to her, not realizing the time was passing. "To the eye doctor in Oakland. We're also taking a walk into the newly opened hospital building."

Jones nodded in agreement to the plan to get into the car. Ms. P looked at him with concern asking how he had been. He sat silently, not knowing how to answer. "School's going okay…" Jones said, sounding regretful. "Well, keep pushing through!" his mother replied, trying to cheer him up. There was a clear disconnect between the two. The music started playing. It was calming and almost formant. Jones was able to relax his mind as he felt at home. The two of them arrived at the newly opened medical center for the eye appointment. Jones walked up to the big glass display doors

CHAPTER THREE – THE INTERVIEW

and began reading about the history of the place, how came into being. There stood another great, successful man. He was wearing a brown hat. Jones laughed to himself, "Not yet."

"What was that?" his mother asked in a concerned tone. "Just reading the history," Jones replied in a quiet tone. He didn't want his mother to know about the secrets that were held in the history display case. Downstairs the two of them entered the eye doctor's office. Jones peaked around the waiting room, then sat sullenly after being told to be still like a five-year-old by his mother. "Sasaki! Long time!" his mother said ecstatically. "How have you been?" she replied, as they smiled. "I'll be outside." His mother quickly exited the room. Jones smiled back, "It's been a while!"

Sasaki, getting right to work, started making idle conversation, "Yes, it has. Did you know there was a mountain lion recently in our backyard?" Jones couldn't believe it, "A mountain lion? That's quite a feat." Sasaki laughed, "Yes! Yes, put your eyes here, and here." Jones did as he was instructed. Focused on reality, the simple tasks kept him out of his mind of traveling. For the moment, things seemed to be normal in his life. After the eye exam was complete, the two of them went downstairs to the optical shop. Jones' glasses needed some adjustments and possible repair. Nightfall was coming soon. "Looks like we'll have to get this repaired another time. The process took a bit longer than expected, but in return, we'll give you a discount." stated the optician.

The front desk person sat there staring aimlessly. The words on the entry window sign read "Eyes Matter." It reflected off the window. Nodding and thanking the lady his mom turned to him, "Odd, they don't normally give discounts here." Jones smiled, "Maybe it's because I'm special?" he said jokingly. The two of them got in the car to drive home. As night was coming, Jones asked, "Hey, mind if I swim?" "Not at all." she smiled. Heading out towards the pool he got ready for his swim. Taking his shirt off in the cold air unaffected him. His mind was set on jumping in. Running towards the water he dove in without a second thought. Swimming towards the deepest parts of the pool, each angle he noticed was slightly lit up more than the rest in the tiny dots that had formed. The triangles on the bottom stood out to Jones. As the pool lights were turned on, the whole pool looked decorated as if it were a stage for a performance under the stars.

Looking up at the night, the bright specks reflected right over the triangle and dot in the pool. There was another triangle of stars up in the sky. Jones noticed that each of the triangles was in a specific order on the pool walls. It was almost as if he was trying to solve a puzzle. Swimming in between the triangles in a patterned angle he started to spin. He spun as fast as he could, just like the time he danced fast. He started to rise within the pool. Almost feeling that if he spun so fast, he could rise out of it altogether, Jones lost traction. "Damn!," he said to himself quietly, starting at the beginning of the pool again. "Everything is perfect chi. Light and dark." a voice whispered to him in his head. Was it his own mind or the galaxy speaking to him?

Jones went back into position at the end of the pool, imagining himself becoming a giant near the lights, his shadow grew from the beam that hit the bottom. A sound came from the distance above. It was a helicopter hovering overhead. Pure black in the sky, as if it was watching him do his antics. He looked up towards the sky holding one finger out to the helicopter. His middle finger as if to say, "fuck you stop watching me." He felt the presence as it simply hovered there almost as if reporting on his every move.

Jones repeated this process over and over until he felt tired. Sitting in the water of what seemed to be warm against the cold wind that drafted above his hair. "I'll try again in a day or two," he said to himself, getting out of the water that now sloshed around from Jones' movements. Jones went over to grab a towel and dry himself off. "One missed call from Ottie"

CHAPTER THREE – THE INTERVIEW

the phone read. Ottie was one of his old producer buddies from the past. He had met him at a few conventions before Jones moved back home to California. "Heyyy! Long time no see bro. How's it hanging!" Ottie said with a happy voice.

"Been good. What do I owe the pleasure?" Jones replied, making sure not to sound too overjoyed even though he was. "Well, I'm struggling here in Ohio… I was hoping to come down." Ottie needed a place to stay and had some debt from his past. Without a second thought, Jones had said yes. "Come on down! It's only $300 for a bus ride!" replied Jones. Ottie agreed to the idea as they were both musicians. Anyway, it could only help his situation. "Alright! I'll pack my things and be there in a couple of days." Jones, in his state, didn't consider his mom or anyone else around him. Without consulting his family, Ottie was already on his way. Hanging up the phone, Jones realized what he had done. However, it didn't affect his mood. Jones had enough fun for one day. He headed inside to take a shower to warm up.

Jones decided to turn on the hot water. While the shower was heating up almost like a steam bath, he eyed the cat shampoo and reached for it, passing over the regular shampoo. "If you use this you will be feeling sleek!" the bottle read. "Wait you?" he thought to himself, taking the shampoo in hand. He took the cat shampoo and put some on his hair. As he closed his eyes with the shower running. He felt like a Warg running through the empty space. Looking like the dark cat in the shampoo bottle picture, it was almost as if a new idea had sprung about in his universe. "Hm, shampoo that disguises people and turns them into animals. Good idea." he marked off this idea in his head as he continued to shower. After thirty minutes of running water, his mom knocked on the door, "You've been in there awhile. Are you alright?"

Jones replied in a normal tone, "I'm fine!" quickly putting the cat shampoo bottle back under the sink. Quickly, Jones got out of the shower and got dressed. He went towards his room and shut the door. Staring at the ceiling getting ready for his sleep that night, he flopped down on his bed. A random text came through his spam mail. Jones would normally ignore them, but he started to pick them up as if they were real businesses. Jones ran his hand through his hair, feeling slick from the cat shampoo that he had just put on it. "Hey, you. Come down right now and you can meet me." the text from the spam mail hit his phone. "I know you're alone." the text continued.

Jones smiled at the thought. He closed his eyes again to go looking for the perpetrator of the text message. A beautiful woman with black curly hair with shimmering undertones appeared. Jones, now within her sights, waved at her. "Yeah…?" he said in return. "Come meet me. I'm over here in San Francisco and going to Club Yow's on Thursday. See you there." she winked. In reality, the spam mail turned into nothing more than an invitation to Singles Online. Jones now knew where the next big artist would be. He had obtained his lead. As he fell asleep, Jones went into his dream mode. He could see Ottie riding on the bus, laying there with no place to go. He could feel the travels that Ottie was experiencing, almost as if he was looking down on the world from an eagle eye's view. Drifting further and further away.

Ottie was sleeping, leaning on the side of the window, comfortable, yet calm. There were very few people on the bus, coming all the way from Ohio. Jones floated around for a bit seeing if he could communicate but to no avail. Giving up for the moment, Jones went back out into the galaxy lying there in the middle of the stars. He could see an orchestra playing. A giant piano flew past him. As his eyes drifted left, he saw a saxophone that man was playing in the middle. Then, a violinist coming next, complementary to the saxophone. In awe, Jones felt like he was in the heavens of the stars, dancing with them, as they played along inside of the hot gas shapes that radiated the light around them. Jones woke up. His dream, though pleasant, started to feel all too real for what he could

CHAPTER THREE – THE INTERVIEW

admire. Ottie was on his way. As Jones got up out of bed, he paced in the dark back and forth for a bit. "I have to solve these world problems." he thought silently to himself. "There's no time."

Finally, due to the lack of sleep building up in his body, Jones couldn't progress further. Just as his thought had finished, he fell right back into the deep slumber he had tried to wake up from. This time the same woman came to him from before. She had a drink in her hand, smiling wide. "So, I heard you had your first interview!" Jones recognized that voice. "Mira!" he shouted in his mind, as he reconciled within himself, now realizing that his soul was back in the dream world. Mira took a step back, "Shh, shh. You're too loud! I can hear your thoughts, you know!" almost losing her temper.

"Sorry, Mira. I'm excited to see you again." Mira gave him a pat on the back, "You know your pirate friend there is causing trouble back home in Hawaii. He's going to all these experts and gathering them. Many of them are quite strong. Neph says it's for his next big hit, a movie and all that… but we know his real intentions up here."

Jones was surprised as he questioned Mira cautiously. He didn't want to lose his newfound friend that was helping him create his dreams. Unknowingly, the two of them had become partners. This made him the acquaintance of the space pirate he felt he had to protect."What is his real intention Mira?" he asked hesitantly. Mira was well built, physically fit and she had full control as they were communicating. "Listen, I told you to stay away kid. Heed my words or you will be locked up. Just not in the way you'd think. Nepharius recently went exploring ancient Egypt for starters. He broke into a sacred temple and stole one of our precious maps. Guess where that map leads?" She said crookedly, 'Atlantis'! He hasn't told you yet, but all these places do exist. He might even tell you who you really are at some point!" Mira slammed down her drink, "You better stick to your lane kid, I kind of like you."

Jones, wary of the conversation, tried to wake up. He couldn't. "Mira, why can't I wake up?" Mira laughed, "You way overdid it, stupid. Stay here so your body can recover. Sit still." Jones sat still in that make-believe space in his mind. His body lying there on his bed passed out in an awkward position. Mira was right. He had been doing too much, too fast and he went too far from reality. Mira also had an agenda. Why else would she help out? "Alright Mira, I'll be cautious. For the sake of world development, I'll work with Nepharius at a distance."Mira smiled back, "Interesting. For the sake of world development, huh? Well, here's the deal, kid. I want to tell you that you're not only going insane, but some of this is also another reality." She cackled disappearing into the galactic night.

Chapter Four - Arrival

Jones woke up after that. The clock read 7:45 AM. Ottie was arriving soon. Walking out into the kitchen, Jones picked up a banana and ate it. "Uh... hey mom, I have to tell you something. Ottie will be here for a couple of weeks. He has a place to go, but he'll be visiting." he lied. His mom gave an exasperated look, "Well this is news. You mean Ottie, that man you met at the convention in Ohio?" "Yeah mom," Jones replied in short, not wanting to accept the fact that he had just lied to his mother. Jones wasn't very good at lying. "Well, you and Ottie be safe. Also, he can't sleep anywhere else in the house, so he's going to have to sleep in your room. So, figure it out." Jones frowned at the idea at first, but then became accepting. "Yeah alright," Jones said in a defeated undertone. Feeling exhausted, he took time on his own. Ottie was pretty damn good at making music. He figured he could learn a few techniques over a couple of weeks that the man would be here.

Having a whole day to himself, he didn't quite know what to do. So, he went out for a quick stroll in the sun. The leaves and flowers, all dressed in colorful green, turned to blue as he passed them. Jones got an ominous feeling as he looked at a large, beautiful dark red tree that stood in the grassy lands all alone. Around the tree, the grass went from green to yellow. Jones' world was changing around him in broad daylight. "Stop it!!" he said to himself, regaining back some of what he had lost of his sanity. Walking further down the way, he passed an old trail line. The train went overhead here. The old BART line had a single graffiti mark written on the wall that otherwise was extremely clean. A sign read, "Do Not Enter, Possible Old Traps." A nearby, former Army Base was surrounded by barb wire fences, yet the old trail line was still welcoming to any newcomer who dared walk it. Jones walked past the Army Base towards town avoiding the old train line trail. Eventually, Jones arrived at the plaza. He sat at the table and watched around him. "Hey, need work?" a voice asked from behind him. Ottie did need work and so did Jones.

"Yeah actually. I've just been working here as a cashier for the juice shack." The tall woman said smiling, "We'll pay you triple." Continuing quickly, "Here's my card." Jones sat there accepting the card. "Hey, I have a friend. Can he come too?" Her smile became even bigger, "Absolutely! We need all the people we can get." Buying a smoothie for the last time at the shop, Jones looked at the people there. This would be the last time he'd be seeing them for a while. Jones started heading back home thinking about his small stroke of luck. He started to drift again. The Veteran's Center building beautifully stuck out, but also had an eerie feeling to it, as if there were graves behind the building. He glanced at it without going inside the building today. Jones imagined running home at top speed again, however, his body was tired. Ring, ring, ring! "Jones! How are you? Nepharius calling in again. Look, forget Truthton. We'll call the magazine Nebulous!" Nepharius seemed happy when calling today, "I got a part in a movie here. Did you get me an artist?"

Jones thought for a minute, "Yeah Neph. I did. I can send the draft over. It's actually a pretty awesome drawing. The artist drew an eyeball in blue and superimposed it over the old logo. It's a novel new logo that hasn't been used before." "So, Nebulous magazine is a go?" Jones inquired. "Okay, I'll send the new logo over right now." Quickly drawing from his data as he continued to walk towards home, he sent the drawings. Nepharius seemed satisfied with the magazine's development and the way it was coming together. Jones had gathered the essential people to start it off. As

CHAPTER FOUR - ARRIVAL

he neared home, he received a quick call from Ottie who shouted excitedly, "Hey, bro! I'm here! I just arrived." Jones replied equally excited, "I'll be right there to pick you up!"

He rushed home, running in to grab his car keys and a few of his essential items for driving. "Where's my wallet?" Jones said to himself out loud, while looking around the room for what else he needed. He was becoming like that — losing his keys and not paying attention to the small details around him. Jones ran out to the car, putting the music at full blast again. He hit the gas pedal and headed towards the BART station where Ottie would be arriving. While driving, the application Waze showed up to show him directions. Jones could see various other Waze drivers and markers, such as Police or hazards within the user database. One of them even said 'biker'. It was as if he was watching a video game in real-time.

A short five-minute drive to the BART station had Jones there in a flash. He slowly pulled up to the rear parking lot where most people usually waited for arrivals. Waiting outside at the bottom corner of the BART station stairs, he could see him. "Ottie!" Jones shouted with excitement. "Hey! Jones! Long time no see." Ottie laughed, as he walked down the steps. Ottie was wearing a big jacket, a beanie, and combat boots. Though clean, Ottie looked like he had been living on the streets for a couple of days. His blonde hair cut short; his aftershave showed with a five o'clock shadow. Ottie went over to Jones and gave him a small hug. Then right hands clapped together and separated, they dispersed. "Hey, Ottie. I've started a new series with a guy named Nepharius. He's looking for a musician to make some songs for his movie. You interested?" Ottie looked back at Jones, "Let me get settled first, man. It's been a long ride. Also, I need a job man... I'm flat broke." Jones laughed, "I've got you a job already. It's not great, but it's something. The offer is $15 an hour for 12 hours a day. It's for a political campaign."

Ottie shrugged at the information he had heard. Though a job was a job, he figured he would make it to be his. Arriving home, the two of them walked through the white front door, portrayed with old Latin detailing. The house, though large, with a pool outside, had an antique feel to it. The wooden floors creaked as Jones moved. "Jones? Is that Ottie too?" his mom inquired from down the hall. Ottie replied, "Hey Ms. P." Not wanting to have a long conversation with Jones' mother, he quickly moved towards the room to unpack his stuff. "Ms. P, thanks for letting me stay for a couple of weeks." She shouted from the other room, "No problem Ottie. Good luck in your job search."

Ottie and Jones laughed together as they closed the bedroom door. "Hey uh, Ottie, I'm kind of tired. I'm going to take a nap." Ottie nodded his head, "No problem my guy. I'm going to shower and get cleaned up." Ottie went into the shower while Jones slept on the bed. For 30 minutes Jones took a nap into a blank space. When the water stopped, he woke up and went looking for food for Ottie. Wandering into the kitchen Jones yelled out that there wasn't much to eat, "There's some Juice Squeeze and String cheese!" "What! Are we fifteen again?" chuckled Ottie. Jones replied sharply, "Well it's pretty damn good. ever heard of juice freshly squeezed?"

Ottie got out of the shower while Jones took some items from the fridge. "Might as well grab some ramen too!" Ottie said. "Now if only I could insta-spark this." Jones thought to himself. There was no reaction. "Damn, the old-fashioned way then." Grabbing the basics, he started microwaving the food. Taking the ramen and juice squeeze to the room, Jones saw that Ottie had already unpacked and was dressed in a fresh outfit. Clean shaved, Ottie noticed the skateboard in the closet. "Know how to skate Jones?" Ottie asked. Jones nodded slightly, "Not much, but in my past."

Ottie said back, "We'll learn tomorrow. Hey. Do you know that famous guy in LA? We should find him. Like we've been talking about." Jones laughed, "Make it a reality and take a trip, you mean? Let's work this job first. Maybe when it's over." The two of them loaded up Jones' computer,

CHAPTER FOUR - ARRIVAL

and Jones scanned his email. "Hey Ottie, I've got a show for us to go to soon," Jones said without hesitation. "It's called Club Red Toys." Ottie knew a lot more about the club scene than Jones looked at him in dismay, "Club RedToys has been going out of business for over three years. You know, right?" Jones, remembering his email, checked the location, "Yeah, but some other guys are throwing a private party there." Jones pulled out the Numark Pro II, "We can practice at home. It's not CD-J's, but it will do. To celebrate, shots tomorrow?"

They both laughed, "The more you mess up, the more you drink." Both of them looked at one another, having an understanding of why Ottie was really there. "Listen Ottie, the man who's at Club Red Toys goes by the name Yow. It's actually his party." Ottie didn't double-check not knowing what Jones meant. He looked at him awkwardly. "Bro, it's called Club Red Toys. You just said that." "Ottie, just listen to me, bro," Jones replied. "There's going to be some big people there you know?" Jones waited while the computer loaded up showing some of the project work that he was working on. "Listen to this," he said to Ottie, enticing him with the music. "Don't mind that, big things are coming soon. Let's get some sleep early. It's going to be a long day tomorrow." Agreeing to an early bedtime after a long trip, Ottie got ready to call it a night. "Hey Jones, I need to put on something, I can't really sleep like this." replied, "Your choice." He pointed to his laptop. Ottie ended up putting on Frozen from Disney. "Frozen? Really?" Jones rolled his eyes. "Well, it helps me sleep…" Ottie put it on low trailing off.

The computer light had kept Jones up, but he dealt with it as he eventually drifted off to sleep. Ottie also started to drift off to sleep on the sleeping bag on the floor. The air was colder the next day, summertime was a couple of months from finishing. Jones woke up to noise in the morning with Frozen playing in the background on repeat. Ottie was fast asleep on the floor. As the alarm went off, Jones went to get ready for work, brushing his teeth for the job. He then woke up Ottie, "Yo. It's our first day." Ottie got out his bag of supplies — a shaver, some cream to go with it, and a toothbrush with non-fluoride toothpaste. He started brushing his teeth while making stupid jokes. "He-he-ayy, get dat, lookin' fly," Ottie said pointing into the mirror. Jones tagged along, "he-he- big boi, you lookin' fly." Getting ready for the job; Ottie, threw on a plaid over-shirt and Jones picked what seemed to be the 'dressed as casual' look. Getting into the car Ottie asked, "So, what's this job?"

"It's a political campaign for a guy named 'Jeez Yazer'. A Campaign management company invited me in, so I asked if my friend could apply too. The woman said it'd be good."After a short, five-minute drive, the two arrived at the campaign office. Jones parked awkwardly at the side of the building, then walking up the stairs, found the office in a small, rented-out room. Inside were all types of people from multiple cultures. "Today you will be educating people on Jeez Yazer. Just sit down and read the script." spoke the woman who had recruited Jones.

Jones and Ottie took seats as directed in front of a bay of computers. A guy named Tennor sat next to the two of them. Tennor's calves bulged from his body as his blue sports pants hung high. Jones and Ottie both logged in to their computers, tested their microphones, and put their headphones on. "Welcome to this shit hole, boys," said Tennor, who seemed half insane. It didn't matter to Jones. He was already there himself. "Thanks, man," Jones said in reply. Another guy sat next to Jones on the other side, this time of Latino descent. "Yo! I think I've seen you before. Did you go to Kelly's College?" he asked. Jones thought for a moment, "Yeah. Actually, I did!" he replied smiling. "Name's Bernz" he said, sticking out his hand to shake Jones'.

Ottie looked over and saw Jones smiling and then got on a call. At least the crowd seemed pleased to be there. "Nice to meet you Bernz, Jones here." Bernz leaned over during their quick meetup, "See that guy over there, Tennor? He and another guy have a good number of buds on them.

CHAPTER FOUR - ARRIVAL

You two like to try a good smoke?" Ottie and Jones looked at one another and shrugged. "Sure!" Jones stated, "No point why we shouldn't have a quick toke during the break,"

Jones, though not big on drugs, was attempting to get himself back to a better sleep cycle. His imagination was running full speed which didn't allow him to focus on the room right in front of him. "Today!" the Woman yelled, even though she was inside the building, "Today you will learn about how to talk to customers over the phone and keep them on the phone to get the full message across. Constantly. All-day." Jones thought to himself, "Yeah, yeah. I can do that." Bernz and Ottie hit it off, talking to each other for a good amount of time during training. The two of them leaned closer as they talked; the Woman continued, ignoring that the two of them weren't paying any attention during her training.

"You will be going out in teams of two. You two!" she pointed. "What are your names?" Jones and Bernz followed the Woman's finger pointed in their general direction. Each of them said his name. "Great! Jones and Bernz, you will go into the neighborhood and drop off these fliers today." Jones and Bernz sighed, "Well ok." each said, getting ready to go outside. As the two-headed to walk down the stairs, Ottie went to partner with Tennor to continue training on the phones. "C'ya later." Ottie waved. Bernz and Jones obtained piles of the fliers in their hands, each wandering down the steps slowly, looking for a common ground to start up a conversation. "So, do you do music?" Jones asked. He brought up the idea to Bernz not wanting to offend his newfound friend.

Bernz smiled, "Actually, I used to use Pro-Tools back in the day! Listen, I didn't tell you this earlier, but…" Bernz opened his car door and sat down inside. Jones followed suit as the two of them drove towards their first starting point. "But what?" Jones asked curiously. "Well, you see, I've been gaming this campaign for a while. All we do is click this button as if we've knocked on this door. We space it out every hour. It's like getting paid to do nothing." Jones smiled back in return. Laughing at the thought that the system had been so easy to game and to make free money on.

"So, just tap it like this?" Jones reached over and pressed the button as they arrived at their first candidate's house. Laughing at the stupidity of the holes in the counting system, the two of them sat in Bernz's car as time passed by. "Hey, Jones. Check this out." Bernz pulled out his laptop pointing towards the movies that the two of them could watch. "Let's pick out something good." Jones laughed again, "So how did you meet Tennor? And when did you figure this out?" Bernz returned the favor, "Actually, it was Tennor who showed me this trick."

Jones now had a way figured out that he could go to Club YOW without worrying about also being at work. And he would get paid for doing nothing too. The way that the days were progressing continued going in Jones' favor. As the day started to move on towards the night, Bernz pulled out his mini pipe, "Want a toke of weed?"

This is how Jones started his spiral of expanding his mind. Knowing that weed would only amplify feelings that he was already having, he took it anyway. "Yeah, bro! That sounds like a good time." Bernz and Jones passed the pipe back and forth. After lighting up the pipe, Jones noticed the bowl was shaped like an elephant. Jones could feel that the spot they parked in was safe and away from others. "So, what do you think of this shithole?" Jones asked, questioning what thoughts Bernz had about the workplace the two of them were in. "Well, it's not so bad and it's free money for us. So, I don't see a problem with it. Do you? Also, try to keep this a secret between us." Bernz said with a suggestive tone. The two of them packed up their fliers taking them out of the trunk. Throwing away 3/4ths of them into the garbage can, they put the rest back into Bernz's trunk. Right under the campaign manager's nose. They had no idea what these two had been up to all day.

CHAPTER FOUR - ARRIVAL

As Bernz and Jones walked back up the small stairs, past the pet center, they saw Tennor and Ottie walking up towards the building as well. "Heyy!" the two of them waved, waiting before walking into the campaign office. "How was your first day Ottie?" asked Jones. Tennor nudged Ottie making him not want to say much. However, he noticed Bernz right next to Jones, making Tennor less tense. "Didn't do jaaaack!" Ottie said with emphasis, stressing that the two of them had done the exact same actions as Jones and Bernz had done. All four of them laughed together as each took small strides towards the main door.

The Woman stared at each of them with piercing eyes, "Let me see your phones!" Grabbing each phone and taking a quick look, she exclaimed, "Looks good. You're all dismissed for the day." The four of them smiled at one another knowing that it would be an easy continuation from the real canvassing that was taking place. Jones went down the steps with Ottie to prepare for their first celebration after an easy day. "Later Bernz!" Jones smiled, as they waved the other two men off.

Heading home, Jones drove slowly wondering what to do. Feeling sleepy, the weed had only made Jones even more tired. "Hey, you wanted to celebrate, right? After finishing up your first day?" Jones asked. Ottie looked over, replying excitedly, "Of course, my guy!" "Safeway is on the way home. We should stop there for some pineapple juice and vodka." Ottie didn't seem opposed to the idea as the cost was minimal. In the silver Jetta, cranking the music up to the loudest possible volume, Jones drove the distance. With the trees swaying and wind blowing into Jones' face lightly, they entered the Safeway parking lot and each tried to figure out where to park.

As they were driving around, Jones spotted an older man standing alone in the parking lot. Wearing a tattered coat and a colorful hat; a disco ball was hanging from the right side of his pants. He smiled as one tooth showed through while the rest of his teeth were covered in black coating. "Jones...

Watchers are looking at you." Jones heard this in a semi-dream state. He had briefly passed out after turning off the car.

Ottie was tapping him on the shoulder to head towards Safeway. "Hey man, if you need me to drive, I can you know"

Jones rebutted, "I'm fine, Hold on a minute." pushing Ottie's hand off to the side lightly. Jones got out of the car and approached the man who had called out to him. The coat that he had on looked soft now, not tattered. Now smiling, the black covers that he had on his teeth started to melt off as a coating. On the inside of his coat was a mini heater. The man seemed surprisingly clean despite his odd demeanor beforehand. "What's a Watcher?" Jones asked out of curiosity, jumping straight into the point. The strange man laughed, "There are people who watch the world. There are people who change the world. There are people who do things in the world and tag along. We're all the same. We're all heading towards the same destination. It's up to you

Jones, or no one really, to take us there." He cackled again as Ottie approached Jones from behind. "Okay, stop talking to this old homeless dude and let's go get something to drink." he tugged on Jones' shirt. Jones left the man in the corner of the parking lot, not sure how to respond to what the man had suggested. Wandering through Safeway, they walked up and down the aisles. "Bah, no discounts!" Ottie exclaimed, complaining about the price being too high in the wine and spirit section. Jones shut his eyes briefly and reopened them, "There." The vodka that he had imagined, now said $6.00. The entire aisle that previously was missing tags now had yellow tags on all items.

"How come I didn't see these before?" Ottie stated a bit astonished, but happy that the price had now dropped by two-thirds. As they headed towards the front counter where hardly anyone was, another man waved from the back catching the eye of the cashier. "Hey! How are you gents tonight? "asked the cashier cheerfully. Jones didn't know how to answer,

CHAPTER FOUR - ARRIVAL

putting the bottles on the counter. Ottie answered for him, "Good. Just about to go home and party!" The man at the counter laughed. "I can see that." Before even starting the transaction, the strange man from the parking lot came inside, pointed towards Jones and Ottie, and then ran out.

The man at the counter scanned in the vodka bottle, "Oh! Looks like we have a technological malfunction. Actually, these bottles are only $3.00, not $6.00. I'll fix that right up for you." Jones and Ottie stood on the other side of the counter in awe, struggling with how to shrug off the feeling that something odd was going on. Could they accept the major discounts that they had just gotten? They eyed each other and nodded. "Okay, cool!" Both of them gave their own opinionated reactions, "Don't understand, but we're not complaining." they said. The man behind the counter asked if they needed a bag.

"No thanks, sir. I mean, thank you, but I'm good." Jones stated in his confusion. Jones and Ottie wandered out of the store. "Man, that old homeless man was pretty weird, huh?" Jones looked over at Ottie as the two of them reached the car. Ottie got in without saying a single word. "Come on man. You never know what someone's situation is, what someone is going through. Don't judge." feeling annoyed at Ottie's response to what had just happened around them. Jones had caught on to the old man's antics. Being a friend of the cashier at the counter, they got a discount because of the old man's signal. Ottie, wanting to lighten the mood, dropped the subject and moved on to the next, "Let's get home. There we can load up my USB and play our game!" almost shouting it with the unsettled feelings he had swirling in mind.

Turning on the car, Jones heard the low humming. Keeping the windows down so he could focus on the road, Ottie hummed along to one of the electronic dance songs playing in the car. In a short moment, they arrived home. "Hey, Ms. P. We're back," Ottie said with a welcoming tone. By this time, Ms. P had already headed to bed and was fast asleep. There was no reply to Ottie but silence. "Shh," Jones whispered. "Let's tiptoe to our room where the Numark Pro II is and shut the door." Ottie put the USB in and powered up the Numark Pro mixing software. "For every song, you mess up, you have to drink." Ottie challenged.

Jones pulled out the vodka and pineapple bottles, mixing them together in some glasses while Ottie used the mouse to click into the software. "Man, you don't have any of this set up properly, do you?" exclaimed Ottie, frustrated. Jones replied quickly, "No, I haven't really had time to set it up." Ottie reached out, rapidly tapping the keyboard and clicking the mouse. He was already halfway done by the time Jones finished his sentence. "Just load this up into the software and it will auto set up. We can midi control it, but there's no point. These guys already did it."

Jones accepted the setup without question as Ottie seemed to know what he was doing. "Okay," Jones said while pouring the two drinks. Closing his eyes, Jones could picture the crowd of people cheering with their hands up in the air. Their fingers holding up the number one sign as if to come together for a bigger purpose. Jones was on stage playing, shouting "thank you" as if talking to the entire galaxy around him. Ottie poked Jones on the shoulder as he noticed Jones holding the number one signal in the air, "Bro what are you doing?" questioning Jones' antics.

Ottie hit play on the Numark Pro and the first song loaded up. Ottie, as expected, mixed the song flawlessly. Jones, in return, took over the controls and tried to mix in the next song. "Drink!" Ottie said laughing. "Try again." as Ottie pulled up the next song. Jones downed a full shot. Jones again tried to mix the song properly but messed up trying to move his hands into a basic rewind. "D to the rink. You, my bro, stiiiink." laughed Ottie. Jones drank again. "It's okay bro, try again." Ottie encouraged Jones.

This time Jones paid attention to the actual timing of the bars. He was able

CHAPTER FOUR - ARRIVAL

to properly mix the two songs. Ottie didn't mess up but drank anyway. "Alright, that's good to see. You got it!" Jones closed his eyes again and the crowd this time was even bigger dancing around as if he had just been booked for the biggest show in the galaxy. Feeling afraid of the possibility that he was actually being watched, Jones opened his eyes again. "Alright Ottie, that was fun." watching Ottie DJ for a bit more.

Jones dropped down on the bed, "Kinda tired man, can we watch something instead?" "Sure." Ottie put on a documentary showing the music-related places of LA, again. "You know we should make an album," he suggested.

Jones perked up for a moment, "Yeah you know what? We should!" He fell back onto the bed looking at the ceiling, viewing a picture of a jeep cut out from a magazine next to a picture of Einstein. "Then we can try to promote the album the right way." Jones got a text on his phone, just then as he was speaking to Ottie,

"Hey, this is Nepharius. We gotta talk bro. I thought we were a team. Listen; I will talk to you tomorrow." The message was heartfelt, but angry-sounding at the same time. Jones knew he had messed up. He thought things were going well with Nepharius and Nebulous Magazine. "Hey Ottie, you kinda know where to go to LA right? After this whole thing's over on this campaign, I'm in for this." Ottie sat down and nodded in agreement, "Hey, uh, I'm getting tired bro." Jones sighed, "Let me guess, Frozen again?" Ottie laughed. "Yeah man, it's kinda comforting just to have something on." Looking over at the laptop Jones didn't complain this time, "Alright, put it on." Jones slowly drifted off towards sleeping, feeling that he was into his own world.

A woman in a green and black dress came up to Jones from behind as he sat at a bar on a tall chair. The stars aligned like an orchestra. First, there was a saxophone flying through the sky with a man playing it. Then there was a piano while a lady in a black sparkling dress played through. Next, a cello soloist and violinist close to one another in the middle of the stars started playing as well. "What is this? Symphonies in the sky?" he asked the woman. As he turned, he realized who it was, "Mira?"

Mira smiled back at him, "Yeah champ. How have you been?" talking to him in a slightly mocking tone. Jones, again wondering why Mira had been keeping in such close touch with him, didn't question her this time. Rather, he nudged back, "What are you? The Galaxy FBI?" This time Mira smiled, almost breaking composure at Jones' comment, "Something like that. Seems Nepharius doesn't want you to be around him for a while," she said, hinting at the fact that she knew what was going on between Jones and Nepharius.

Jones replied quickly, "Yeah. See Ottie and I are making an album together. I don't know what it's about yet, but Nepharius sounds like he wants to cut connections with me for a little while." Mira laughed at the idea. Holding her hand up to her mouth to stop her chuckling, as if she knew what was about to come, "Oh, you poor guy. You'll learn soon enough not to stay too close to Nepharius. For now, you have this ability. Don't lose it." Jones opened his eyes. The time read 3:00 AM. Feeling exhausted, he wanted to go back to sleep as the wind rustled the bushes outside the windows. Ottie was fast asleep, snoring in the sleeping bag on the floor. "We are going to be so hungover in the morning," Jones said to himself as he slowly drifted back off into his deep slumber.

Chapter Five – Splitting Journey

The next day Jones awoke to the bright sun on his face. Ottie was lying over on his side, sleeping quietly, almost as if he slept like a king. Barely breathing, but healthy, Jones could see that Ottie was feeling comfortable and at home here. Jones rolled out of bed as the clock read 10:30 AM. Having an adequate amount of sleep, Jones got up to prepare for his day. After throwing on his casual clothing for work, Jones poked Ottie on the side, "Yo! It's almost 11:00 AM. Get up!" Ottie rolled over, "Hey, that's like 11:00 PM for me, still. Too much fun last night, bro." intending to go back to sleep. Jones, frustrated, poked him again, "Bro, you said you were going to teach me today." Ottie rolled over again, "Alright. Give me five minutes at least to wake up."

"Alright, alright," Jones said in return. Jones went out the front door to check the weather. The sun was shining with a completely pure blue sky. As he looked behind him, a cloud appeared. 'YOU CAN' was written in big letters directly behind his house. Jones could see the cloud letters slowly dissipate. "Yo!" Ottie called as he came outside. Finding Jones, looked directly at him from behind, "What's going on?" Jones turned around shouting excitedly, "Hey! Finally, you're awake!" Ottie tossed Jones the skateboard with his foot. "Here just get on this and ride back and forth until you get it," he said, not wasting any time in idle chit chat. "We both still have work, bro". he said, noting the time was 12:00 pm. Jones put one foot on the skateboard, slowly waddling back and forth, as it rolled down the minor hill of the driveway. He almost fell off, somehow regaining his balance in time.

"Okay. I got it!" Jones remarked to Ottie. "Great! Now take that board and start practicing by going down the hill a little further." Jones hopped on the board. The board started to catch speed as it was rolling towards the steeper part of the driveway. This time Jones lost his balance, flailing as he landed hard on his side. The skateboard traveled solo further down the driveway. "Left foot first if you're about to fall," Ottie shouted from a small distance away, watching as Jones practiced. "Hey, let me get a skateboard too. Then we can ride together. Fear is the only problem in skateboarding. Get rid of that, and you'll be able to stay on the board." Jones said in return, "Got it. Let's do this." Getting on the board again he found his footing. This time Jones was able to ride fully down the hill and not crash into anything.

Jones looked down at his phone taking note of the time moving by, "Yo, we have to get off to work." he said towards Ottie. Ottie agreed as Jones picked up the board. Opening the trunk of his silver car, he put the board in, "Let's stop at the skate shop before work." Jones turned the music all the way up. Both enjoyed the music loud, as it played through the car with the windows closed up. It didn't matter to anyone around them because they could not hear it. It was as if time passed by with nobody noticing. As they drove down the street towards the skate shop, passing a CVS,

    Jones never paid much attention to his surroundings before. Now he started to notice in detail each building. He spotted the parking lot in front of the skate shop. The word "SKATE" is painted in bright blue, with an entryway up into the store. There was a stairway behind the store going downwards into a narrow curvature.

Ottie got out of the car with Jones following directly behind him heading towards the entryway. The man behind the counter waved them in politely. Immediately the store walls popped out at Jones, tinted in bright yellow.

CHAPTER FIVE – SPLITTING JOURNEY

The store had beanies, skateboards up top, and stickers of all the well-known brands. Jones joked with the man behind the counter, "Professional skater I see." laughing at the idea. "Yeah. Actually, we have a small team." the man replied seriously. Jones was surprised, "A small team? I don't believe it. That's pretty cool." "So, what exactly do you do?" the man said back to Jones wondering why he and Ottie were in the skate shop. "Well… I work for the Yazer political campaign, along with my buddy here." keeping it short and to the point.

Ottie, after looking around, pointed towards the top shelf where the skateboard was that he coveted. It had a rainbow bottom with a man holding two snakes. Around him were six arms on the design. A few stickers were placed towards the bottom which gave it a full length. "That one's pretty sweet, dude," Jones said as the deck came down off the top shelf. The man behind the counter nodded his head in agreement. He pointed out the window behind him towards a flight of stairs. "See those stairs? That was probably the biggest thing we've jumped since." the man said with a bit of humbleness in his voice. Ottie became excited at the thought, "My Dude! That's crazy!" he said, reaching out for some tape deck to put over the newly found board. "New trucks with that too?" Ottie jokes. "Actually…" not giving it much thought, the man agreed, "Yeah, why not? I'll throw it in as a discount and tighten those for you."

After a few minutes of taking a screwdriver to the board, both Jones and Ottie now had functioning boards. They would be able to skate to work and back, continuously getting some exercise. Ottie hopped on his newly purchased board and headed off to work. Jones retrieved his board from the trunk and scrambled to catch up to Ottie. He figured they could skate back to the shop, picking up the car later. Jones went off each curb struggling to catch up with Ollie before reaching the next. Glancing back and seeing Jones, Ottie joked, "Do a tre-flip, bro!"

They skateboarded past the veterinarian pet hospital towards the steps of work that day. It was exhilarating. But Jones knew that work had to be done before they would be able to make Club Yow's that evening. That wasn't the only problem bugging Jones — the message he got from Nepharius was still ringing in his mind. A space pirate from a faraway galaxy telling him that he wasn't exactly pleased with his recent decisions didn't sit well.

Walking up the stairs towards work, they opened the main door, trotting down the old red carpet to that plain brown room once again. Ottie and Jones saw people on computers this time, headphones and jacks connected, voices blaring about the man of the hour that the campaign was promoting. They were taken by surprise, wondering what was going on in that tiny brown room. The woman came up from Jones' left side, "There's donuts and punch on the counter for everyone. This time you two will be making telephone calls to the public. You're late!" Ottie and Jones looked at one another giving the signal as if to say, "What in the flying fuck is going on here?". Each of them cautiously went over to the counter with food.

Ottie reached out for a donut right as Tennor patted him on his shoulder, "Welcome back to the shit hole boys. Seems like we're actually going to have to do some real work today." Jones laughed, "Yeah, It's unfortunate right?" Scratching his head, he attempted to figure out what the purpose of all this promotion was. After a few minutes, the woman walked up to the three of them, "All of you, go sit down next to Bernz over there." She pointed, making sure that work was going to go smoothly for all the hours the company was paying them. The three of them walked over towards the brown table and proceeded to sit down at workstations. A little circle with a voice chat and green dot showed on the screen with a basic script that each worker had to follow as if they were robotic drones in a factory. Jones loaded up his screen, half paying attention to the instructions regarding the phone calls he was about to make. Beside him, Ottie and Tennor were getting ready to make their calls.

CHAPTER FIVE – SPLITTING JOURNEY

Bernz waved from the end of the table, "Hey good to see you again!" smiling as if he was going about what seemed to be the easiest job in the world. Tennor added to Jones' frustration, "See all these people around you? That BART guy over there? He has been here for a while. He's been retired for 30 years since driving for trans and then BART!" Laughing in his short-sided laugh, he threw in a joke, "Fuck this shit, I'm going to go teach English in China." Tennor started reading from the script. Jones loaded up the microphone with his headset on. He felt hollow as his first customer answered, "Hi. Is this Mr. W-?" Jones paused for a minute, trying not to burst out laughing immaturely at the name. "Mr. Weener?" "Or is it Mr. Winer?" He tried to announce it without laughing, but he couldn't. The man on the other end shouted back, "It's Weener!!!" Jones hung up, bursting out laughing uncontrollably.

"What's so funny?" Ottie said to Jones, prodding him, wanting to know what he was laughing so hard about. "Give me a moment," Jones said back, half able to get through his sentences as he tried not to fall off his chair. "Mr. Weener called — "

Ottie immediately cut Jones off of his conversation, "Must have had a big dick to hang up on you so fast." The two of them started laughing, trying not to fall out of their chairs. Tennor and Bernz each ignored their conversation, instead of focusing on making their calls. But they couldn't help notice them laughing hysterically. The woman couldn't understand what had just happened from afar, but looked at them, "Do I need to separate you two?" Ottie snickered, "No, N-o it's alright. My guy is bothering me. I'll willingly move."

Throwing Jones under the bus as Ottie decided to go towards another table, Jones rolled his eyes. He put his headphones back on avoiding the fact that he was thrown under the bus. His mind started to drift as he relentlessly made his calls out to the voters for the Yazer campaign answering on the other end. "Focus." a voice ran through his mind, briefly telling him to go back into the brown room.

Jones knew that if he started daydreaming, people would be able to find him from the other end. He had to control his mind, control his thoughts, to keep himself in his own space. Tennor was looking right at him, along with Bernz, "Hey man. Bernz and I were going to go smoke after this. You in?" he whispered, after seeing what had just happened between Ottie and him. "Sure Tennor, why not?" Jones replied.

Tennor pointed towards another man drinking a bottle filled with green health juice. It seemed he was messed up on some sort of alcohol, hiding himself away in the corner at work. "My friend Jack's coming along too." he laughed pointing at him, "Yeah, that dickhead." Jack was a close friend of Tennor's who had grown up with him. Jones and Bernz shrugged it off going along with the idea. For the next four hours, the five of them sat there making outgoing campaign calls with the rest of the crowd. The woman yelled out to everyone, "Good work. Now put your computers away. Take some leftovers from around the corner if you want. The food is going to go bad otherwise." She eyed the five who had become friends under her watch and smiled at them. "Get on home, I will see you all tomorrow." As everyone else was leaving the room, the five friends decided to do so as well, heading down the cement steps, across the road towards the Burger King. Jack took out the joint and rolled it up while Tennor, Jones, and Ottie stood in a circle. Ottie and Jones both had their skateboards in their hands ready to start riding towards the Skate shop to retrieve the car, and then home. On Jones' mind was Club Yow. He had to get there in time for his interview.

Jack spoke up first, "Who wants this one?" He said offering the joint, as the rest of them were wondering what would unfold. Jones took it in his hand and lit it up. "I'll take a puff then hand it off to you Bernz." lighting up the joint not caring about the fact that it would be amplifying his astral state of mind. Jack took another big sip out of his container of bio mixture,

CHAPTER FIVE – SPLITTING JOURNEY

"Pass that shit Jones." he said, clearly wanting to smoke too.

Instead, Jones passed the joint off to the right towards Tennor who had been talking to Ottie about the day regarding his callers, "Man, people here are so weird. I swear!" laughing at his own comments. Bernz seemed to be getting bored, "Hey guys, I think I'm going to head home. I've got family stuff to take care of." Tennor passed the joint to Bernz, "Puff this shit and then hand it to Jack. We'll all go." Ottie and Jones had to prepare for the show tonight. The five of them dispersed to head home.

Jones and Ottie skateboarded back over the curb towards the building which they originally started at. Ottie looked at Jones for a brief moment wondering when he would mention the club again. The sky had turned into a beautiful pink, mixed with orange, as the sunset behind the mountains. The wind, lightly brushing up against Jones' face, as if it was egging him on in the direction he was supposed to go. Ottie and Jones reached the silver car, left untouched, "Hey free parking!" Jones made a silly joke as the two of them opened the car door. This time Ottie rolled his eyes, "Start the car bro., Let's get on with it. Isn't the show in a couple of hours?" he said, questioning the time.

Jones had no idea as he was high off the joint that the five of them had just smoked. Well, it didn't matter much as long as they showed up at least nearly on time, he thought. "Yeah, let's get ready." Turning on the car with the music blaring, the two of them drove towards Jones' current living place. Ottie and Jones arrived back home in five minutes. Taking both skateboards inside with them, Jones rushed to his room where he received a call from Nepharius. "We're going to have to split for now. You need to go on your own Journey." Jones, surprised by the call, responded with concern, not wanting the connection to end, "What do you mean?" He paced the room back and forth with worry. "You didn't consult the team. You and Ottie want to make an album together. You did not even bother to tell me about it. You need to go out and explore first. Clearly, you know our mission. I have nothing more to say to you for now."

The phone clicked off. Jones heard the basic dial tone. Jones, feeling bothered by this call, went to check in on Ottie. He was getting ready for the show, dressed in plaid. "Yooo! So, you put on cologne like this, because when you walk past a woman's head, they will smell it," he said looking at Jones in the reflection of the bathroom mirror. Jones joked back, "Yeah, I bet all the ladies at Club Yow—. "

He got cut off by Ottie, "Why do you keep saying that? It's the RedToys Club." "Right!" Jones said as he threw on his overcoat over his nicely-made wool pants. Ottie looked back at him, "Umm…Okay…?"

"Come on. Let's go. It's getting late." As the two of them headed out towards the car, Jones threw the keys to Ottie. "Bro, all I have is my expired Ohio license," Ottie said. Jones shrugged, "Well you're good at driving, aren't you?"

Ottie replied with a quick, "Alright dude, but it's your head if we get caught." This time another CD went into the car and the first EDM song started playing. "So where is this place exactly?" Ottie asked. Even though he knew about the place, he hadn't actually been there and he had never driven in the area.

"Downtown Oakland. It's down one of the main streets towards the center of the city. I'll pull it up on my GPS." Jones replied. Driving down the street, Ottie made a quick left while speeding up going around the first corner. A truck with the label 'Good for you, better for us' drove by as Jones started drifting out into his own world. As they got close to the club, Ottie prodded Jones. "Hey bro? Are we close?" Ottie prodding Jones awake.

Jones opened his eyes and looked down the street. He spotted a line of people across the double sidelines. There was a man on the other side of the street who seemed to be homeless. He was wearing a mini lightbulb and

CHAPTER FIVE – SPLITTING JOURNEY

mumbling to himself. Jones thought about connecting to the galaxy world but decided against it as the man wearing the mini lightbulb disappeared between the alleyways. "Yeah, alright. I think it's that place." Jones pointed towards the line of people dressed up in various outfits.

They parked the car across the street and walked briskly towards the other side of the road. The wind flowed slightly behind Jones as if pushing him to the place where it wanted him to go. They walked up to the security guard and passed the line.

"Hey, we're here for Sawn's party," Jones said as the guard stopped them. "Woah, see that line? You need to come in that way." said the security guard sternly. Jones insisted, "We are on the guest list." Sawn saw Ottie and Jones standing outside, "Jones! Glad you could make it!" Waving the two in. "Alright; you two are good to go." the security guard said, letting Ottie and Jones skip the line. Jones got a stamp on his left arm from a woman with long hair who was checking in people. Ottie followed shortly after. "Come up to the bar. I'll get the two of you some drinks tonight." Sawn said in an excited tone. The stairs, showing a purple color of lights in a small hallway, lead upstairs into what seemed to be a rave of people. Jones and Ottie started walking up the stairs, noticing that there were two more big rooms and entryways.

Jones looked around. The bar had glowing green lights all across it with another bar filled with labels. This time he ignored the idea of whether something would be healthy for him or not, trying to control his mind to stay within the realms of reality. Sawn patted him on the shoulder, "See this tattoo?" showing the Aquarius on his arm, "I've been doing these shows for years. Just enjoy yourself." Jones noticed that Ottie had already taken a drink and had run off to chase after a taller woman with pink hair. The lights were blaring out crating multiple designs on the dance floor. Jones took the drink out of Sawn's hand, saying thanks, and wandered towards the corner. Massi had sent him a text prior, but Jones had missed it, "Yo, Jones!" he wrote. "See you tonight?" As Massi had gone to the show as well on his own, Jones realized Massi was walking up to him as he was reading his text. "Hey man. Been looking all over for you!" Massi smiled, as more and more people slowly flowed onto the dance floor.

"This place looks interesting. Let's go outside for a moment." Jones didn't know what he was looking for at this show, but he figured he would find the next expert to interview. Outside people were smoking cigarettes and talking. A strange man with a beaded mask came up to Jones. "Yoooo! How are you?" he said cheerfully. "Well, I uh? Make music. I'm here to do an interview." Jones responded. The man took off his beaded mask, "BRO! I MAKE MUSIC TOO! COME DOWN SOMETIME. GOT A STUDIO!" he said. "Name's TY-Man!!" "Excuse me one moment," Jones said, not knowing quite how to react. The people flooding the outside space seemed amplified in his senses.

"This is Massi," Jones said, gaining his composure, trying to make sense of what was going on. Another taller man in a big coat came up to them. The man leaned over towards Jones, "Hey man, need anything?" Jones said, "No thanks, appreciate it." but keeping a straight shot view, looking over periodically towards the taller man he had spotted in the crowd. A woman was sitting in the back, smiling, with a group of people all dressed in black with logos on their shirts. "Hi! Name's Sunshine! Heard you were here to do an interview?" she said happily.

Was this who Jones was looking for? "Actually, I am... It's a little embarrassing, but Nepharius and I aren't talking right now." Jones replied. Sunshine laughed, "Well, it doesn't matter. does it?" This is E-J and DD." She said pointing at two of the crew members. Jones smiled at the general friendliness of the person, "So, this is why you're named Sunshine?" Jones thought to himself as he drifted out. She replied to him out loud, "Yes!" knocking Jones back into the reality of where he was. Massi, still conversing with TY-man, came back over to Jones. Ottie, who had also walked outside, found the two of them.

CHAPTER FIVE – SPLITTING JOURNEY

"Yooo, who's this?" Ottie asked, wondering what Jones was up to. By then Jones' senses were honed in. "This is Sunshine," he said pointing towards the woman who had green hair and a mashup of colors with a black logoed shirt on. "Sunshine, huh? That's cool." Ottie said, thinking more about the taller woman with pink hair that he was interested in earlier. Sunshine leaned over to Jones, "Uh, your friends don't know, do they?" Jones slowly shook his head as Ottie went back through the crowd. "Sorry about that." Jones said with a basic response, "It's just the way they are." Massi started smoking a cigarette nearby with TY-man, who didn't seem to have much interest in the conversation. Jones turned his attention back to Sunshine.

"So, aren't you going to ask me some interview questions?" Sunshine inquired. Jones felt that the time wasn't right, "You all have emails, right?" he said in return, hoping that he could send the questions and write it up later. Jones was not prepared to take her information down, not with Massi by his side, nor with the entire universe secretly watching Jones's every move. He had to be cautious. Sunshine replied, "Well I don't normally email, but I like your style, so alright." "Send your email to me through here, @ Jones T.H. Galaxy," he said, giving his email address to Sunshine.

The conversation ended abruptly as Massi came up to him, signaling him over. Massi, whispering into Jones' ear, "I just saw my really old-time Ex. Here on stage. She's kind of in a gang, you know. If she sees me, I swear, she will have me killed." Massi started to freak out as Jones briefly scanned the area. "I think you're overreacting there a bit, bro," said Jones trying to calm Massi. Massi raised his voice another octave, "No! Jones, you don't understand! It's really like that." Massi turned and headed into the crowd and went towards the exit. "What was that about?" Ottie said to Jones coming up from behind. "I don't know." shrugged Jones.

As Ottie and Jones walked towards the front past the bar, Sunshine walked by as well towards the next room. Jones pointed her out. "Let's go this way. I feel like the show will be much bigger here for some reason." surmised

Jones. Ottie had already been satisfied, as he was enjoying the music and the sights within the club. Jones and Ottie followed Sunshine into the next room where the music and lights were much different. This time Jones shut his eyes knowing what might possibly be coming next. "Please take me there" Jones whispered to himself, as he started to picture the place. The reflection of water flowed into the ceiling as multiple colorful lights reflected from below. Around Jones, the walls turned into purple and pink fluff with cotton candy holes sticking forward as if one could simply pluck them from the wall. Yellow and green M&M's spilled onto the floor. The music, formerly inaudible, was coming to life in 3D throughout the room, popping out towards his face.

Ottie gave Jones a little shove forward, "Holy shit! That's one of the famous artist connections from the documentary. Those guys own their own record label." Jones slipped back into reality seeing M&M's spilled on the floor. As man dropped them, they rolled across the dance floor, and now they were being crunched by people's feet. An '80s visual was on the big screen, playing on repeat. It showed cotton candy sticking forward in the same way that Jones had visualized it. "If you won't talk to them, I will bro," Ottie said, pretty tipsy off drinks. Jones walked off to talk to Sunshine. As the crowds got bigger, a strange-looking man walked up behind Jones and tapped him on the shoulder. He was wearing spikes on his coat with a black jacket. A punk rocker Jones thought. "Name's Onny. Come with me." Jones was reluctant at first, then said "Where're we going?"

Onny replied, "Shh, doesn't matter. Sawn told me about you. Let's get out of here." Onny walked with Jones. The man had a much bigger build but a soft voice as he was calm, cool, and collected. "Crazy night, right? I heard you were talking to some of our crew about music earlier." Onny began. The two of them were now outside. An Uber was waiting close by. "Listen, where we are going doesn't matter. You'll never see me again, but I've been asked to do this. I'm moving soon anyway." "Where are you moving to?" Jones asked curiously; feeling no intent of a threat, but some

CHAPTER FIVE – SPLITTING JOURNEY

sort of acceptance. "I don't know," Onny said, "Probably Ohio." "Oh, my friend Ottie's from there!" Jones said in return.

Cheery in his response, Onny lightened up, "You know, thanks. You're pretty cool after all." Onny dropped them off at a house with a plain gate that one could almost hop over if they tried. The outside had a small yard. The yard's grass hadn't been cut for a while. Outside people were waiting. "Hiii!" A woman called, half-naked, after making out with a taller man. Both had pure black hair and black coats, the same coat as Onny's. "We hear you two have been really cool lately. Come on in." Their eyes were big as if they had just snorted cocaine. Inside people were holding cups. To the left, others were snorting the snow that had been left to the sides. The musical feeling had surged through Jones as he explored the house. Plain in white, Onny took Jones down a corridor to a green door that was broken part-way. On the couch, there was a man with spiky hair, looking like he had just come out of a fight. Another man was sitting next to him with blonde flowing hair, dressed in a white coat. The coat had spikes on it as well.

"This the guy?" the man on the couch inquired. Onny nodded politely. "Thanks, Onny." the man surveyed Jones thinking of what to say. A beautiful guitar in red lay above his head. "Sit down man. There's space here. Make yourself at home!" A magazine sat in the middle of all of them with snorting candy on top as if it were cocaine. Jones, feeling less tense, poured himself a drink. He sat down on the black couch and shook the man's hand. "Hey, thanks for secretly inviting me here. Nice to meet you." Jones said respectfully. Jones had stumbled upon a band's house, filled with punk rockers and gangsters, who had grown friendly towards him.

"Onny said that you are kind of a musician yourself. Name's Jasper," he replied calmly. "This is Joey and the guy with dreads over there is Noe. That man's guitar skills are something else." "Can't sing. To be forward, but I can try." Jones said, expecting to be shot down as the man with dreads stood up and grabbed his guitar. "Yeah' probably not." the others said laughing in agreement.

Jones felt as if music, being the universal language, would take him wherever he needed to go. He just needed to start following it. Jasper got off the couch and took the red guitar from above the stand. He started playing chords in succession until it seemed like it was becoming a song. "You're pretty good at that. How come you guys haven't had any record deals?" Jones asked, knowing that seeing talent was a specialty of his, after all. Jasper replied, "Well, we did, but some things got all messed up see. So, you know, we're just going our separate ways soon."

Jones felt the deep sorrow in Jasper's voice. The man had a soul for music and he could feel it resonating from the man through every inch of the air. Trying to cheer up the mood, Jones attempted to sing again, Noe followed along as Jones came up with the words on the spot. All dressed in a black sweatshirt, Noe moved his hands in ways Jones had never seen before. Wondering if the man was another galaxy player, he didn't want to upset the flow that Jones was hearing. So, he sat back down. "Hey, you want some beer?" Jasper threw Jones a can. The can this time was a pure gold can. Written on it was 'beer up!'

Following the same rules from before, Jones believed it was healthy and started chugging it. "Man can chug boys," Jasper said cheering up. "Listen, if you ever need any help, let us know. We're around," he said, knowing he'd be there for a while. A text hit Jones' phone just then, "Yo. This is Ottie texting from Massi's phone. Where in the hell did you disappear to?" Jones looked back up, "Hey Jasper. Where exactly are we anyway?" Jones said not even realizing he didn't know where he was. Jasper stood up again in his white jacket with a V in the middle, all in red.

Jones hadn't seen it until now, but it was clear that if these men didn't accept people it wouldn't be pretty. "No problem, we're at Stacy's drive,"

CHAPTER FIVE – SPLITTING JOURNEY

replied Jasper. Jones texted the address to Ottie. Massi had come back to the club as his fears of consequences about meeting his Ex had left him. Jones walked down the hallways in the house at Stacy's Drive. Black clothing and makeup started streaming off people's faces. His thoughts were placing him back into reality. He spoke, "I am Jones! Listen up, Universe! I'm changing everything, one by one! Starting with this world! All I have to do is prove these things actually exist!"

Jones started getting responses. Everyone, but Jasper and the crew in the back room, was staring at him. The guitarist heard Jones' words and started playing even more delicately. Right then another car pulled up outside near the gate. The old brown gate had turned into the shiny metal with holes inside of it as if Jones had stumbled upon a small castle with a fancy gate. Jones smiled as Ottie and Massi showed up at the house, "Alright Jones, time to go bro." The two of them were not trying to stay around any longer than necessary. Jones gave a rebuttal, "C'mon man. Come inside." Ottie took one look inside, as some drunk people floundered down the street, while the rest of them waved goodbye. "No man. It's late. Let's go."

"Alright, fine. "Jones got into his car with Massi driving, while Massi put on Grime music. Jones, feeling irritated by his lack of sleep, turned towards Massi, "Hey man, put on something else. This is too dark for me. I can't listen to dark music right now." Massi laughed, "It's just music, man. It's not a big deal." Jones said it again louder, "Change it, bro." Ottie stayed quiet, surveying the situation. He suggested something else. "Yeah, man. It's alright. How about playing some rap or something simple?" Ottie reached over to the CDs in the car and picked another CD up, "Here, this is good."

Massi didn't argue as he puffed another one of his joints. Jones started to drift off to sleep from the music he was now hearing. The three of them were on their way back to Jones' house after a long night. Not knowing where his journey would take him, Jones was taking more risks by the day.

Massi turned left back towards the forests that surrounded Jones' street. A little triangle painted on a blue school sign popped out in more detail than before as Jones came closer. "What about your car Massi?" Ottie said in the distance. "Don't worry about it. I'll take an Uber back to my car. Let's just get Jones home." Massi started with a worried voice. Jones, in his altered state of mind, didn't care to wake up fully as he droned off to the music. Massi opened the door that Jones was lying on. As the door opened, Jones fell out, catching himself before briefly hitting the cement. "Massi, what the fuck?" he shouted in anger.

"Wake up Jones," Massi replied, laughing at what had happened. Jones rubbed his eyes and got off the ground, "Whatever. I'm awake now." Jones headed towards the front door, wobbling, as he waited for Ottie to join him. Massi called an Uber while taking another joint in his hand, "Hey, what a night huh? There's a beach party coming up soon. You in?" Jones turned around and stuck his thumb up in the air, excited until the next party came up. Ottie followed right behind waving Massi away as the Uber pulled up. "Ay, we better get some sleep. Yo!" Ottie said, wondering what type of reply he would get. "Yeah, we should," mumbled Jones.

Their trip to LA was coming up soon and Ottie wanted to be sure they had enough cash for traveling from the campaign job. Jones passed out on the bed. As he looked at the ceiling again, he wondered when the patterns would end. It felt as if he had started to crack the code of his power slowly when he projected his thoughts. Ottie had no idea what would be coming as he got into his sleeping bag on the floor that night. "Hey, Jones!" Nepharius this time appeared in his dreams, "Champ, did you forget the mission?" Jones floated for a moment. "Don't worry, I put a shazaktu seal around you from manko'tonnen in the old days. Nothing will be able to hurt you in this world or hear us if we don't want them to. As long as we are connected."

Jones's jaw felt weak, a bit as if he felt himself slipping back into a

CHAPTER FIVE – SPLITTING JOURNEY

comfortable position. "So, what do I owe this to you? I thought you wanted me to go on my own journey?" Jones replied. Nepharius put his hand up, "This is why you need time to go on your own journey. You need to be able to experience life, so you understand what being a team means. I'm here to tell you where to go next." Jones tilted his head back, "All right, what's going on?" Nepharius replied, "I'm glad you asked. There's an honor seal and school by an old Army Base close to your house. I want you to go to the school, past the Iron Trail. Talk to them about Retragrammatron. Take note though, they won't take kindly to you. If you mess up, you can never return there. Security will be tight, up and down those roads. When you reach the lemon trees, try to reach me."

Jones scratched his head for a while wondering what the point of all this was. "Why go there? Some kind of family connection?" Jones inquired. Nepharius rocked in his chair. He was wearing a costume that was blue, green, and shiny, representing his Ethiopian heritage. "You'll figure it out. Remember we are collecting experts out there. I have to go. This guy's an expert costume designer, hence that's why I'm wearing this shiny outfit. I don't plan on texting or calling you until the next mission, by the way. Oh, and keep your head down, but your eyes open. A lot is about to happen!"

Nepharius disappeared from Jones' dream, leaving him floating there in galactic space. All colors from what looked like to be the magazine's pieces, floated by his head as the giant eyeball that the artist had created now floated behind him. "Just say 'protection shield' when you need to feel safe in your mind. You will feel a bright white light and warmth as the energy goes through you. You will feel an invisible circle that no one can see or feel, but you." said Nepharius' voice, now fading into the distance. Nepharius' protection was surprisingly warm. Despite the warnings, Jones started to feel as if maybe the gentleman wasn't so bad. Drifting, further along, his mind wandered back to the beach where a beautiful woman with curly hair was. The scenery that was connecting their minds, the galaxy, had now left, leaving the sky filled with colors as water trickled alongside Jones as he lay there.

"You're getting closer," she said. Jones reached out towards her, waiting for her signal to come closer as she wore her bikini. Jones thought through his mind, "This is the right timing. It must be, as no one has stopped me yet." he said to himself, waiting for the general response. Nepharius's voice rang in his mind, "All these people want to do is just play. You need to focus." Jones smacked his face in his dreams as the whole viewpoint went away from him, "Damn... I guess..." The time struck 9:30 AM as Jones woke up from his dream. Ottie was hovering around the computer, already making a new song out of the other one that the two of them had started a few days earlier. N"Hey, so before work each day, I figured we'd get started!" Ottie exclaimed as Jones rubbed his eyes. "Bro, come on...." Jones mumbled. "Feeling tired as it is."

Jones heard hard Dubstep coming through the headphones. He hadn't slept well during last night's dream episode. "At least let me grab a coffee or something," he said, wondering what he had slept through. "Bro I almost got it. Our first song in a while. I took the melody you made and edited it. We'll call it 'Burnout', Cause I'm feeling burnt out." Ottie said. A fun melody with a heavy bassline ran through the song as it rang in Jones's head. "Cool, so... I'm going to grab a coffee," replied Jones.

Jones went into the kitchen. His mom waved at him, "Jones, what time did you get in last night? You guys were out late again, weren't you?" she said, questioning what was going on. Jones replied in an easy manner trying not to have her dig deep, "Well, we've been out at a friend's birthday show." Jones said, dropping her worry a little. "Alright. Sounds like you had a lot of fun. Aren't you two going to work today?" Ms. P said looking outside, "It's a beautiful day, you know."

As Jones sat there sipping his coffee, he looked into the mug. Details started to take shape as if he had supervision. He saw the molecules in the

CHAPTER FIVE – SPLITTING JOURNEY

coffee moving around. Jones blinked and reverted, "Yeah. Uh… yeah." he said distractedly. "Are you okay?" his mom said worried. "I'm fine, mom," Jones said, retreating to his room where Ottie was finishing up mixing the song. Jones finished up his coffee. "Hey, Ottie, we have to go. Grab the boards." Headed out towards the front door, Jones yelled, "Bye mom!" The two of them hopped on their boards and rolled down the street.

Jones had gotten better at skateboarding since Ottie arrived. "Woah, look at that view!" Jones said, pointing at the mountain." "I wonder what's up there with all those blinking lights from the towers." Ottie shrugged, "Who cares bro. Let's get to work." Ottie pushed his foot against the ground pushing the skateboard further upward on the road. Jones followed behind pushing harder uphill. Each of them went faster as cars passed them. Jones couldn't believe he was able to stay on the board as the both of them headed towards the school with the little blue sign. Jones looked over at Ottie, "Hey do you think we can mob it down that hill?" Ottie laughed, "Yeah if you wanna die. Let's try it." Ottie went first down the hill, picking up speed on the right side of the freeway, pebbles scraping up against the bottom of the wheels on the board. Now moving faster from a short-stopped roll, a bigger pebble was in the middle of the highway. Trying to swerve left, Ottie was unable to move the board in time. He put his left foot first to try to stabilize, as the board flew out from under him. He rolled over twice towards the curbside, running forward as he tripped over himself continuously.

The board stopped by the side of the curb as Ottie laughed out loud, "Bro try it." He said proudly. Jones yelled back, "No way! Not after what I just saw happen to you!" Jones went slowly down the hill on his board, slowing himself with his foot as he rolled down the hill. They pushed their boards under the bridge where the BART train went overhead. The rusty old fence looked inviting to Jones as if the curvatures of the barbed wire didn't make a lick of difference. Jones ignored his temptations to walk along the path that said, 'Holes or minefields may still exist here.' Ottie waved Jones forward, going past the Community Garden and the Veterans Center building. At last, they made it into town. "Hey Jones, we're kind of late today," Ottie said as they skated towards work.

"Yeah, we are. We'll be fine." Jones said, already coming up with ways to combat what the campaign manager might say. "Hey Ottie, do you think you can crack a joke as we go inside? If we lighten up her mood, she may not yell this time." Ottie raised his eyebrow "Alright, I'm on it." They sped even faster, trying to reach the stairwell of the building where they would be stuck inside the small, brown office again. As Ottie and Jones moved towards the cement steps, Jones took one last look at the sky of another perfect day. Ottie went ahead towards the main door. "Ayyy, What's good my G?" Ottie said, nodding towards the woman. She looked back at Ottie and rolled her eyes, scoffing, as Jones slid inside following right behind Ottie. "You're late! Where were you two?" she said in a scolding tone.

"Well… ay, just look at these computers. I can update them for you. Can I be your techy?" Ottie said, trying to change the subject. Jones quietly went towards a desk, sitting down in the back. Another man with a black afro eyed Jones wondering what Ottie, his friend, was talking about. "Hey, the name's Gio". he said, reaching out his hand towards Jones. "You guys skated here?" Jones replied quickly as he was coming up with a plan to save Ottie from the wrath of the woman that was about to dock the two of them. "Well shit, yeah we did," Jones replied. "Come skate with us, man," Jones stated in an inviting tone. Ottie took a rain check, "Alright. I'm sorry miss, can I get you a coffee?" he said trying to get on her good side. "Ugh!! Ottie! Sit down, already. Hop on the computer and get some work done." she ordered. With her mood hardly improving, she walked off towards her office door. "So Gio, after work, we can skate a bit in the area towards the garage. You down?" inquired Jones.

Gio held his thumb up and got to work. Bernz and the rest of the crew were bickering in the back of the room as they were about to be sent off to

CHAPTER FIVE – SPLITTING JOURNEY

do more of the door-knocking portion of the campaign. Jones logged into his computer, hyper-focusing this time. After hitting the green light on the computer that told him "go". This time, instead of laughing, he picked up the script and read it. Again, there were donuts in the break room of the small campaign office. A woman sat across from Jones, close to Gio. She kept eyeing him over slowly as if interested to start a conversation. Jones focused back on his computer, not noticing the basic advances that she started. Meanwhile, Ottie sat next to a bigger man. He had a beard and seemed to be high off of weed. His eyes were red, yet no one seemed to notice. "Styles," he said to Ottie, as he sat back in his chair making calls. "Nice to meet ya, Styles." The two of them hit it off in conversation, immediately getting along. "So, the scene is set." Jones thought to himself. "We know pretty much everyone. Now we can go ahead and get away with what we want." Making a plan in his head, Jones hoped to continue screwing the campaign: everyone got paid for minimal to no work, while still covering everyone's ass in case anything spiraled out of control.

As the day passed by, the campaign manager woman stopped everyone who was working on their microphones, "Alright. It's time to go out and drop off more fliers. This time, Ottie you're with Styles. Jones, you're with Tina." Tina was the woman who had been eyeing Jones earlier. She just grew more interested. "Hi, I'm Tina." She said kindly as Ottie walked out the door with Styles. Jones reached out and formally shook her hand, "Jones. Nice to meet you. So, what do you do?" "Well, I'm studying pets." she joked as the two of them headed towards her older car. Something about older cars and Jones always seemed to click. The beige car color lit up in Jones' side glance view as they were walking outside. "Hey cool car," Jones said casually, not knowing how to converse to the opposite sex.

They started to drive towards their territory to door knock, drop off fliers, and take surveys for the Yazer political campaign. Jones didn't want to work that day, but didn't want to break his word either. An oldies song played in the car that he didn't recognize. "So why do you want to be a vet?" he asked. Tina drove to an area where Jones could be dropped off, "Well animals, they're great. They can figure out how you're feeling about others from miles away." Tina said. She moved around in her seat, adjusting to it to be more comfortable. "So, what do you do Jones, besides the campaign?" studying him for a moment, then put her eyes back on the road. "Well, I make music. It's kind of my thing." Jones said in return. "Hey, we're here. Drop me off at this corner." Jones got out at the corner, noting the first house to walk to. "See you later," Tina said as she headed off to her territory.

"Yeah" Jones replied, as he pulled out the company phone that the woman from the campaign office gave him. Jones fake marked the first address and quickly went off to grab some food. As he started walking down the road enjoying the scenery, he started. feeling bad for doing no work. So, he dropped off fliers at the second address. Jones continued down the road in the unfamiliar area. He saw a park close by and decided to take a seat watching the clouds go by. He started surveying the people passing and watching the way they walked.

"I bet everyone that walks by here, walks across the same pathway at least once." he thought to himself, laying down in the grass. A woman smiled at him from a distance, wearing a brown hat. She was walking her dog and stopped to stare at Jones. It was almost as if what Tina had told him earlier was coming to life. Jones could feel the energy around him. He smiled back at the lady as she and her dog moved right along. He wondered how Ottie and Styles were doing. Jones picked up the phone and gave Ottie a call. It rang four times, Ottie finally picked it up. "Yo, I'm skateboarding. Eating some Fritos. What's good?" Ottie said. "You didn't tell Styles yet, right? We should tell these guys. Don't you think so?" Jones asked.

"Yeah! Styles is pretty dope. He used to deliver drugs for a guy driving Bugatti's and shit. Of course, he stopped that since high school, but his story is cool. The man won't say a word." Ottie said as he came up towards

CHAPTER FIVE – SPLITTING JOURNEY

his next door to canvass. Ottie started taking the survey. "Listen, I'm pretty bored, so I'm doing some work today." The phone clicked off. Jones got up from the park and slowly walked down the pathway back towards the urban road. Feeling hungry, he thought of grabbing some food. Reaching into his right pocket, he found a small bag of chips and started eating it. "I better tell Tina." Jones thought to himself. "After all, why not? I can get away with more this way. I mean the worst that could happen is the entire place finds outright?" Hearing laughter in his head from the Galaxy, Jones shook his head in an attempt to get his mind to stop wandering. "Well shit, I just thought that thought and now it's going to happen." Jones instantly looked down with his hands in his head, as if he could have done a lot better with his thoughts. "Damn! I mean, really? Damn! I need to think only good thoughts and ideas. This power is too much for me to control. Okay, calm down." Jones said as he mumbled repeatedly to himself.

Jones clicked back into action. He decided to go and knock on his first door so that he would be able to tell a bullshit story to the woman back at the campaign office when arriving there. "Hi, Mr…" Jones scrolled the list as he looked for the house number. He had already been fake checking them off every hour. "Mr. Trin. I have a few quick voter questions to ask you." Mr. Trin smiled, "Why, certainly." Jones went through the interview process asking Mr. Trin what he thought about Jeez Yazer. At the end of the interview, he shook his hand. This time there seemed to be no connection to the galaxy involved. Somehow, if the music came up in the conversation, the galaxy might have peeked in to view what Jones was up to. Tina came back around the corner texting Jones as he waited by the roadside, "Jones, I've been trying to reach you for the past 20 minutes. What in the world are you doing?"

Jones replied quickly, "Just work. What in the world are YOU doing?" he teased. As he got back into her car, she replied, "Just roaming." Jones pulled out his phone, "Hey. Tina, listen, I think we get along, and… I want to do nothing. So… if we just mark these houses once every hour, it will look like we're working." Tina stayed quiet for a moment, then smiled, "Well, why didn't you tell me sooner? I can do so many other things!" Jones let out a big sigh, feeling glad that Tina agreed to not tell anyone. But he thought that she would eventually tell someone else. "Alright, let's return to the campaign office where we can report back to the campaign manager woman." "Great," she said, "Hey, want to grab a Burger King or something later?" inviting him to some food for telling her the trick. "Sure," Jones said.

For the rest of the ride back, the two of them were mostly silent as Tina had done work during the day. She pulled in her car around the Vet Hospital place as there was meager parking around the campaign office. "Alright, hop out Jones. We're here." Tina said with a smile. They walked up the steps towards the red carpet. Tina grabbed onto his arm, briefly with interest. Jones shook her off. "Hey, listen. You know we're kind of at work, and I don't know you that well yet." Jones said. Tina replied, "Oh I see. Okay." waiting for a moment to figure things out. Ottie came back with Styles. They were already talking in the room, sparking up an interesting conversation about Styles' past. "Good work today, everyone." The campaign manager woman said, not questioning what was happening under her nose. Bernz had already left, along with Tennor. Gio walked over to the group that was forming. "So, Burger King guys?" Gio asked.

The group agreed and walked over together. The clock had already struck 6:00 PM. It was getting dark. "Man, I gotta have that pie," Jones said, as Ottie went up to the counter. "It's all about that burger meal, boi." teased Ottie. Styles brought out his weed pen as he took a puff, "So I heard you guys easily game the system from Ottie. Is that true?" he asked. Jones and Ottie looked over at one another, "Yeah. It's pretty easy, but you know if we let this get out of hand, things could get really bad really quick." Jones said with a worried look. Gio walked up from behind, "What do you mean by game the system?" Ottie and Jones gave one another that 'Oh shit' look as if their worst fears had just come true. "You ready to go, Gio? We'll

CHAPTER FIVE – SPLITTING JOURNEY

tell you later." The two of them said in unison. Gio put his skateboard on the ground. Jones and Ottie waved goodbye to everyone as they followed behind. The night sky showed, as the three of them went in and out of curbs, stopping near a garage off to the right. The empty residence spoke out to Jones as if it was a nice place to stop to rest; where not much had been going on.

Ottie pulled out his iPhone and put on the song that he and Jones had been making together. "Yo, what's that?" Gio inquired. "A song we've been making," Ottie replied. "I rap you know," Gio said in return. He started up over the beat and spit some bars as the other two listened. Gio, rapping in perfect sync with the beat had caught Jones' interest, "I knew there was something about this guy." Gio pulled out a blunt and started smoking it under the garage. "Blunts too huh?" Ottie said as the two of them rolled through the garage. Gio was wearing a grey sweater with pockets as he puffed the blunt again. "Alright, yeah, maybe we can get something going here." Ottie thought. As Ottie talked about the tune, the three of them continued to skateboard, eventually coming to a gutter. "Hey bet you can't ride down that cement!" Ottie said, challenging them all as Gio went full speed into it. Ottie followed without hesitation. Jones closed his eyes for a moment, working up the courage. It was as if his foot stuck to the board as he went down the gutter. Through both sides of the open half ends, each skateboarder went up and then back down, pressing through the cold night before coming out on the other side.

All three started laughing as their motions flew by. Jones thought about what Ottie had said about getting closer to heading to LA. Based on the way work was going, it was almost time. Jones and Ottie told Gio that it was time to go home, as they picked up their boards. "Hey, want to grab some more drinks later?" Ottie asked Jones. "Let's grab a creampuff. I could use one of those." Jones responded. Ottie scoffed, "Alright Jones, we'll get your fucking creampuff." Jones laughed, "We can get some drinks too man." They headed back towards Jones' house, skating on their boards through the quiet night by the trees. Jones started to notice some differences as the two of them were going back up the final hill. A small trailer, with a satellite stuck out on the side, was parked on the road. Slowly this town was changing, but Jones only started to notice the small details, growing curious day by day about the world around him. Looking down at his phone, Ike shot him a text. Ike, being Jones' old friend with whom he constantly made music, asked him if he was free. Jones shot him a text back, "Yeah around Saturday I should be free. There's a beach party coming up soon if you're not busy." he said in return.

Ottie looked over at the phone wondering who Jones just talked to, "Who was that?" he asked in idle curiosity. "A good friend of mine who has a personalized studio. You should come with me." Jones said, inviting him along. Ottie was still at his house and almost a week had already gone by. He was taking his time as he struggled to find a more permanent job. However, Jones covered for him every time his mother asked.

"How's the job search going?" Ms. P asked, attempting to be supportive. "Ottie's doing his best. He's just using my laptop. I mean, we both have this temporary campaign job, for now, right?" Jones responded in return. Ottie went out to greet Jones' mother, "Hey Ms. P, thanks for letting me stay. I appreciate it!" After taking a little time to make some ramen, Jones and Ottie went back into Jones' room and closed the door. "What are we going to do?" Ottie asked, wondering and waiting for an answer. Jones thought for a moment, "Well, let's go to that beach party. Maybe we'll find some leads there." Jones, feeling tired, lay down on the bed as Ottie played a mix on the website. Then Ottie loaded up a video game, looking for ways to make money. "Says here I can create weaponry through their small coding. People will pay me $5.00 for the look." Ottie said.

Jones replied, "Hey, I know that game. Some guy was trying to get me to DJ some London-style Dubstep there. He kept raving about the video game. He said he was a bass player and would pay me a small amount to

CHAPTER FIVE – SPLITTING JOURNEY

play sometime." Jones sounded shaky, "The man's a little off his rocker though, I think, otherwise, he's overly excited about music." Ottie raised his eyebrow, "Contact the dude. It sounds interesting." Jones loaded up the video game and messaged the man through his PC trying to contact him. But Jones' character wouldn't load as the PC they were on couldn't handle it. "Well, there goes that idea." Jones frowned. Ottie tried to optimize the computer, "It says I have to wipe everything. Can you back up all your stuff?" As Ottie went through the basic procedures, Jones sat back in thought.

"Well, I haven't cleaned it in a while," Jones said, not realizing how messy his computer had become. The folders were all out of place, scattered like Jones' mind. The folders need to be put together in order, along with all of the ideas that had been rapidly flowing through Jones' thought processes regarding how to change the world. Jones passed Ottie his external drive, looking for a way to clean the computer without losing all of its data. Ottie seemed knowledgeable about working on computers as he had mentioned this to the manager woman back at the campaign office. Determined to be able to properly make music and connect deeper with the vibrations of the world, Jones trusted Ottie to proceed. While Ottie loaded up the music programs onto the external hard drive, he reviewed the mess, "Holy shit! Dude, how much did you take?" Jones replied, "Keep this on the down-low, but I stole millions worth over the years. Not like I'm making money off it. So, it doesn't matter." Ottie shook his head, "Well you'd buy them if you were, wouldn't you?" Jones nodded, "Of course. I mean, a bunch of people would freak out if they knew. And we were making money on it."

Jones and Ottie stared at the computer for a moment after the PC finished making copies to the external hard drive and then reformatted its hard drive. "Hey Ottie, it's kinda getting late. We have to work tomorrow." yawned Jones. Jones was feeling better during this week. He had made it a point to get an adequate amount of sleep to control himself and his mind. He also needed to keep a normal persona for work, after all, he and

Bernz were becoming good friends. Ottie went over to Jones' laptop and put on Frozen while the personal computer optimized. Jones laid back down on the bed. "Do you think we'll be able to make this album?" he asked, questioning his abilities to use his skill sets towards the differences of the music. The computer beeped twice right as Jones said that. The PC was logging off and restarting itself. Ottie loaded in the repair disk and then turned towards Jones. "Bro, you have the marketing skills and I have the musical abilities. We've got this!" Jones looked over towards Ottie feeling reassured. "Now let me just re-download everything else onto the computer." Ottie reached over, taking the external hard drive and the USB stick and started installing whatever he could.

"Awesome! It's up and cleaned out. This should make our life a lot easier, and for one another in the music world." Ottie said smiling. Ottie installed the screen dimmer along with the musical programs. Jones loaded up the digital audio workspace and started making music. As the weed hit Jones' body, the screen dimmed yellow. He loaded up the drum software in the workspace, creating multiple drum loop patterns by clicking on and turning the software knobs on the screen. Jones felt as if he was making music with the gods and the galaxy in his mind, creating gold. Jones sat back and watched in disbelief as Ottie took over, blasting through making each section. Although the focus of each drum had not been mixed down to fit the ears, it didn't matter. Each sound and pattern went through perfectly. Jones closed his eyes, calling to the galaxy, as he floated there listening to the sound. A simple piano melody went directly from his brain right into the computer as he imagined himself creating it right there. Laying back in the chair, an orchestra mixed with electronic music playing through his head. Jones had fallen asleep in the chair while Ottie stood by.

"Uhh... Bro, you gonna get that?" Ottie asked, shaking Jones. "You hardly moved the mouse." Jones woke up out of his slumber. "Oh, uh... Yeah, ha... Sorry man." Jones got to work on the drums, slowly selecting them

CHAPTER FIVE – SPLITTING JOURNEY

as he heard them playing in his head. After three hours, Jones finally came up with a basic small drum loop that Ottie could work off of. "Thanks. Let's take your old melody and we'll work on it from here, Bro. Get some rest." Ottie said, slightly peeved that Jones was unable to focus. As Ottie went in to start mixing the song, Jones went back into the galaxy. "More! More! We see what you're up to." three men in brown hats surrounded Jones. They stood next to a bright yellow Jeep. "Who are you guys?" asked Jones. "Why we're the guys who will take you on a long journey." said one smiling at Jones as the other two men stood looking back at him. "Hop in. We'll go for a ride!" Stars and dust came out through the tailpipe of the yellow jeep as music played in the background. In a beautiful purple and blue hue, they made a U-turn landing back towards the platform from which they started, dancing upon it by driving in circles.

Getting out of the bright yellow Jeep, the elder man, who spoke to Jones earlier, stood there with a cane in his hand, "You'll be able to ride in a car like this Jeep one day too, Jones. You were meant for this. The next decade of change, the change of ideas!" The three old men laughed as they got back in the car. Before Jones had a chance to rebut, the men had already gone. He could feel the power surging through him as he felt like he was recharging in his sleep. Ottie kept working through the night on the music that he and Jones had started creating. "Man, leaving me to do this stuff," Ottie mumbled to himself. Looking at the laptop still playing Frozen, he had forgotten to turn it off. "Well, I better put on something." Ottie took the laptop and switched it off. Instead, he put a different Disney movie on the main computer. "Alright, that's better. Time to get to bed." Ottie went around to his sleeping bag, laid back on the floor as he looked up at the ceiling. The two of them slowly went towards dreamland together.

Chapter Six – A Day's Job

The next day when the alarm hit, neither of them woke up on time, not caring if they would be late to work. Bernz threw out a text at Jones as his phone buzzed in the morning. "So, I hear Berkeley and the A's game is going on tonight. My friend Jaime and I are going to meet up after work. Are you down to go?" Bernz texted. Jones read the text message from his phone as he rubbed his head. Due to the dreams Jones had been having lately, he hadn't been getting much sleep again. Jones replied, "Yeah." then fell back asleep, not caring. The clock now reached 10:00 AM. Jones woke up slowly, rolling out of bed to the left side. His hand hit the drawer. "Ow! Fuuuuuck!" he said silently to himself, trying not to wake Ottie. Ottie, undisturbed by the sound, continued to lightly snore. "Ah well." Jones yawned, as he went over in his pajamas towards the restroom. He put the water on light and kept rinsing his teeth not paying attention to his surroundings. The day felt bright and sunny, as sunlight peeped through the glass skylight down onto the tiled black and white floor. Putting on his two slippers, Jones slowly walked back towards the kitchen. "Hey mom," he said in a light voice.

Ms. P stared back at him wondering what Jones had been up to. Looking at him with questioning eyes, she asked, "Where were you the other night? I'm worried, you're getting that exhausted look." He glanced back at her, recalling the night of crazy dreams he just had in his head — a man with a fur coat, and a superman dressed in a tie, both talking to him at the

CHAPTER SIX – A DAY'S JOB

dance party. The man with the fur coat was wearing jewelry, claiming he was with the British Secret Service. He said, "I'm still married to my wife and I'm part of English royalty blood." Superman had a crew cut. His tie flowed down to his chest. Jones had shaken his hand. Then Superman pulled out his iPhone, wanting to take a picture together as if they were good friends. "I've just been going to show mom, nothing special," Jones replied. Jones's mom sighed, "Be careful Jones. You know how it can get if you're out too late too many nights in a row." Ottie, waking up, joined Jones in the kitchen. "Hey Ms. P!" Ottie said cheerfully. "Time to go to work." smiling at Jones.

Ottie went over to cook some ramen as he put in a mixture of Thyme and Capri. He didn't notice the intensity of the conversation that had been going on between Jones and his mom. "So where did you guys go the other night?" she asked again, this time questioning Ottie. Ottie casually replied, "Oh yeah, we went into Oakland to Club Red Toys. It was really fun." Jones's mom seemed irritated, "Alright, be safe next time. As long as you guys had fun." Ottie and Jones headed out the front door after eating, "Thanks, Ms. P!" Ottie shouted as Jones got in the car. Ottie checked to make sure the skateboards were in the trunk before he got in. "Dude. What was that about? Your mom seems to hate me." Ottie said, wondering where the irritation came from. Jones shrugged, "Nah, she's just worried. If she hated you, you'd probably not be allowed back in the house."

Turning up the music volume, they drove towards work. Racing up the stairs that led to the office, neither of them picked up any available food for the campaign workers. "Hey Ottie, my boss man from Animal Beats is coming into town. Can you cover for me?" Ottie looked back at Jones, "Sure. What do you mean? And why haven't you told me?" he asked, wondering what was going on. "Well, you see… my boss and an EDM artist are coming into town for a day, and I have to drop them off at the airport." eyeing back and forth between his screen and Ottie. The campaign manager woman walked up to the two of them, "Anything you'd like to tell me, boys? You're late again. Seriously, you can't keep doing this." The entire room looked over as the woman scolded the two. "Bro… she's got a stick up her butt today," Ottie whispered.

The woman looked at Ottie, "I heard that Ottie. I do need some tech help, so I'll let that slide IF you can optimize the computer systems." she said, rolling her eyes. Ottie happily agreed as he got up and hopped on the computer in the small office. The rest of the crew sat back watching the show, as Tina stared at Jones, then started waving for him to come over. "Hey… how are you today?" Tina said in a loving tone. "I mean…" Jones sat down near her and got to work calling. "Hey, let's grab food and go up to a spot. I have something to show you." Jones said as he thought of the area close to his house. Styles waved at Jones as well as the rest of the crew. "Ayyy," Bernz said from behind. "Me and my friend, Jaime, are going out, remember? Joining us tonight, right?" Jones shook his head up and down indicating to say yes, "Yeah, probably. Sometimes a little later! Sounds exciting!"

Tina eyed Jones and reached for his hand under the table. "First I have something to take care of." The woman called out to the room, "So, we've got a complaint that someone has been eating Fritos and skateboarding throughout the neighborhoods while taking surveys. To all of you here, DO NOT eat while taking surveys. And especially, DO NOT skateboard." The whole room questioned why she was telling them the obvious as if she needed to make this announcement in the first place. "Ottie especially." She said, singling him out to make an example. "Dude, the guy was old and I'm just eating Fritos." Ottie shrugged his shoulders, trying to defend himself. "Ottie get out of here! Go do some surveys." the woman screeched, as the rest of the room giggled to themselves. "This campaign is such a joke," Tennor said from the back as he prepared the fliers for the day.

Jones felt in his world with Tina as she held onto his hand under the table. Jones pulled away and whispered, "Not during work. Outside of work it

CHAPTER SIX – A DAY'S JOB

is fine, but not here." He was adamant, not wanting to draw attention to their small attraction to one another. "This time you're going out with Tennor." the woman said nodding towards Jones. "You'd better keep Ottie in check. I understand his situation, but we cannot keep him here if he keeps acting up." Jones put his hand on the back of his neck and smiled, "Right. Ha-ha. I will!" nervously thinking about what might happen if Ottie lost the job. Jones started walking out the door as Tennor followed behind. "Yo, butt-face. I'm with you today." as he laughed with a twisted smile. Tennor's way of expressing his closeness seemed to be that of insults. Jones replied, "Yeah" then questioned, "So why are you on this campaign anyway if you dislike it so much?" wondering what Tennor had to say.

"The money is basically free, stupid." laughing. "Let's hurry up and get out of this place. These people make me sick." Tennor ran down the stairs as his muscles bulged from his legs. "Do you run a lot?" Jones asked, noticing the fitness that Tennor had gained. "I used to," Tennor answered. Jones quickly replied, "Ahhh… so what's your plan after this?" Tennor looked back over at him, "I'm out of this bitch when I can. I'm going to go teach English in China." laughing as the two of them got into Jones' car. Jones drove towards their designated suburban neighborhood trying to get oriented. Tennor looked over at him, "Stop here, man. We'll just walk." "Alright sure." Jones parking where requested.

Tennor jumped out of the car and headed towards the top of the hill. "Hey, shitbag. Let's climb up here." Reluctantly, Jones followed him as the sun shined down on the spot where he was standing. Tennor pulled out a joint and started smoking it. "On the job?" Jones queried. Tennor laughed, "What work? What job?" throwing it back in his face. Jones, growing tired of Tennor's high energy and sassiness replied, "Well I think I'll go and do some actual work today." Jones started down the other side of the hill feeling the wind on his face. "Have fun, shitbag," Tennor replied. Jones went down the hill thinking through his many thoughts. He wondered why he was stuck in this never-ending loop of finding jobs and then not wanting to work. Feeling tired, he laid down by a large rock in the grassy corner of someone's property, staring at the sky. Not caring that this was another person's house, he closed his eyes.

"Jones, you know you're supposed to be focusing on this magazine." a voice trailed off in the background. As this echoed through his head, he wondered what would come next. Jones sighed, as he drifted in thought. "Hey! I thought you were covering the Poulici guys over in Berkeley?" Nepharius's voice rang in his head. "Also, you're at work. So, what the 'F' are you doing?" Jones woke up, getting up off the grass. An old man was standing over him with a hat on. "What are you doing on my lawn?" the man blinked twice as the drool from his head fell on Jones' face. "Sorry, sir. Just taking a quick rest. We're doing a campaign survey." said Jones cautiously. "Well come inside. But first, can you help me catch this bird? This poor little bird is stuck in the corner of the yard by the rock."

Jones went around to the rock to check it out. There was a little bird in the corner with ants ridden all over him. Jones chased him over the grass as he went over to catch the bird. Instead, the old man reached over and picked the bird up in his hands. "Sir, I think the poor little guy is gone," observed Jones. As life slowly went out of the bird, the ants began walking on the old man's hands. Then slowly moving red bugs came out of the man's shoulder. "I'm going to clean the little guy now and put him back in his birdhouse," said the old man. Jones slowly backed away from the man, "Shit." he said to himself. With his thoughts scared back into reality, Jones went running fast back up the hill towards Tennor. "Whoa. What's the rush, fucker?" sounding disturbed. Jones smiled, "Just shut up. Let's go. Hop in the car." Tennor, laughing, started running along with Jones. Jones didn't know why he felt so intimidated by this. Driving back, but way too early to return to the office, Tennor suggested they stop and eat first.

"I'm starving," Tennor said without remorse. He failed to notice Jones' expression; it was as if he had seen a ghost. Jones pulled into a burger

CHAPTER SIX – A DAY'S JOB

shop. He was munching down food as he marked himself down on the application. Tennor looked over trying to lighten the mood, "China! Man, I'm telling you. That's the place to be." He stared up at the sky for a moment waiting for a response from Jones. None came. Ignoring Tennor, Jones sent a text to Bernz, "Hey, let's go out tonight". Bernz responded right away, "Yeah! I'm so down, bro!" For some reason, his nerves calmed down. Jones smiled, "Yeah, China seems like it would be an awesome place to visit one day. Are you getting a teacher's certificate?" Tennor sighed, "Yeah. Anything to get away from here. Anything to get away from home. Maybe my cousin can get you a certification too. Let me know if you're interested."

"Alright Tennor, I'll do that," Jones said. As the time went slowly by, they hung out in the car, laughing and making jokes. Jones wanted to get home to prepare for the night with Bernz and his friend. After all, Jones had a little time to kill while Bernz was at the A's game. He turned on the car to head back to the office. Tennor lit up a joint as Jones drove slower than normal. "I'd puff that, but then I couldn't drive." Jones chuckled. Tennor gave him a little jab and then zoned out, staring into the streets. As they pulled up into the parking lot, Ottie, Styles and the rest of the crew were pulling up as well. Up the steps they slowly walked, chatting about their days and the brief adventures each of the teams had. As Ottie headed over to Jones, Jones went over to Tina.

Everybody went into the room where the woman was standing waiting. "Alright. Good work again today. We got no complaints this time and the campaign numbers look good." the woman taking a light-humored jab at Ottie, seemed satisfied with the work. The whole room was gaming the system now without anyone in management notice. The entire crew walked out towards the red carpets leading outside to where the cars were parked. "Hey, want to go for a drive?" Jones asked Tina. Ottie who was getting the memo eying Jones walked back over to Styles. "Styles and I are going to go for a smoke.", said Ottie as he reached for the door. "We'll catch up with you later. Remember the stuff happening with Bernz tonight." As the door closed leaving Tina alone with Jones, Tina nodded her head as she latched onto his arm.

"Where are we going?" She asked, questioning Jones' antics. "Hop in the car and I'll show you. Let's go to the hillside close to my house where we can view the stars together. They are out tonight you know." Jones said, turning on the music in the car. Jones drove the car through the pine and wood trees. The colors of the leaves changed from yellow to red filling the air. The air however felt warm rather than cool. A spiral road curved up the hillside where a home sat alone on top next to a water tower. The house had pearl flooring and metal gates, resembling a castle. The place was rumored to be previously owned by the Mafia. Jones drove off to the left of the rock wall driveway leading up to the large house. Parking, the view was vast. You could watch over the entire town. Jones lay back one of the seats, opening the top of the sunroof so they could see the stars clearly. Tina also moved her seat back, cuddling up towards Jones. She laughed as she tried to position herself.

"Ow, I can't cuddle like this, you know!" she chuckled. Jones ended up laughing along, "What curfew?" Tina fell silent. "Well, no but my mother's alone. Come over sometime after work and check out the house." "Okay." Jones didn't pry, respecting Tina's boundaries. "Well, it's getting close to 7:00 PM and I really got to get going," he said as she nodded her head. "Yeah, you're right. Let's get going." Jones put the directions to Tina's house into his GPS. Retracing their way down the spiral hill and across town, it was not long before they arrived. The house had an older tint to it with a slow-moving gate that was secure. Inside, a little wooden pulley hung down to pull the gate open. A tiled walkway next to the garage appeared to have stones by it. Tina walked down the path after hugging Jones. "See you at work tomorrow!" she said excitedly.

Jones thought to himself, "Okay, the next plan succeeded. We're safe from

CHAPTER SIX – A DAY'S JOB

problems." As he started back towards where Ottie and Styles were, he grabbed his phone and called Ottie, "Yooo! Let's go to Berkeley! Also, I got invited over to Tina's house tonight, but I'd rather go with you guys to Berkeley." Ottie replied quickly, "Alright my guy, get that!" excited for Jones that he was starting to date again. "Nah, it's not like that," Jones said, playing it down. "I'll pick you up at the Burger King." heading back down the road towards where Ottie and Styles were. Ottie and Styles were bickering over who could make the best burger. "It's all about that double cheese!" Ottie said as Styles took a puff of his weed pen. "No! It's obviously about the quarter pounder!" Styles said in return. Ottie turned towards Jones as he walked in the door, "Quarter pounder or double cheese?"

Jones looked at the menu. "Pie!" he retorted with a wry smile. "Alright Styles. We gotta go, but we'll catch you later" Ottie and Jones went out of the Burger King and got back on the road. Bernz called Jones, "Heyyyy Jones! What's up? We're going to explore Berkeley tonight. Wanna come?" Jones said in return, "You bet. My friend is down too. Mind if we meet by the skate park there?" Bernz replied ecstatically, "Yeah no problem. We're just getting back from the A's game." Ottie and Jones headed to Berkeley, blasting music and talking about skateboarding. Ottie yelled at Jones, "Gonna do a tre flip boi! Heh heh." They arrived at the skate park in a few minutes. Bernz pulled up right behind them and parked his car."Yooo! 311 in the quad!" Ottie shouted. Jones and Ottie looked at one another. "What the fuck you on about?" Jones asked, wondering where that came from.

"311 in the quad is from some stupid meaningless video on YouTube. A man runs up and just yells it." Ottie explained. He started laughing, "HEY EVERYBODY, IT'S 311 IN THE QUADDD." Screaming it. "Have you ever heard of the Cream in Berkeley?" Bernz asked with delight. "The Cream? Ottie asked. Like Ice Cream? Yo! Let's go." Everyone piled in Jones's car. Bernz put on trap music and off they went. Jones yelled, "So is there 311 IN THE QUAAAAD at the Cream?" Ottie took on the joke adding in, "HEY EVERYBODY! 311 IN THE QUAD AT THE CREAM!" Bernz laughed as he put the weed pipe to his lips and gave it a puff. Turning the trap music even louder. The Cream was packed with a line reaching almost out the door. Ottie, Bernz, and Jaime got out of the car as Jones' parked behind the Cream.

"Yo! This place is poppin'." Ottie exclaimed as he got in line. Jones replied with a simple, "Ayy yee." as he joined them "So, what can I grab you boys?" asked the cashier. "A chocolate cookie cream and a mint," Bernz replied quickly. Ottie stretched his hands and yawned, "I'll have the same!" Jaime thought for a moment then said, "A double scoop of chocolate with sprinkles on top." Jones said, "One mint milkshake." The man behind the cashier smiled, "Great! Today's a Creamer discount too!" Jones wondered if these discounts were becoming a coincidence or were a special discount due to his working with Nebulous magazine. With ice creams in hand, they walked over towards the Berkeley Town Square enjoying their meal. A blue mini-van showed up on the side of the town square with four people dressed in hippy clothing. The main guy in the front looked right at Jones. "What's up?" he asked.

Jones replied, not thinking twice about it, "The sky and the stars." looking up at the sky. "You seem chill. Want some acid? I have leftovers and need to get rid of it." said the hippie. Hesitating, Jones took it. "Thanks, my guy. So, what brought you out here?" questioning them as he put the tab under his tongue. "Well, we've been out here for a while. I play a lot of guitars." Ottie jumped into the conversation, "Sick dude. That's a nice acoustic brand guitar." Jones looked behind him. He could swear he could hear his friend Trexor's voice saying, "C'mon, let's go Jones." In Jones's mind, his friend Trexor had formulated by the blue minivan that edged him away from the possible danger they might have gotten themselves into. Jones looked up at the sky, now seeing an orchestra assembling like before in the stars. This time it was both vivid and blurred. Jones and his friends walked towards a bar that seemed to have a lot of action. People

CHAPTER SIX – A DAY'S JOB

were shouting and a couple of men paying a bunch of money for drinks. Jones sat down next to a man with a beard; tan and brazen.

"Hi!" the man said, shaking Jones' hand.

"Hi!" Jones said in return, shaking the man's hand twice as fast. "What do you do?" Not wasting any time. "Well, you see, I'm a battery chemist. Working in the Berkeley Labs up the top of the hill. Trying to solve how to make batteries last much longer. I came down to do a presentation on campus." the man said, smiling back at Jones. Feeling impressed by his expertise, Jones felt he would like to interview the guy for the magazine. He asked him if he would be interested. The men behind them overheard their conversation, "A chemist? We've been looking for one." Jones turned to the man who spoke, "Oh cool. And what do you do?" He replied, "All those vape juices you see over there, I created them with one of the biggest labs." The Chemist seemed intrigued, "Alright, I'll see if I can." Just like that the men were gone, tab paid, and out the door. Jones looked around for Ottie and the others, not seeing them anywhere. Jones asked the chemist to wait a moment and went towards the door.

Jones found Ottie outside among a group of people. A lady on her skateboard was talking to him with a garnered interest. "Yooo, Jones! Come meet Ley!" Ottie said, beckoning to Jones. Jones went over and waved hello, "Hey Ottie. I've got to go with a chemist up to Berkeley Labs, man. I'll be back in a few. It's a short trip." "A chemistry lab? Alright, whatever." Ottie said, not thinking about any possible repercussions. Jones walked back inside the bar as Ottie began to toss a tennis ball with the skateboarder Ley, seeing how far they could chuck it. The two seemed to be getting along well enough. Waving at the Chemist, Jones asked if the offer still stood for him to visit the Berkeley Labs with him, "Hey, so can I come to see the Labs?" The Chemist shook Jones' hand, "Absolutely man. Let's go. I'll show you the city view too!" Now the acid had kicked in even more. And Jones couldn't drive anyway because his car was parked behind the Cream near the bar where they were, so Jones asked the Chemist politely if he could drive. "Sure. Here's my car. Hop in." the Chemist said smiling.

The world around Jones had been amplified again as something major was coming. Yet Jones couldn't predict or depict the world changing around him this time. He viewed the curb that had yellow and black striping, as the lights danced everywhere. He wondered why the signs on the side of the road didn't have electronic signals of happy or sad faces to easily show when people could park there rather than the confusing, unreadable words suggesting street cleaning between 7:00 AM -10:00 AM on Thursdays. They drove up a hill where the Chemist showed his badge to the guard at the gate. Berkeley Labs sat towards the top overlooking the city. Jones followed the Chemist over to the Berkeley Labs' main door and up the steps, feeling as if he was right out of a spy movie. "Woah, this place looks crazy," Jones said with eyes popping wide. The walls were covered with different scientific documents explaining how atoms broke down. "Uh, so what's this screen show?" he asked. The Chemist turned to him happily, "I'm glad you asked. See this chart of all these little droplets? These are showing the holes in which the battery is leaking energy and converging over time."

"Oh, I see," Jones said, trying to make sense of the grey chart that looked more like an edible sandwich. The Chemist took him down the steps towards, what seemed to be like, a laser for separating material. "This is the caudle. We use this to separate the materials as we sift through which ones are matching. If there is a match, we can separate one energy from another. This is how we can make batteries last longer, by closing the leaks in the material." he explained. Jones sat quietly for a moment, idly watching the green laser go by. "Hey, what's outback?" Jones asked as the lesson went through his brain and sunk in. "And you know, maybe this will be used by an electric car company someday." The Chemist's face brightened up, "That would be pretty awesome if I could work there." They walked outside and sat down on the white curb staring across the

CHAPTER SIX – A DAY'S JOB

city. "Woooooow! Jones exclaimed as the entire city lit up from under his gaze. The world started to spin. "You know man, I make music with a big company. Let's meet again sometime. I'd like to show you some of my musical work."

The Chemist smiled, "Let's get you back to your friends." Jones replied, "Okay." He looked down at his phone. He had received a text from Bernz, "Hey Jones, it's getting late Jaime and I decided to Uber back to our car. We'll see you at work later." Jones and the Chemist walked back down to the car as Jones started to stumble. Almost falling over, the Chemist caught him, "Woah there. Too many drinks, I take it." not knowing Jones was on acid. Jones opened the door and got into the car as the Chemist got into drive. Slowly Jones's eyes closed. He started to imagine Trexor again. "Yo, you need to find Ottie and get home before this stuff kicks in, Trexor warned. This is boomer acid you know. You can die from this stuff." Somehow Jones' consciousness had portrayed a realistic version of his friend. The Chemist slowly drove down the hillside, showing his badge again as the security guard let them out. Jones really felt there was no turning back. It was time to go to LA. He couldn't shake the feeling that his alternate reality was now becoming one with himself. Enough of the drugs had fully altered his mind to the point that the galactical energy had merged with his.

The Chemist shook Jones' hand and turned off his car parking next to the bar, "Let's meet again sometime! This was fun." Jones smiled, "Sure, the Kav's Bar is pretty interesting!" Arriving back outside the bar where Ottie and Ley were, Jones found them still throwing tennis balls as far as they could. One went over the gate and bounced off a car. To Jones, it was a sound bouncing off from afar. "Oh shit! Jones! Let's get out of here." yelled Ottie. He told Ley, "Give me your number. Quick!" holding out his hand. Jones yelled out at the top of his lungs, "311 in the Quaaad!" as the two of them started running away, back towards the car that was parked behind the Cream. Taking a second look back, Jones saw Ley all beat up from falling when she and Ottie were messing around.

Hopping in the car, Jones pointed the general direction of his house and shouted to Ottie, "Go, go, go!" Ottie stepped on the gas pedal and sped away from the curb towards the freeway. Jones passed out due to the acid. Ottie looked over at Jones for a moment but kept on driving through the trees and roads. Back and forth they went until rounding the final corner leading up to the house. "Jones, wake up man." Ottie shook Jones' shoulder. Jones fell forward to the right of his seat thinking it was Trexor behind his shoulder. "Wake up," Ottie said again. Jones slowly responded, "You know what would be cool?" Jones mumbled, "It would be cool if I wrote down everything that I'm seeing right now." Ottie looked over at him, "What are you talking about?"

Without responding, Jones opened the car door and waddled off inside. He went straight to the computer and started typing:

A Musical Warrior and Your Friend in the Universe.
First, I'd like to start by describing one of the toughest things that I've ever had to say out loud to the world —Psychosis. Yes, psychosis, a form of mind control, originally set out as the war on our imagination. The control now is released for a free mind to fly like the birds in the sky. However, we must remember to be grounded in the realities we live in. The universe revolves around all gods and includes me, you, everyone really — just wanted a good friend in my mind.

Ottie reached over as Jones hit the 'save' key, but Jones saw Ottie acting as Trexor in his mind. "Yo! This is some weird shit. Chill on this." exclaimed Ottie after reading what Jones had just written. Jones laid down on his bed and began describing the geometrical shapes and sounds he was experiencing. He described going into ancient temples as the patterns repeated in his head. "Water! Ottie, I need water." gasped Jones. Ottie went into the kitchen and grabbed the water thinking Jones wasn't going to come out of his state. He gave him a glass as Jones chugged it. "I need

CHAPTER SIX – A DAY'S JOB

to sleep this off," Jones said. Ottie replied sarcastically, "Yeah, Brooo, I think you do." Jones rolled over on the bed and laid on his stomach, feeling bitten by the cold air of the open window. "Hey man, I'm going to go off to that skateboarder girls' house, Ley. Call me if you need anything." Ottie took the car keys and drove off leaving Jones lying there on the bed. Jones drifted further into his psychotic state hearing the bushes rustling in the corner outside the window. "Must be the Warriors, the Musical Warriors." Jones smiled as the bushes rustled to his response. "Who is there?" Jones quietly asked. Then he shouted, "GO AWAY."

The bushes rustled again as he sensed the Warriors moving on top of the house. The room formed into blank spaces as he fought for his sanity. "We need ideas… new ideas." a whisper shouted in his head, "Your imagination is being stolen!" Another said, "Jones, we need you." The whispers continued as Jones got up and walked towards the corner of the room in his boxers. He stood next to the window. A car passed by the neighborhood shining its headlights on him as he stood there not moving. After a minute Jones noticed he was — in the corner of his room, standing. Shaking his head, he went back towards his computer. Jones could hear the shouts of war up the street. "Get 'em!" Jones walked outside of the house after putting on his shirt, shorts, and slippers, not feeling the cold. Up the hill, an orange light showed along with what sounded to be a motor, as if an army tank were there. Jones started walking towards it. Halfway up the hill, something clicked. He didn't know if it was the cold cement or if it was the coldness of the frosty air. "It's okay. You're fine, Jones" he said, consoling himself.

Jones ran back towards the house as fast as he could, testing out his consciousness. He felt free as he ran, it felt like his body was lighter. The deer stopped in their tracks to watch Jones intently, stray cats and animals around him came to follow him, rather than running away. Operating at a high spiritual energy level, Jones closed the front door. He slowly tried to calm himself and fall asleep. Getting back under the covers, he hid away, smiling cheekily, like a little kid haven been given an ice cream cone. "This is not going to go over so well with Ottie, is it?" he questioned himself. The voices raced through his head from the universe. It was time to go to the beach party. Jones was ready for everything the universe had to throw his way, as he drifted off into blankness.

Chapter Seven - Static Beach

The next day Jones woke up with a major headache. Jones' car was nowhere to be found as he looked over for his keys. Not remembering that Ottie went over to this random skateboarder Ley's house, Jones reached over to the nightstand, searching everywhere for them. "Shit! Where the fuck's my car?" he asked confusingly. Jones read his phone. There were 20 missed calls on it from Ottie and two texts. "Hey, I'm going to be late, but I'm coming back down today." Ottie's texts read. "Son of a bitch." Jones replied to himself. Jones picked up his phone and called Ottie feeling irritated that his sleep wasn't restful. "Hey bro, when will you be back? We have to work today." Jones said, annoyed. Ottie whispered in a low voice, "Shh, the girl's sleeping next to me. She's kinda cool and I don't want to wake her. I'll be there in a few." Jones couldn't believe what he just heard. "What happened last night?" he asked Ottie, trying to retrace his steps. "You went off with some dude to Berkeley Labs. I don't know what happened, bro. You tell me?" Ottie responded. Jones' mind was blank, "Well, whatever. Let's just get off to work. Get down here so we are on time."

Ottie complained not wanting to leave, "Look man, I'll be there. Give me a few alright? Let me enjoy this for just a bit longer." Then he hung up the phone not waiting for a response. Jones went over to the shower and brushed his teeth. He didn't really think about much except for the cat shampoo. Seeing it, Jones quickly took the shampoo and started to put it on. His hair spiked up and felt silkier, feeling as if this would add camouflage to himself from the rest of the world. His mother shouted from around the corner, "JONES WHERE'S THE CAR?" Jones replied as quickly as he could, "It's coming back. No worries." His mother, not feeling up to a bullshit answer, shouted back, "WHAT DO YOU MEAN THE CAR IS COMING BACK? HOW? WHEN?" "Ottie has it. He's on his way back," Jones admitted, caving in not wanting to continue the discussion further. Already almost 10:00 AM, Jones was going to be as late as Ottie for work. Drying himself off quickly with a towel, Jones headed back to his room, got dressed, and grabbed his skateboard.

Running as fast as he could towards the front door his mother stopped him, "Don't you want breakfast?" "No mom. Thanks though, I'm really late for work." Jones said as he closed the front door behind him. Hopping on his skateboard, Jones rode it like a musical instrument swinging back and forth. Jones bombed it down the hill almost as if he had sprung into mania. Dropping the skateboard at the top of the hill he started a smooth run down it, noticing the small details beside him. As he rode towards the bottom, a group of runners that Jones passed gave him a wave. Jones waved back and smiled. "Nice board bro!" said one of the runners. It seemed the runners were of A-class as a GTX car pulled up next to him. "Where ya headed?" two guys in the car said as Jones moved forward. "Work! I'm late!" Jones replied. The two men looked at one another, one with brazen blonde hair and blue eyes. The other with pure black. "Yo hop in. We'll give you a ride!" they offered. "We see what you've been up to, bro!"

Jones got off his board and got in the car as the door opened. One guy turned back towards Jones as the other stepped on the gas pedal speeding through the city zipping with the car. The car had an older tint to it and a brand-new look. Jones felt relieved that he would make it to work on time. "So, what do you do?" Jones asked one of the younger men upfront. "We're linguists. We translate 12 different languages." Jones thought about it for

CHAPTER SEVEN - STATIC BEACH

a moment, "So, do you ever say full sentences in 12 different languages, all within the same sentence?" The two men upfront laughed and started practicing it, "No, not really. You're a funny one."

Jones pointed towards the Burger King, "Alright we're here!" he said, signaling them to stop. He waved thank you as the two of them sped off. Running up the stairs towards work, the Campaign Manager woman was again staring at Jones. This time she did not have a happy expression on her face. "Where in god's name is Ottie?" she inquired. Jones dropped his head for a moment scratching it, "Well uh... Ottie said he'd be here." The woman eyed Jones, "Listen, I understand Ottie's situation, but if he doesn't get his ass over here on time, I'm going to fire him." Jones went towards his seat quietly and sat next to Tennor. "W's up fuck face?" Tennor laughed, "Bro, get here on time." Jones, half ignoring him, started to make calls. Styles sat right across from Jones this time.

"Jones. Where's Ottie, bro? We're paired up today." Inquired Styles. Jones replied, "He's at a girl's house and is on his way, so I last heard." A few minutes later Ottie got up the stairs, "Ayooo. Woman, I'm here." The Campaign Manager turned towards Ottie, "If you're late again, we are going to have a long talk, Ottie." she said not leaving any headroom. Ottie mumbled, "Well okay," rolling his eyes while looking at his buddies. The woman turned towards him again, "Ottie! What was that?" she asked. Ottie turned back but said nothing in response. "That's what I thought. Sit down and get to work." The truth was that under the woman's harsh demeanor, she had taken a liking to Ottie's antics. Jones started to feel bored at work and got up to go to the restroom. Tina saw him rise and decided to follow him towards the soda machines. She grabbed onto his arm, "So, coming over tonight. Right?" Tina asked hopefully.

Jones nodded his head, "Sure. It could be fun!" As the two of them got to talking, Jones pushed the button for a candy bar. Tina smiled, "It will be fun. My mother might be there though." Jones walked back with Tina towards the room saying nothing as he was laser-focused on getting through the day. He had all sorts of ideas running through his head and the upcoming beach party interview was on his mind. Sitting back down, Jones picked up the phone and started making his calls, following the pitch that was given to him. Gio sat in the corner with his hoodie on waving hello at Jones. Jones smiled and waved back. "Hey man, let's go skateboarding after work," Gio suggested. Jones replied, "Not tonight, man. How is tomorrow?"

Jones had already made plans to go to Tina's house tonight with Ottie and Styles. The three of them would be showing up for a mini-exploration. Gio nodded as if to agree, "So I do graphics design too. Know anyone in need?" Jones shook his head, "Cool that you do that though." The clock struck 6:00 PM and it was time for everyone to leave. On a seemingly normal day, Jones was ready for the night again. He went over to Styles and Ottie signaling them down. "Hey, guys! Ready?" Jones queried. Styles and Ottie bro-fived one another as Tina walked towards her car. "Hell yeah! We're going to grab some beers and we'll all show up together later," they said. Styles left his big SUV in the parking lot, all decked out in gold color.

Ottie gave him a compliment, "Tryna is flashy for the ladies?" Ottie smiled at Styles. Then when Jones appeared, "Jones, let's take your car. I'll drive if you want and we'll wingman." suggested Ottie. Jones replied, "Nah, I can drive, Bro." Styles and Ottie started making jokes as the two of them pumped up the conversation, "So, you and Tina are getting it on tonight? Huh?" Jones heard them, but he didn't participate, "I don't know, let's just go and see." waving the idea out of his mind. Shortly afterward they arrived at the Safeway close by. "Yo, obviously this beer is the best," Ottie said, pointing out a 16-ounce bottle of Sierra Nevada and then a Shock Top. "Let's also grab a can of beer!" Styles said pointing at the tall cans further down in the aisle.

CHAPTER SEVEN - STATIC BEACH

The two of them bickered again, challenging one another, "Yo I bet I can chug this one faster than you can!" Styles boasted. Ottie laughed, "Yeah. Just wait till we get to Tina's." joking back. Back at the car, Jones gave Tina a call, "Hey um, we're on our way and we will be there briefly". he said to her. "Okay. No problem! See you soon!" said Tina gayly. Jones stepped on the gas and floored it. Ottie and Styles didn't seem to care as they were deep in conversation. Shortly after, as the trees flew by changing colors from red to blue, Jones arrived at Tina's. The black gate slowly opened, creaking. Ottie and Styles commented, "Woah, man. What is this place? Looks like an old castle." "I know right? Damnnnn." The two of them got out of the car as Jones sat in the driver's seat for a moment. Jones texted Tina, "We're here."

Tina came out through the black gate and over to the car, "Hey! Come on in." Passing back through the gate, they walked over the hedge stones placed in the ground where a water bird fountain sprouted out from the middle. Towards the side of the courtyard, koi floated in a mini river. The first thing they saw when they walked into the house was that it was painted all pink. Sticky notes were posted on everything. 'Don't forget.' one of the Post-it notes said. "Um." Ottie and Styles eyed one another feeling uncomfortable. "Yo Tina. What's with this doll on the counter?" asked Ottie. The doll was beaten up, almost as if it hadn't been moved in years.

Styles proudly proclaimed, "Fuck it. We've got beeeer!" Styles took out a knife and stabbed the can, shotgunning it down. "Yeah! Beeeer!" yelled Ottie. The two of them shook the idea of the house and went back outside. "So, uh Tina, can you show me further around?" Jones asked, watching as the antics played out with his two friends. Tina, feeling calm, took Jones downstairs to a couch. Happy birthday was written on the pink wall far above with a ladder that still stood there and hadn't been moved in a while. "So... got any pets?" Jones instigated the conversation as Tina cuddled up next to him. "No, I haven't had them for a while." as she stared at the happy birthday sign. Another sticky note was posted on the bookshelf. "What's with the sticky notes?" Jones asked, trying to be polite. But Jones was feeling creeped out by the yellow Post-it notes found on every item. "Well, it's…" Tina fell silent for a moment. "My grandmother is trying to remember my grandfather. You see, he died recently." Tina stared at the floor. Jones didn't know how to respond, "Well, happy birthday, right?"

Tina said in return, "Actually, I was 6 years old when my grandfather passed away and we haven't taken it down since." At this point, Jones felt too out of place. "Let's go back upstairs," he suggested. The uncomfortableness of the place sent a weird feeling down his spine. Tina started towards her room, "Jones, meet me back in here." Jones went over to Ottie and Styles as the two of them didn't want to leave Jones for very long. "Uh, we'll be over here in the kitchen." Styles said, chugging another beer. Ottie whispered to Jones, "Bro, get some, but let's get out of here." Jones went into Tina's room as she lay there on the bed staring at the ceiling. It was still filled with things from when she was six years old. Jones went over to the bed and the two of them kissed. She rolled over on top of him saying no words. "Wait! Tina, honestly… I can't do this." Jones felt too scared to continue.

Tina didn't object as she fell back on the bed right next to him, "Are you going to go?" Jones said shakily, "I think so. I'm sorry." Picking up his shoes as he left, he went into the courtyard towards Styles and Ottie who were waiting outside. "So, did you…?" they both asked, waiting on an answer. Jones replied right away, "Nah, I can't. This just isn't right and feels weird." Both Styles and Ottie egged it on, "Oh my god, that doll and the Post-it notes everywhere. This is freaky, Bro. We're glad you didn't." Wandering back to the car, Jones drove slowly back towards the workplace where Styles' car was parked. Jones knew that after this moment, most work moments would not be the same again. Ottie and Jones waved Styles off home. As Styles took one last puff of his hash oil pen, the two of them then got into Jones' car. Jones cranked the volume up too loud trying to figure out what he's going to say to Ottie.

CHAPTER SEVEN - STATIC BEACH

"So, my boss is coming in tomorrow from Animal Beats. I have to take him to the airport. Don't tell anyone, okay? We're also skateboarding with Gio tomorrow, Bro." Ottie turned towards him in agreement, "Alright bro, sounds good!" Heading back home in a hurry, they rushed through the front door and tossed their skateboards on the bed. Ottie turned on the PC. "Yo, Jones! Cook us some ramen and grab some squeeze. We're going to go ahead and contact that guy for some money." Loading up the game, Jones attempted to contact the guy who would pay them through MixlR, a digital music site. Every mix had a specific touch to this guy's ear. "Hey man, I think we've got it." Ottie started to code his character into the game. Jones saw another character walk up. This other guy's character was a complete mess showing that it wasn't worth their time.

Ottie looked at Jones, "Yo! This is too weird. Let's get out of this, dude." Jones agreed as the two of them logged off, MixIR. "So, what do you want to do?" Jones asked Ottie, wondering what music he would be making next. Ottie loaded up an old melody, "Hey, how about this one? Let's just edit it a bit and drop it down an octave. It can be our second song. Ottie dropped some anime voices over the old melody and started formulating music of what he thought sounded good. Jones sat by idly watching and making suggestions on each piece until the clock struck 10:00 PM. "Hey, I think it's time we both get some rest," Jones stated as Ottie nodded off feeling tired. "Yeah, I think so as well." Ottie turned off the computer as he headed towards the restroom. Jones sat on the bedside thinking to himself about what he was going to do at work the next day. As the two of them drifted off to sleep, Jones started to imagine again.

In his own thoughts, he saw another woman on the beach with curly-blonde hair. She waved towards him as she threw rocks. The rocks were crystal clear as the two of them sat together. "Hi. I'm Jones. You?" She looked surprised, "I'm Layla." she said laughing. "Take my hand. I've heard a lot about you." She took Jones' hands in hers and walked over the crystal rocks in the sand as the sunlight glistened over them. Walking over towards the water, the two of them danced, laughing as the crystal rocks around them spun. "Jones, what did I tell you?" Layla smiled. "What?" Jones replied, not knowing a thing. "This is Nepharius. I told you to focus. Why do you insist on not listening to me?" Layla was now Nepharius standing right next to him. "I just went to the Brazilian temples. I could feel you were in trouble lately. What happened?" Jones explained about the universal car and people who were following him throughout the galaxy.

"You know you're being hunted," Jones warned. Nepharius replied quickly, "War is fun! Why not?" he laughed as he disappeared. Jones woke up with that last thought brimming through his head. Thinking he might have to be careful of Nepharius. Ottie poked him as Jones became conscious. "Yo, don't you have to pick up one of the artists from the airport?" Ottie asked. Ottie looked over at Jones. Jones couldn't make heads or tails of the differences between dreams and reality around him. "Ottie, can you cover for me?" Jones pleaded. Ottie nodded his head as the two of them went over to the car. Racing down to where they worked, together they ran up the stairs, just as the woman announced they were canvassing today. Jones requested to go alone. The woman nodded her head as Jones eyed the room. Tina was there, sitting in the call center, but she had paid no attention to him. Running back down the steps, Jones' picked up a call from his boss at Animal Beats.

"Hey man, we need to get to the airport. Can you drive us? his boss asked. Jones put on some EDM music and drove the car as fast as he could, heading towards downtown SF. He would pick them up from the city and then head to the airport. Jones spotted his boss near a BART station on Market as he walked out wearing a T-shirt with an animal logo on it. An EDM artist with purple hair was vaping as he waited by his side. "Yo! Good to see ya, Jones. How's the marketing been?" his boss asked. Jones shook his boss' hand. "Oh, you know. It's been alright. Going to LA soon." Jones said mentioning the trip. Jones switched gears as they got in the car, "Hey can you start marking off these houses?" pointing at his phone. "Just

CHAPTER SEVEN - STATIC BEACH

press one house address every 30 minutes." His boss looked down at the phone, "Sure, why not." In the back, the artist was vaping, "I can't wait until the next song finishes. It's going to premiere soon." Jones and his boss both smiled, "Yeah! It's going to be big, man."

Driving in towards the City there was a lighthouse on top of the hillside. Passing through San Francisco they blasted the EDM artist's music in the car. People gave the car a weird look as if to say, 'What is going on in there?' Jones dropped them off at the airport, "Alright you two, safe flight." Jones rushed back towards work driving as fast as he could. Calling was about to start within the hour. Thinking in hyper-mode, Jones went into his mania mindset. Using the same trick that he had witnessed earlier, Jones started to speed through the cars on the highway, dodging them as they went through. While thinking of WAZE, the road warriors on the WAZE Icon stopped the policeman from pulling over Jones, as the road warrior bikers were being pulled over themselves. Almost in record time, Jones landed back in the work area. Making a hard turn and stepping on the brakes, he stopped the car. A bit of smoke came out from where the tires came to a halt. Jones ran back up the stairs right as the clock hit 4:00 PM. He took the seat next to Bernz and Gio. "Yo guys, what's up?" Jones said, smiling as he waited for a response. Gio whispered, "Bro, the only good thing here is the food."

Jones laughed as he got to work making his calls. After a few moments, Tina nudged him with a text, "Hey meet me in the hallway." Jones went out into the hallway walking towards the red carpet. "Hey… So…" Jones looked at Tina, feeling guilty about the time at her house. "I'm sorry, but this won't work." Tina latched onto his arm, "Please don't." Jones said again, "I'm sorry, but it's not a good idea." He shrugged her off, walking back towards the company door. Jones closed it behind him as he left her alone in the hallway. Jones took a seat next to Gio, "Yeah, so skateboarding tonight?" Jones questioned. "Hell yeah!" Gio said. Ottie sat back in his chair smiling.

Ottie and Gio bickered back and forth, "Do a tre flip." Ottie whispered into Gio's ear laughing. Jones made some more calls during the day, trying to stay focused on the walls around him. The workplace had been on his mind. One of the employees had told him that they sat at Starbucks earlier as the Woman Manager congratulated him for canvassing 300 houses in two hours. Jones felt that the workplace might come crashing down on them. Soon the white walls would be closing in as it seemed the Woman Manager now knew what was happening in the workplace. Jones could sense it within the four walls. As the clock hit 6:00 PM, the Woman Manager called everyone up, "Good work today, everyone. Tomorrow we will have a long talk."

Jones cowered away towards the back of the room, realizing what that had meant. The entire workplace had been caught gaming the system. "Yo, Gio!" Ottie shouted from the side of the room, "Ready to go skateboarding again?" Ottie egged Gio on, "Do a tre flip, Bro! 311 in the Quaaad!" Bernz shouted, "311 in the Quad!" as they all left out the door. Ottie ran down the steps, hopping on his board. Gio and Ottie skated over to the Burger King across the street. Going up and down on the curb, Jones followed behind. "Hey, let's go back to that one neighborhood again," Gio suggested. "Yeah man, I'm down." as Ottie focused on trying to do an actual tre-flip.

They all got on their skateboards. Ottie went first — up a small ramp holding onto an overhang. There was a tall building with a garage and one security camera. Gio followed as there were no cars in the lot. Lighting up a joint, Gio gave it a puff and passed it over to Ottie. Jones followed suit right behind them. A can of unopened paint sat on the corner of the parking structure. Ottie pointed it out, "Bro, what is this?" tossing it over to Gio. "Looks like a can of paint." Jones said with caution, "Gio, take that can of paint and put it back, man." Jones had a bad feeling about the paint. Ottie jokes, "Yeah if you can't jump over the can just leave it." Gio took the can and was about to put it back. However, for some odd reason in his mind, it clicked for him to pour it out instead.

CHAPTER SEVEN - STATIC BEACH

"What are you doing, Bro?" Ottie gasped, as Gio upended the can onto the blue, disabled, parking spot. The red paint color seeped over the blue disabled symbol, covering up the whole corner of the parking structure. "Why the fuck did you do that, man?" Ottie shouted in anger. Gio shrugged, "I don't know, Bro. There Are no cameras here anyway. So what?" Ottie pointed straight up at the ceiling "It's right fucking there, Bro!" Gio defended himself, "It's not a big deal. Let's get out of here." Ottie and Jones skateboarded out of the building garage towards the corner next to the gas station. "Hey man, it's getting late. Let's go home." Gio agreed as he walked off towards BART. Jones and Ottie turned to one another, "Yo, if the cops come, it's totally his fault." Ottie said to Jones.

Jones nodded, "Way agreed, Bro. We did warn him." They started skateboarding back towards the pathway that led to the Army Veterans building. Under the bridge, there was graffiti written along with a picture of a face. Jones, still feeling as if he had some sanity left in his mind, played along as he hummed a melody in his head.

"Man, we got the rest of the day to do whatever. Isn't that beach party tonight?" Jones asked for reconfirmation. He figured he could find it by checking his spam email as a text came up. "Still coming over this weekend to my house?" Ike's words were on Jones' phone. Jones had completely blanked on everything due to the crazy life that had been happening around him. "I don't know if we can make it this weekend for the production, man. It'll have to wait until we get back," Jones messaged back. "Alright. No problem. When you get back from LA!" responded Ike.

Jones thought for a moment more before heading into the house. Ottie entered first and put his skateboard on the bed. "So, what's this beach party about anyway?" Ottie asked. "Well, remember my friend's birthday party bash over at that other club? Apparently, they are having a privatized beach party in the City. There's supposed to be a lot of people there." replied Jones. Ottie's eyes lit up in excitement, "Yo that sounds amazing!

We gotta go!" Jones threw on his better separates, dressed in all black with a beanie. Ottie followed suit putting on his plaid clothing. "What are you a lumberjack?" Jones teased as he threw on his overcoat. "Yeah, I'm always out pickaxing back in the woods, boi." Ottie joked. The two laughed as Jones raced Ottie out the front door to the silver car. After settling into the car, Jones put on some EDM music to prepare for the night.

"I heard Static might be there tonight," Jones said. Ottie replied excitedly, "No way! Static?!!" They headed out towards the direction of the beach. Ottie had grabbed the USB, just in case, from the computer. "What's the USB for?" Jones asked Ottie, wondering why in the world he had it on him. Ottie laughed, "Well in the case Static is there… I've seen it in documentaries — some of the guys get big by throwing their USB during a set or by giving it to the main stage artist to listen to." Jones laughed with him, "That's pretty insane you know." While in the car Jones got a text from Nepharius, "Paging all Jones." Then the phone rang twice. Another text, "How's your journey so far?" Jones replied right away via voice text, "The journey's been fine, man. What do I owe you? I thought—."

Nepharius cut him off, "Look, I just got a brilliant idea despite your disservice to the team. We should throw a show. It'll be called the pirate theme. You'll go around town and post wanted posters of us to generate interest. Lots of people will show up." Jones thought the idea sounded brilliant. "You mean, you'll put on costumes and post it around town to fake being wanted?" he asked Nepharius. "Yeah! The party location would be on the bottom of the poster. The galaxy would go nuts." texted Nepharius. Thinking for a moment, Jones felt like it would generate a lot of interest. "Well… Alright. I've got to go for now. I have a beach party to attend." Jones replied.

Nepharius left it on read, texting back, "You already know." Ottie saw the minor stress on Jones' face. "So, what do you think will happen at work tomorrow?" Ottie inquired. Jones shrugged as another car passed

CHAPTER SEVEN - STATIC BEACH

them on the freeway, "I... I have no idea. Let's party and forget about it for now." Jones felt as if he was being toyed with. Forgiving as he was, everyone always wanted to jump into his emotions only if they needed something. The life he lived was never about him. Jones felt that this party was one way to bring about the love that he had to give. Mainly for his own well-being.

Arriving at the beach, Jones walked up to Sawn high fiving him. His courage was brimming, lighting up the sand as the people watched him wearing lit-up hats. There was a giant wooden tree with a DJ booth not too far off. People were sitting there half-dressed. "Heaven!" Ottie shouted while he slid down the hillside towards the scantily, half-dressed women. Ottie took note of the girl closest to him. He was instantly entranced. "I'm telling you, Jones. This is heaven!" Ottie admired again. Jones shrugged as Sawn came up from behind. "Jones! Ottie? Glad you could make it!" Sawn slung his arm around Jones as if they were buddies from the start. "Yo, as a promoter, you have to be at every party, everywhere!" Jones smiled, "Everywhere?" questioning what Sawn meant. "Yeah, see this chica, this is GG. Take a seat and cuddle." Sawn pushed Jones down onto the blanket. As he lost his footing, Jones found himself sitting next to GG.

She was smiling at him with full interest, "Hi Jonesy! I've heard so much about you." Jones focused on Ottie instead of GG, eyeing the giant tree in the middle of the beach. He knew that the giant tree was his ticket out of the beach party's action. Ottie went over to the DJ booth where a guy was playing. Jones watched someone sit in the tree, so he asked GG if he could share the blanket. There was a man with golden hair standing nearby, posed next to his girlfriend as he looked out over the water. "So, we heard there's supposed to be a main event tonight," Jones said loudly, looking at the guy. "Yeah, man. I'm excited!" he said standing on the blue blanket, not caring about the weather around him. GG smiled as she cuddled up against Jones trying to stay warm. She laughed listening in as Sawn also got under the beach blanket.

"Well now we have to get up and dance, don't we?" Jones said getting up following the energy of the party. He could feel that there were plenty of musicians around. He saw Sunshine hanging from the tree. "Hey, Jones! Awesome to see you here!" Sunshine's eyes glistened a fiery red for a moment. Waving at Jones, he waved back. Jones was ready to wander off to find Ottie, but turned back towards the man standing on the blue blanket and asked, "So, do you do music?" It was all about following the music at this point. This was the only consciousness Jones had left. The cold night sky and wind picked up making Jones shiver. Sawn came by again, "Here's another blanket, man!" From a distance, Ottie waved Jones over with the USB grasped in his hand. "Bro! We gotta throw it. Static is here!" he shouted. Jones looked around, "What do you mean?"

The man standing on the blue blanket smiled, "What USB?" Jones smiled back, "Well it's for this artist we aspire to follow." The man laughed, "Pass me the USB. I'm Static." Jones waved at Ottie to come over. Ottie was with another woman heading up the hill. "Bro, this IS Static!" Jones exclaimed. Ottie lit up, "No way! Man, I love your work." Ottie tossed the USB by Static's feet. "I'll listen to this later," Static said as he picked it up. "Come down the beach and watch me play a little." Ottie and Jones high-fived one another, nodding their heads towards Static. They started making their way to the front of the beachside. A bunch of people were dancing and smiling, lit up by the glowing wind. Plants sparkled in the air as the night sky went down on them. The sound system and lights set up behind the DJ started coming up into view from behind the sand dune. Hidden away, the music blared through the crowd showing colors. Jones could see the vibrations of the music in colors red and blue for the rich, deep sounds. Then Jones saw the music wave marks of yellow and pink crossing through the people towards the other side of the sandy cove. Jones could pick out people with feathers on their clothing. Though Jones couldn't find anyone to interview, Ottie and Jones made their first move of attempting to become recognized.

CHAPTER SEVEN - STATIC BEACH

"Yo!" a man said from behind. Jones looked around as a photographer walked up to them. "So, I hear you met Static. And you two are musicians. Need a picture done?" the photographer asked. "I do it for all of the current bigger guys." Jones and Ottie were both flying higher off the energy that kept coming their way. "No, man, but tell us more," Ottie said humbly. "Nice to meet you. I'm True." True said as he shook their hands. "Truly nice to meet you," Jones said in return, making a joke. "Hey man. We need to disperse soon. I hear the cops are on their way to shut us down. For now, let's enjoy." warned the photographer. Jones and Ottie laughed, "Yeah, whatever." As the three of them kept dancing in the front, another man danced right in front of them going all out. "You know, if that guy had air boosters on the bottom of his shoes, he could be doing flips," Jones remarked.

Static played his first song and the crowd went crazy. As if souls were rising off the sand, heading towards a dance floor. The room spun in Jones' mind. Jones felt as if he was dreaming, floating through the galaxy again, as the crowd started changing. Crazy suits and costumes formed around each person. The large tree lit up from the inside as leaves sprouted, twisting forward and backward. "Jones?" someone whispered into his dream. Jones caught himself, "Yeah?" he said as Sawn's eyes were on him. "You alright?" Sawn said with concern. "Never felt better!" Jones replied. The beach came back to normal. The dance floor dispersed as Static walked down the stage steps.

"Looks like we have to go, guys," announced Sawn. True went up to Jones and Ottie, "Let's go." As they started walking back up the hill, 15 cops were waiting to try to grab people. True shouted, "Told you! Guys, come! I know another way!" Trekking back around, Ottie and Jones ran down a pathway climbing up rocks towards the top of the hill. A barn lay in their sights next to a fence. An animal made a sound. "Horse!" True shouted. "Lay down low guys." All three of them watched from afar as the 15 cops separated with people dispersing in chaos everywhere. "Shh..." True said to the horse while petting it. He had a carrot in his bag. The horse then quieted down. "Ottie, want to pet the horse?" True asked. Ottie took over, nuzzling with the horse. "You've got a good heart, man. Hey, listen. I need a ride home if you guys don't mind." Said the photographer. Jones replied quickly, "Nah, I don't mind."

As the last of the cops sped away, they left the barn and ran across the rocks towards Jones' car. Jones turned right out of the parking area to drive them away from the commotion. "Shit! I have to grab some gas." Jones exclaimed, putting on the GPS. The Waze app showed the road warriors again, clearing a path. "You'll never see me again, but you guys have been super helpful." remarked True sincerely. Jones pulled up to the gas station. As he filled his tank Ottie walked down to a burger fast food restaurant close by. From afar you could hear him, "There better not be any sausage juice on my pancakes. I'm vegan, you know." Ottie was irritated, after being drunk and then having to run across the hill. "Time to make it on home." Jones called, after finishing filling his gas tank, "Let's go, Ottie."

Stepping on the gas, Jones floored it again. His car left a dent in the gravel on the cement road as the car sped down the highway. After thirty minutes of driving, they were close to where True lived. Twelve chickens were crossing the road as Jones tried to drop off True, getting stuck in the traffic of the animals. "Chicken!" True scoffed. Jones looked at the chickens, sensing them stop in the middle of the road to look at him. "Jones! Oh, thanks for stopping for us." the chickens communicated towards Jones. "Oh great... now animals are talking to me." Jones thought silently to himself, "Then get out of the road." The chickens started moving, right as Jones requested this in thought. "Whatever you require!" the chickens clucked. Jones continued driving slowly as True joked, "Man, what type of traffic was that?" Jones shook his head, "I don't know, but we're here." True got out of the car thanking Jones and Ottie profusely for the ride. He stumbled off towards his house. Ottie lightly jabbed Jones, "Bro, what a night. Huh?" They both laughed, "Throw a USB! Pet a horse."

CHAPTER SEVEN - STATIC BEACH

Jones turned the car around and started to drive towards home. He saw a man on the side of the road wearing a tinfoil hat with a necklace around him. The man was waving a hairdryer in the air. "Clean air is a necessity." he kept mumbling. Jones tried not to engage the man as the man looked up to stare straight at Jones as he drove by. Passing other strange people further down the road, Jones felt the sand in his shoes. "Damn, maybe we shouldn't go to work tomorrow," Ottie said, still slightly drunk. Jones replied, "Show up late? I think we'll do better." Jones pulled up to his house as the sun was coming up through the night. Ottie drunkenly walked towards the front door. Falling asleep on his bed immediately, Jones relished the thoughts of what had just happened that evening. Yet Jones had no idea what to expect next, as life was going to push him in a brand-new direction.

Chapter Eight - Fall

The next day Jones rolled over with three new texts on his phone. "Where are you? The cops are here." The Campaign Manager Woman said texting Jones, "They are looking for you." "Shit" Jones moaned. A knock on the house front door happened a few minutes later. Ms. P opened it. "We need to talk to your son. We got a complaint regarding a garage and a few skateboarders." Ms. P knocked on Jones' bedroom door. "Are you awake? The Cops want to talk to you. They are in the living room." "What happened is the cameras caught you guys pouring some red paint on a disabled parking spot in a company garage. It's going to cost you $360. You'll need to go to court." said the police officer. "Wait, sir." Jones started to explain, "We told our friend not to pour the paint. He didn't listen to us. Review the security cameras and you'll see that we weren't involved." The cop looked at him sternly, "Okay, do you know the name of the guy?" "Yeah." Jones said, "His name is Gio."

The cop went out of the door thanking Jones for his time. Jones texted Ottie who was at work, "The cops are looking for you, man. Gio too." Jones grabbed his phone as he got ready to watch for messages. He quickly got out of his pajamas, freshened up, and headed out to work. The woman stood at the campaign office door infuriated. "What the hell is going on? The cops were here!" she asked as she let Jones enter the office. "Well, it doesn't matter. "Everyone, circle up!" We noticed everyone's not properly doing their work. We had to fire half of you. We will be getting a new

CHAPTER EIGHT - FALL

system installed tomorrow." Jones piped up, "Man that's crazy." Acting as if he didn't know. The woman eyed him, "Your friend told me you went to the airport. Also, Tina had to be let go." she said bluntly. In Jones' mind, his plan of using Tina to keep their group safe worked. Ottie had thrown Jones under the bus but pointed fingers towards Tina.

Tina got fired on the spot. Bernz had also not shown up to work. The worker who had just been rewarded for 300 houses was also gone. Jones sat there silently in the circle as the woman rephrased her wording, "We are very disappointed in the entire workplace and should fire all of you. However, some of you have done some actual work. Therefore, we are keeping the rest of you on board." Jones looked at the floor in guilt knowing that because of their group, the word got out. There were only two weeks left in the campaign. Somehow Yeezy was still in the lead, keeping the chance for redemption. "We're looking for a Gio?" one worker asked in a semi-concerned manner. The woman shouted, "What's going on here? Can't you mind your own business and just work the campaign?" Earlier, the cops had come to the office to interview Ottie. They took down names and went straight to the Campaign Manager woman. Gio never finished the campaign as he was fired on the spot. After the cops showed up at the office to talk to Ottie, they chased Gio down and fined him the $360 for property damage. "The woman replied to the worker, "Yes, one of the workers said to be here has to go to court."

Jones felt remorseful. He had befriended Tina. She started copying his group. Was it for when the time came, that she would be the one to take the fault? "What a devious plan." Jones thought to himself, as he quietly mourned. Now the employees were scot-free to finish up the campaign for extra money. Jones didn't have to worry about losing the job. "Okay, listen up. Here are the new phones with built-in trackers. We will know if you're working or not in the last two weeks. Dan will be taking over the daily campaign operations." With that said, the woman stormed off the other way, not wanting to look at the rest of the room. Dan, a man with red scaly skin came out and sat down on the desk. "You two. Jones and Ottie, right? Come here. Tomorrow, you will go out and do the first test run of the new phones."

Ottie and Jones shrugged at one another and came forward to pick up the phones, "Well alright." they said. They had to take their job seriously now that word had gotten out. There would be no more Bernz. Tennor got fired on the spot and Jack quit. The group was back down to two. As Ottie walked down the stairs with Jones he smiled, "Well, work's going to be a lot different for the last of it, huh?" Jones replied, "At least we get to see this through and finish it." Jones chilled by the side of his car taking the fliers in his hand, "Hey, I've got an idea… delivering these fliers sucks, right?" Ottie turned and nodded in agreement. "Instead of hanging each flier individually, let's just drop a pile in front of some driveways." Ottie laughed, "It would save time, Bro."

The two of them sped over each speed bump, dropping off the fliers as they waved towards the people in the street. Ottie turned towards Jones waving his hat, "It's almost as if we're going through an election or something." he laughed as the wind flew past. After a few hours, Jones and Ottie had nearly run out of fliers with only a couple left. Most of the people on the street were now holding their campaign's marketing materials. In just one day out of an entire week, they had covered a lot of ground. Driving back towards the office, Jones felt a feeling of accomplishment. "You know, we should pack up to be ready to go next week. Los Angeles isn't that far and we both have enough money." Jones said. Ottie smiled, "Bro, I'm all for it. I'm so excited that this is finally going down." They got back to the office, hustling up the stairs, headed towards the main office door. "Good work today. Did you run delivering the fliers?" the Campaign Manager Woman teased. Jones puffed as he caught his breath, "Yeah! It was a great workout."

The woman waved them off as if it was nothing, "Well you two are in early.

CHAPTER EIGHT - FALL

Go home and get some rest." As the call center was full and Jones and Ottie covered all the canvassing ground; there was nothing left for them to do. "Let's go to this show tonight. It's kind of random, but it's in the City." Jones said smiling, looking over towards Ottie as they headed home. "Alright, we'll go into The City again. Do you know Club Temple? I've emailed the guy who's playing there tonight. He's pretty cool. Do you want to go there?" asked Ottie. At first, Jones waved the idea off, "I'm not sure." Then Jones thought about it again, "Well maybe." Ottie looked at him with intent, "C'mon, it will prepare us for LA." Ottie was right: They could use some prospecting experience. After all, this could be another shoot for the magazine.

"Alright Ottie, let's go to this place. Don't expect anything though." Jones said acquiescing. Ottie went back down the stairs right behind Jones. Ottie tripped on the first step as he made his way down to Jones's car. Styles was standing by his gold SUV, just about to leave. "Crazy what happened today, huh?" Styles said, initiating a conversation. Jones waved in agreement trying to get to his car. "Yeah." Ottie replied, "A little too crazy." Ottie shut the car door, not wanting to associate with Styles for the moment. The whole place almost lost their job because of Jones and Bernz. Weighing on Jones' consciousness, Jones wanted to go out and party off the stress. Jones checked his email, "You're not doing your work! How could you? You pirate liar! Headlines all about it!" The headlines in Jones' spam email attacked him from all sides.

You said you would fix our universal problems! LIAR!" Jones had no idea how to respond. Out of panic he went into his head and shouted from within his mind, "Okay, look! I'm working on it!" The noise in his email calmed down, "I'm improving the world slowly! Give me time!" Jones said, begging for the noise to stop. An email popped up on his phone, "Come to Club Temple. Stay focused on yourself, Jones." the message read, calming him down. Ottie eyed Jones not knowing if he was asleep or stuck in deep thought, "You cool?" he questioned, wondering if Jones was okay. Jones replied, "Yeah, I'm fine man, let's go to Club Temple." They freshened up and changed their clothing to be more set for the night. "This is the last show we will attend before L.A.," Jones said excitedly. "So, let's enjoy it!" This time the focus of the party wasn't to find an expert to interview. This time the party was simply to have fun. Jones felt like he would be able to relax for a moment at the club.

After turning on the radio to the max in the silver car, they headed out for their night of fun. Arriving at the Club, parking lights lit up in pink on both sides of the road. However, only Jones noticed the feeling. Inside, there were women in skimpy outfits, dressed like the men with no shirts on. Lights of all colors flashed around the people, who were wearing strands of lights and holding various tools in their hands. A man sat on the sidelines hammering in the last nail with a hat. The man then put the hat on his head, having the tool disappear. Jones questioned what he had just seen, but let it go. From behind him another man came up and poked him. "Hey. Saw you at the last two places. What's your template?" he asked. Jones turned around, "What do you mean?" The man shook Jones' hand, "Name's Sao. The CIA's been after me for a while." He was wearing a red shirt and a red hat. The hat looked just like the brown hats that successful people wore. "You know some people wear red, black, brown, or other kinds of hats to define who they are. At club shows it's hard to decipher their meaning, though," Sao continued.

"I see. Excuse me." Jones said, trying to break away from the conversation. Jones walked around a bit more. A man with lightning earrings sat down nearby. "So, do you like old cars?" Jones asked him, trying to make conversation. The man growled, "I hate old cars." Jones backed away and over towards where Sao was standing. "See, some people can be kind of a dick around here," Sao said, glancing over at the man with lightning earrings. "So, I hear you're trying to play. Let's get to the music and make something sometime. I could be your way out from the CIA." Jones looked Sao up and down a few more times, "Alright." he said as he passed him

CHAPTER EIGHT - FALL

his phone number. Jones found Ottie dancing in the middle of the floor. "Man, this is fun!" smiled Ottie. Feeling like a fugitive on the run, Jones put his hands up in the air, "Not going to get us!" Jones shouted as he ran through the crowd. The crowd randomly started following him holding up a number one finger sign. "Go Jones go!" they chanted.

Clothing changed into futuristic styles. The people around him were now speaking French and puffing purple smoke from lit e-cigarettes. The people kept leaving and coming out of the door at a high rate as if Jones' consciousness had put him on the other side of the world. "Does Jones always dance like that?" Sao asked Ottie. Ottie shrugged, "What? Like an idiot? Yeah, kind of." Putting his hands up, Jones spiraled them in and out while spinning in circles. "It's kinda weird and different, but I like it!" Sao observed. 'Extra! Extra! Jones comes up with a new quirky dance.' The newspapers outside of the Club began to change. And a dance instructor was shown teaching Jones' dance steps to a class of students."Damn Jones, you have a lot of influence," Sao said, patting him on the back. "What exactly do you do again?" Sao waited for Jones' response as a man serving drinks came towards them.

"I make music. That's all." Jones replied. Sao cautiously said back, "Listen, you have my number. This place is almost done for, so let's get out of here." Sao pointed at the exit door as images, lights and music came out into the space in 3D. As the next song came up the world quickly changed, being created from the ideas Jones was communicating in his mind. Jones fell towards the floor trying to focus and control his thoughts. Ottie patted Jones on the back, "Bro you good? You disappeared for a bit." Jones checked back up from the floor that now moved like a conveyor belt. Drinks were being served and thrown from the ceiling. The shadows of people danced as the drinks fell into their mouths. Jones laid on the floor and made a snow angel, viewing the ceiling. "Look!" he said laughing as he pointed towards the ceiling. "A shadow angel!" Ottie looked over at Jones, "C'mon dude. Get up off the floor. People are looking at us funny." Jones smiled,

"If they are judging me, fuck 'em." Sao watched Jones from afar, "Kinda like that kid. He might just go far."

Turning towards the security guy at the door and nodding, Sao walked out quietly. Jones got up from laying on the floor. Spotting a wet area on the dance floor, Jones walked over to it and started dancing. "You know, dancing like this with water — we'll call it water dancing!" Jones laughed, sparking another idea as he slid across the floor. Ottie rolled his eyes, "Alright Bro, you're out of control. It's time to go outside." Jones slid over towards Ottie, but half off on his aim. He fell on his butt continuing to slide. Jones sat up quickly, "Alright, you're right. Out for a cig?" he inquired. Silently he thanked Ottie for bringing him back to reality. They walked outside where most of the party-goers smoked cigarettes. Ottie took a cigarette from a gentleman's hand as the man stared at Jones. Jones went over and took a beer off the counter and began drinking it. "See! No one cares," Jones stated as he looked back at Ottie. "That was someone's random drink you know," Ottie warned.

Ottie began talking to a random stranger, losing sight of Jones. Jones decided to go back inside, retracing his steps that had taken them outside the Club. Once inside the back door, the stairs glowed a fluorescent purple, marked as if splashes of paint had been tossed on them. For a moment Jones lost sight of his purpose. What was he doing trying to go to shows without a target in mind? Was meeting these people really all that important? Jones sighed as he slipped on the stairs.

Ottie, who had followed behind, caught him from falling. He started dragging him out by the arm. "Yo! Alright man. It's time to go. You are way too much right now." he said sternly. Jones struggled a bit and then slowly accepted. Sitting down by the front step Jones puked not remembering what had just happened. "How many drinks did we buy?" Jones asked Ottie. "Bro, you've had one drink," Ottie said, looking at him confused. Jones wasn't sure why he had puked. The energy against his

CHAPTER EIGHT - FALL

body made him feel drained as if he could feel what the souls inside were saying. A man in a black T-shirt walked by and read, "I'm cooler than you". Apparently, the trend in town was to wear exactly what you were doing for work. Jones wanted to ask the man about his T-shirt, but let it go. Sao texted him, "See you soon with that template. The CIA are after me, so I had to go." Jones peaked at his phone as his Notes smiled back at him.

"Well... To LA!" Jones shouted as Ottie opened the door to their car and helped Jones into the passenger seat. Jones put down the window and let the cold air drift in. He needed to catch his breath from what had just happened in the Club. Ottie put on some loud music. "I can't listen to this right now, man. It's hurting my ears." Jones whimpered. Without realizing it, Jones' hyper-focusing on the people around him had made music hurt in his head and his ears. The music was starting to drive Jones crazy. "Bro, it's not that loud." Ottie objected. "Just turn it down!" Jones shouted.

"Okay, fine. I'm turning it down." Ottie said slightly annoyed that he couldn't listen to his rock music on the way home. Jones laid back in the seat trying to relax. Had this encounter not happened, Jones would've never learned about the agents from the underground. Sao was right, someone was monitoring Jones. However, what did Jones expect after pairing up with a known diabolical space pirate who starts wars? Jones and Ottie arrived home. Throwing his coat on the bed, Jones had a disgusted look on his face. Ottie paid no attention to it as he hopped on the computer. Ms. P called out from the other room, "Jones can I speak with you a minute?" she asked.

Jones went over to his mother. "Sit down Jones, Ms. P stated quietly, Ottie needs to leave. He's overstayed his welcome. I'll give you guys a little extra time, but I want a plan." Jones sat down without question, but his mind was elsewhere. He rebutted loudly, "Mom, where will Ottie go? He has no place to go!" Ottie overheard them. Seeing his mom's look, Jones quieted down, "Okay, I will tell him. Give us time to sort this out." Ms. P shook her head in dismay, "Alright, but he had better have his life sorted very soon. He can't keep staying here."

Jones went back into the bedroom and lay on his bed as he scrolled through his spam email. There was nothing new popping up — the night was silent. He needed to think quickly. "Ottie, let's go to LA tomorrow. We have a break in the campaign work right now with this whole firing thing and the new system being tested." Jones eyed Ottie wondering if he'd agree. Ottie's eyes lit up, "Hell yeah! I'll start packing first thing in the morning." Ottie slipped into his sleeping bag and put on the music documentary to remind himself of the spot they would be driving to. While Jones fell asleep, Ottie got back up. Loading up the computer, he graphically designed himself a new stage name, 'Allorium'. It now said the new name on the front screen.

Ottie was determined to finish his song before going to Los Angeles so that they could promote themselves as artists and music promoters. Making an EPK along with a poster was guaranteed to give some credibility that they as artists knew what they were doing. Loading up another DAW (Digital Audio Workstation), Ottie got to work. He stayed up all night to make a new song, while Jones was asleep, tossing and turning. "Jones. Jones, what are you trying to accomplish?" a person asked him. Jones didn't have an answer. He tried not to let his thoughts race. Only "I don't know." came out from his mind as he tossed and turned. "You don't know?" the voice said from far away, "I'm an expert. Come find me soon." After a short moment, Jones' world fell silent.

Chapter Nine – Depression Trip

The next day as Jones woke up, the weather was predicted to be a warm 70 degrees, as if another day of perfection rolled in. Ottie was already up and packed before Jones had even gotten out of bed. Ottie had jumped on the bed excitedly causing Jones to bounce twice up and down due to his weight. Ottie laughed, "Yo, this is fun. Isn't it?" he asked, as he watched Jones sit up with an annoyed look on his face. After the fiasco with the Yazer campaign, who had apparently won the election, they had enough money to stay in Los Angeles for a couple of weeks. There was a campaign congratulations party but neither Jones nor Ottie showed up for it. Due to the insane amount of calling and dropping off of fliers completed in the last two weeks of the campaign, Yazer had gotten his money's worth. Jones yawned, "Give me five more minutes, Bro. I'm hardly even dressed or ready to leave."

Ottie showed Jones a USB that he held in his hand, "Our songs are done. We can more effectively promote ourselves now. I've got a few friends in Los Angeles too." Ottie said, already thinking about the trip. "It's a long drive you know," Jones replied, slowly rolling over. This time Jones sat up and rubbed his eyes as his mother shouted from the kitchen, "Breakfast's ready!" Ms. P yelled. Ottie went in and sat down at the kitchen table as Ms. P. stood there with a spatula in hand, "Eggs and bacon, Ottie?" she asked. Jones joined Ottie at the table, after putting on his pajama bottoms so he could be semi-presentable around the house. "Thanks, Mom. I'll take them scrambled with ketchup." Jones requested. Ottie looked at him weirdly, "Ketchup? Is that like a California thing?" Jones chuckled, "Not even. I swear it originated in the south."

Ms. P put the eggs, bacon, and toast right in front of Jones, turning to get the ketchup from the fridge. Jones sat in front of his toast slowly eating it as he thought about the long journey ahead. Driving to Los Angeles was an easy feat, however, they had no idea where they were going. The first stop was in Orange County to see one of Ottie's friends. "Is something on your mind?" Jones' mother inquired. "We have a long trip ahead of us, that's all," Ottie replied. Jones didn't answer as he finished his eggs. He went to his room to put stuff in the suitcase. An old war veteran's cane lay in the corner of Jones' closet. Jones picked it up gathering its details. The cane was made from black coral with a bronze handle at the top. The design was simple and light, easy to hold with each step. Jones quickly put it back into the closet as he felt a weird aura coming from it. "Alright, done! Let me take a shower and we'll be off!" he shouted to Ottie from his room. MS. P took the plates away as Ottie had his last bite of toast. With a backpack and suitcase in hand, they were both ready for the four-hour drive to LA to start their new careers.

Jones took the driver's seat looking over at Ottie, "So where do you think this famous artist is at?" Ottie thought for a moment, "Well, you see, in the music documentary, there's a food place shown. The food place is one place that he visits a lot. However, I have no clue where it is. I believe if we find an old factory, we should be able to find him."Astounded by Ottie's deduction skills, Jones shrugged his shoulders,

"Okay! No problem. Let's go then." he smiled. Jones turned the key as Ottie popped in a CD chock full of their music. The first song came on through the car's sound system yielding decent results."Hey when we find the place, let's hand out these fliers. I'll make some!" said Ottie with glee. Jones laughed, "Alright, that sounds decent. I believe we'll get pretty far if we happen to stumble across the right place." As the forest slowly

CHAPTER NINE – DEPRESSION TRIP

dissipated, Jones got on the highway headed towards Los Angeles. The desert and farmlands to each side didn't give much room for scenery on the long drive down there. Ottie made his first call, "Yooo! Garne! How have you been my dude?" he asked. Garne's voice ripped through the phone, happy to receive the call, "Down in Orange County! Dude, I was just at the office of those well-known guys! I'm in close with them. It's pretty amazing down here!" Ottie feeling hyped by being on the road shouted back, "I know! I can't wait to check it out. We'll probably be there by night. You work at a grocery store, right?"

Garne replied quickly, "Yeah! It's an outlet store!" he said happily talking about Orange County. A cow passed by outside the window as a farmer picked the grass around him. Nut trees sprouted from the side of the road. A little gas station appeared as Jones noted the car had gotten low. "Hey, I need to stop and get some gas. Want anything from the inside of the store?" Jones asked Ottie as he pulled up to the side of the station. "If they've got coffee, yes," Ottie said in return. The two had eaten not too long ago, but both felt tired from last night's escapade. Walking on into the gas station, Jones went over to the cashier. "One donut and a coffee please!" Jones requested. The cashier eyed him, "Alright it will be a moment." she said in return.

"Is there a restroom I can use?" Jones asked, peering around the corner. "Yeah, that way." the cashier pointed towards a door leading around back. Jones happily started to walk that way. However, in the back of the gas station near the restroom there sat fifteen, bulked, strong men. Many of them had tattoos across their body as they sat in little chairs watching T.V. The whole room in this part of the gas station was wooden with brown wood around it, almost as if an old schoolroom had been remodeled into the gas station. Jones stopped in his tracks as the men looked up, taking notice of him. One of the men turned towards him, "Hey traveler, come join in." in a surprisingly warm tone. Jones pointed to the restroom, "Alright, after I use the restroom." Jones replied, buying himself some time.

These men were serious bikers or truckers, some sort of travelers. Jones didn't want to upset the crew as he washed his hands then sat down. "So, where ya headed?" the man with the mustache asked.

Jones eyed the T.V., zoning out as country music played in the background of the gas station, "I'm headed to LA." he replied. The man with the mustache laughed, "Better get going then. Sounds like your coffee's made. We'll be seeing you on the road, maybe." Jones studied the tattoo on the right side of the man's arm. It read 'Road Warrior'. "Hey, you know if you tattoo your arm, it doesn't go away. Don't do the hands or it will fade. We're watching out for you buddy." Jones did not ask the name of the burly man with the mustache. He got up out of the chair, thanking the man for the tip, grabbing the donut and two coffees. While munching down Ottie asked, "Hey, what took so long?" Jones smirked, "Coffee takes a long time to brew. Did you know that tattoos on the hand fade the fastest?" Ottie wondered what had happened inside, but didn't question further, "Yeah, I read an article once where a lady cried purple cause she had tattooed eyeliner too close to her eye. Stuff is scary, man. Gotta stay away from it." Ottie signaled Jones to start driving. Jones pulled out of the gas station as the 15 bikers peacefully started to roll on their way. He supposed the group knew one another from past travels across the country. Feeling confident in his safety, he revved up the car, and off they went down the highway towards LA.

Ottie, bored out of his mind, looked out the window towards big gates and fences that lay outside of the grassy fields. Over the long stretch of road, there wasn't much to do except listen to music. The wind replaced empty air and filled the car as Ottie slowly fell asleep. Jones was feeling hungry but didn't want to stop the car. "Guess we'll just sleep when we get there," Jones said to Ottie trying to keep himself awake by talking aloud as he plotted out their journey. "So where will we stay?" hoping to get a proper answer from Ottie as the two of them drifted into their dream state from driving. Ottie opened his eyes and turned up the music just as the two had

CHAPTER NINE – DEPRESSION TRIP

driven past a burger shop. "Hey, let's pull into here," Ottie said pointing at the sign. The two coffee cups sat in the middle console of the car from the last stop. Jones had moved from feeling hungry to feeling sleepy. "Alright, we'll go through the drive-through and continue our journey," Jones said, biding his time. Ottie asked for a vegan sandwich with just eggs on a bun, "There better not be any of that sausage juice on there." he said jokingly as the man in the burger joint started his order. Jones laid back in his car looking up at the sky through the sunroof as it passed over. There wasn't much to think about. Ottie's vegan burger was finished as the two went around the corner of the drive-through and got back on the highway. For the next two hours, Jones and Ottie didn't say a word, waiting for the time to pass.

"Nothing but trees," Ottie said finally, breaking the silence. "Yup," Jones said in return, not knowing what else to say. It was still sunny when they arrived in Orange County. Jones and Ottie both felt tired from the drive. "Hey, give Garne a call, won't you?" Jones asked, hoping to be able to stay in a friend's house. "Alright. I'm calling" Ottie dialed Garne's number not expecting an immediate pickup. The phone rang several times but there was no answer. "Leave a message if you're a cool boy!" Ottie shouted into the phone, "PICK UP BOI." "Let's pull in somewhere where we can park," Jones suggested to Ottie knowing that they couldn't simply stay on the streets around Buena Park, Orange County without being noticed. They found a burger place and pulled into the parking lot. A big green sign hung above the old building. Written on the top of the sign-in faded paint was 'Welcome to the New Land' as a giant cow hung from below. A man holding up a milk sign smiling with a mustache stared right down at Jones."Good ol' capitalism. I'm going to take a nap while we wait," Jones said as he laid back his driver's seat. Ottie, also feeling tired, agreed. Jones felt the sand underneath his feet. The water was climbing up to his neck as a woman's hands rubbed the back of his. Playing with his hair Jones felt in bliss almost as if he was floating.

"Heaven?" Jones mumbled aloud as a passerby peered inside the car window. "Hey!" the passerby said, trying to catch Jones' attention. He knocked on the window. Ottie was startled awake and opened the door making the car alarm go off. "Shit!" Ottie yelled, waking Jones woke up out of his reverie. "Uh, what's going on?" Jones asked, fishing for the keys to press the alarm button off. The man in the window held out his hand, "Got any spare change, man?" he asked while scratching his beard. "We really don't have anything," Ottie said standing on the far side of the car. The man walked off, "Fucking posers." mumbling under his breath as a chain hung low from his pants. The chain glistened in the sun as if it was there to ward off attackers. "Well, that was exciting," Jones said looking down at Ottie's phone. "Bro look, you have five missed calls." Ottie realized that Garne had been trying to reach them. Ottie picked up his phone as the messages played through. "Yo, I'm here! Got work until 6:00, but we can meet for a bit." Garne's message played on. "Um, guys?" The last message was a text. "Alright hit me up when you get this." Ottie dialed the number.

After three or four seconds of ringing, Garne picked up, "Yo! Where have you been? Where in the hell are you guys now?" Ottie spoke immediately, "We're in Buena Park, next to some sort of museum, and parked in a weird burger shop parking lot." "Alright, I know where you are. I'll be right there." Garne said as the phone clicked down. As Jones sat there listening in, a big smile crossed his face. He realized that they had successfully made it, completing the first step of their journey to Los Angeles. Ottie turned to Jones, "Yo, while we wait, let's go check out the museum over there." pointing the building across the way. Jones turned on the car, feeling excited about the overall situation, "That sounds pretty damn cool."

Jones pulled up to the curb parking his car next to a sign that showed a gigantic wave. The old museum had the look of a child's castle as if it were a model blown up to adult size. The mixture of grey and orange filled the outside of the building façade as box crevices stuck out. Almost as if to say, 'come on in', a deserted red rope on metal polls snaked around outside in

CHAPTER NINE – DEPRESSION TRIP

front of the entryway. Golden ribbons hung down from the rope on each side of the polls as if to say 'get in line'. A sign that hadn't been touched in years hung from below the red rope saying 'closed on Sunday'. Ottie went over to the building attempting to look for a way in. "I don't think we should go in there, Bro," Jones warned. Near the museum was a grassy field with a lone tree that sat in the middle. Jones climbed to the top of it. "What do you see up there?" asked Ottie. "I don't know, but I'm sailing!" Jones shouted, trying to distract Ottie from the museum. Noise from a nearby amusement park roared in the background. Jones was attempting to keep them out of trouble, but to no avail. Ottie was determined as he walked from the grassy field back over to the museum.

"We could scale this wall easily," Ottie suggested. Jones shook his head in dismay, "No, I don't think that's necessary. Look, I can see the castle drawbridge is open from the backside." Peering inside the museum, they were unable to see around the corner. Jones tried peeking even further and noticed an old mushroom water fountain. A voice yelled from the back, "Hey! The museum is closed guys."

Ottie shouted back, "Sorry! On our way out." The man guarding the museum seemed sleep-deprived, almost as if he was a zombie, ready to attack at any moment. "Hey let's go, man," Jones warned, feeling bad energy from the man guarding the rundown museum. After all, an old mushroom fountain that shot out water from the cement didn't seem like a good place to wait around anyway. "Alright." Ottie finally agreed walking away from the museum.

"Stay out, will you? This galaxy is full of poachers." In his head, Jones heard another voice, but this voice sounded like the voice of the man guarding the museum. Jones tried to ignore it and focus on Garne coming to meet them. Jones looked back at the museum and spotted the main sign 'The Titanic' and read a sign underneath 'Permanently Closed'. Jones couldn't comprehend why anyone would guard a closed, rundown place. He figured there may be a connection, but this was no time for exploring.

After all, Jones was being watched, right? Jones rationalized this in his head, trying to stay on task for what the two of them had come to Los Angeles to do.

While waiting by the sidelines of the giant sign with ocean waves up top, Garne arrived with music on full blast. He was playing EDM bounce house.

Wearing a T-shirt with an animal on it Garne shouted at the top of his lungs, "YOOO! GIVE ME A HUG, BRO'S, GOOD TO SEE YOU!" Ottie reached out and gave him a one-handed high five as Jones followed behind. Jones didn't know Garne, so stood cautiously behind Ottie. "Don't be bashful, my dude." Garne smiled as he went up and hugged Jones as well. "Where do you guys want to go to talk?" Garne asked. Ottie looked around still trying to make the realization that they had arrived in LA. "How about a coffee spot?" Ottie suggested "Yeah, we can head to the one 10 minutes from here," Garne said as he pointed towards his black car that was still playing EDM bounce house at full volume. "So, I recently came back from the office of Cat Beats! Dudes, if I can get you in, we have to go." Garne shouted as Ottie and Jones went back towards their car. Ottie shouted, "That's sick, dude!"

"Also, there's this other cool guy I met. I'm going there later to their house party. Do you guys want to go? Ah, just get in your car and let's mosey on outta here. We'll talk at the coffee shop." Garne said. Jones and Ottie went back to Jones' car. As Jones peeked in, he saw the two coffee cups sitting there. He reached in to clean them out and heard Ottie's voice annoyed. "Let's go, man. Garne's waiting." Ottie said rushing Jones. "Alright. Follow the loud music, right?" chuckled Jones. Garne stomped on the gas making sure that his car revved up before letting the clutch go. His bounce house music traveled off as Ottie dodged quickly around the corners trying to keep up. Jones felt almost as if the streets had welcomed them to LA as there were hardly any cars on the road. Ottie went around the first car speeding down the highway as Garne honked his horn jokingly from ahead.

CHAPTER NINE – DEPRESSION TRIP

As another car slowed exit right, Garne went around it into the left lane. This blocked off Ottie from getting ahead of Garne. Jones had the coffee shop in the GPS. A road warrior sat on the side watching them as a cop was pulling him over so that Jones and Ottie could get to the coffee shop peacefully. Looking down at his GPS the biker beeped at him sending a simple text that said, "continue on". Ottie opened the sunroof as they whipped around the corners towards the coffee shop. "We're here guys!" Garne shouted.

Jones had almost lost Garne in the car chase. He wiped a bit of sweat away from his forehead. Ottie quickly pulled into the parking lot next to Garne. "So, are you more of a latte guy?" Garne asked with disregard of his ridiculous driving. "I'm more of a macchiato type," Ottie said as he had previously been motivated by the coffee left in the car. The coffee shop had the same tint of color as the museum. There was hardly anybody in the actual place as they went to order their drinks. Ottie and Garne sat down chatting away as Jones looked out the window. "So, what did you guys come to LA for?" Garne asked, wondering. "Well, we found out where one of the big artists lives and we were going to try to send him a demo," Ottie replied without hesitation. Garne's eyes lit up at the thought of the adventure, "Alright! I'm in." he said with excitement. Ottie replied quickly, "Hold on Garne. Let's find the place first, at least. Then we'll text you." Garne looked at the two seriously, "Listen, there's a guy I know here who is making moves. We're planning a big get-together. Come meet me after I get off at work today. Meanwhile, you two explore LA a bit."

Jones's eyes went back over to Ottie as if to say, 'why not?' After all, Garne was currently their only link in the LA Journey adventures. "I'll meet you guys in your hotel later!" Garne said as he chugged the remains of his coffee. Jones and Ottie walked outside as the two of them were hyped up on the idea of experiencing beautiful LA. "How do we get to the Motel 6 hotel?" Ottie asked Siri as he put it in the GPS. Jones questioned this idea, "Let's make a plan first. We don't even know what we're going to do." "Well, first let's grab this hotel," Ottie repeated. That's a plan, Bro. Jones put in a CD as he drove off, "Ugh this traffic." Jones complained. As he made a left turn onto one of the main streets Jones asked, "So where does Garne work anyway?" Ottie, being distracted, looked back around, "Woah! Did you get a look at that building?" An all-black sports car pulled out of the building with a logo design on its side. The building had glass walls that changed with the angles as mirrors showed the cars back to themselves.

"Hey, Ottie! Where does Garne work? We need to know where to meet him." Jones asked again, trying to get a straight answer. "Uh, a grocery outlet, Bro. Don't worry. I got us." Ottie said, totally distracted by the fancy streetlights and lit-up overhangs. "It's beautiful here," Ottie exclaimed. The GPS mentioned for them to turn left. Just as Jones was about to turn left into the hotel, another car came out from the hotel into the middle of the street. It was a solid-yellow color and went head-on into traffic. "Jones watch out!" yelled Ottie. Jones hit the brakes as the car who made a quick turn honked at them. With the windows up Ottie quietly gave them lip. "Fuck you too, buddy." he cursed and rattled. Jones tried to laugh about it, "Ah good old Los Angeles." Jones turned into the Motel 6 parking garage. "Well, it ain't pretty, but it does the job and the price is right."

The rundown building lay off the side of the main two-way road in Buena Park. As Jones pulled into the garage to park, there was a triangle sign with the word 'caution' posted on it. The triangle sign was bright yellow with a black border. It stuck out at Jones. 'You can get energy here.' the sign read under it in secret. Jones opened the door to the Hotel Lobby and the two of them walked in. With no one else around, the lady stared at them. "What do you two need?" she said, smiling politely. "Just a room for us for a night or so," Jones responded. She smiled again, "Certainly, would you like your premier discount with that?" Ottie looked at Jones and shrugged. "I guess so?" said Jones, forgetting that the galaxy was watching him. Jones pulled out his credit card and handed it to her, "Okay. Sure, run it." She

CHAPTER NINE – DEPRESSION TRIP

took the card from him and ran it as it beeped twice. "Alright, you're all set. Here are your card keys for the room," she said.

Jones and Ottie headed back out to the garage, then took their luggage out of the car lugging it towards their hotel room. "I'm going to open up the computer," Ottie said to Jones. "I need to finish my Allorium track in case we run into anyone." "We're pretty close to finishing, right?" Jones asked as Ottie loaded up some of his newer songs. "Yeah, I'm almost done connecting this all together." Jones walked back outside noticing the Caution sign in the glass mirror. He touched it for a moment before going to his car. A jolt of energy rushed through Jones' body. He almost felt completely renewed just by touching the sign itself. Nepharius pinged him, "Jones, see everything for what it is." the voice echoed through his body as the world became brighter. "Is that what that statement meant?" Jones thought to himself out loud. Jones took one more piece of luggage in his hand from the car and ran back over towards the hotel. Back in their room, he found Ottie cross-legged on the bed. He had connected the computer and was loading it up. "Well, this is reality, huh?" Ottie said. "Yeah, I suppose so," Jones said in return. "So, we're going to explore this town, right? Let me GPS somewhere. Remember that old factory in the documentary? We should start looking there tomorrow."

Ottie nodded his head in agreement, "Alright just give me a second to figure this song out. We'll go scout out the area tomorrow, after making a flier." As Ottie focused on the song, Jones put a GPS on the old factory. "An hour. Looks like we have to drive through Alhambra or something." Jones said in a non-excited tone. "We will get over it I suppose, it's just an hour's drive after all," he said complaining, trying to reassure himself that this was a good idea. Ottie started mixing down the track as Jones went back outside. There wasn't much to look at as he checked down the street. "Well, I guess I'll get some air and see what's up in the town." Jones thought to himself. A man waved at him as he sped through the hotel garage touching the Caution sign that said 'get energy here' underneath. The man sped away almost as if he was moving at inhuman speed. Jones watched from the sidelines attempting to comprehend what was happening. "Maybe I'll stay inside today," Jones said back to himself, not wanting to interact with the world around him. After a few hours of sitting around in the hotel, Jones saw Ottie close the laptop. "It's done. We might stand a good chance with this." Ottie said proudly holding up the USB. Static had already taken their first USB. There was a possibility to leave their music elsewhere. Ottie ejected the CD as Jones texted Garne. "Yo, are we meeting you here or at your work?" Jones texted. Garne replied, "My work. Then we're gonna meet up with Eyd."

"Well alright, sounds good." Jones texted back to Garne acknowledging that this idea made sense. But neither Jones nor Ottie knew who this new guy was. A few minutes later Ottie closed the laptop taking the USB with him. "Yo, Jones. It's time to go, Bro." Ottie said, excited about his new track that he just finished. Jones and Ottie raced out of the building as Ottie ran ahead, "I'm going to beat you to the car!" Ottie said laughing. Jones shouted back, "Oh no you aren't!" Jones ran towards the sign that said 'Caution' on it and pressed it feeling the energy surge in his mind. He ran over to the car beating Ottie by a hair. Ottie didn't seem to notice as he jumped in the car. "Bro, alright you win," he said laughing. Jones turned on the car ready to head off to the grocery outlet where Garne was working. Ottie rolled down both windows blasting the music as loudly as he could. "No one cares right?" he said as Jones did some headbanging in agreement. After a few minutes on the road, they pulled up to the grocery outlet. "Yo, we're here!" Jones texted. Garne immediately responded, "Come inside. I'm in the back!"

Ottie and Jones walked in as some food crates stuck out into the aisle. Garne was putting away a pair of grapes right as Ottie waved to him. "Yo, Garne! Nice grapes, my dude." Ottie said jokingly, giving him a pat on the back. Garne joked back, "Only the freshest, Bro." Garne and Ottie got right down to talking as Jones walked around the store. "So, who's this Eyd

CHAPTER NINE – DEPRESSION TRIP

guy?" Ottie asked Garne, wondering about him. "Oh, Bro. This Eyd guy is awesome. He throws weekly shows and festivals. Maybe he can promote you?" Garne said with interest. Ottie replied, "My dude, that sounds like a good time. Can we get out of here though?" Garne laughed, "I'm off in a couple of minutes." Garne took off his black apron and put it in the back of the store as Ottie and Jones went back outside. "Starfruit is the best. I swear." Jones said to Ottie. Ottie replied, "Starfruit? Those yellow-looking things?" Jones laughed, "Yeah, imagine a starfruit smoothie!" As the two of them wandered in the parking lot. "Oh, here comes Garne now," Jones said. "Yo!" Garne shouted "Let's go!"

Jones shouted back, "Don't speed this time!" Garne sped off first again with Ottie and Jones tailgating right behind him through the streets of LA. Garne signaled with his left hand to pull into Eyd's neighborhood as he slowed down to a stop. A weird man with a party hat and glasses flagged them down. The sun beamed down on the white house in the plain urban neighborhood. Ottie and Jones got out of the car to greet the gentleman standing there. His flashy hat and scarf blew in the wind. "These are my friends," Garne said, inviting them into the house. "Oh… alright!" the man said, "Name's Eyd". The four of them walked down the stairs where a fish tank was. "Hi, I'm Brenger and this is my crew." The man smiled with a scarf tied on top of his head. Taking a big swig of whiskey, Brenger offered Jones a sip. "So, what did you all come here for anyway?" The rest of the crew asked, looking at Ottie and Jones in curiosity.

"Can they even DJ?" Eyd asked Garne wondering as his party hat glittered towards the ceiling. "Oh Bro, these guys are something else," Garne said, as he hopped on the decks and put up the first song. A ping pong table layout to the right in all blue. Ottie grabbed a paddle, "Serves up, Bro!" he said as he hit the ball to the right. Eyd's friend joined him, hitting the ball back and forth. As the song played, Jones listened carefully, taking the music in. "Now this is forward-thinking," Jones said to himself listening to the crunchy sounds as Brenger went headbanging to the song. "Jones?"

Ottie shouted, signaling him over to play. Jones didn't hear Ottie as he felt like he was in a trance. The music surrounded him as he took in the scenery of the DJ set built under Eyd's house. "Scope will release your stuff if it's good," Garne said moving over to the decks. He started to test out his mix. "Only five more hours until we reach touchdown." the song shouted as Jones made a pose. "Almost as good as a T-rex with short arms," Ottie said from the back of the room, throwing out an insult towards his ping pong player. Everyone started to laugh as the next song came on.

"So, so far we've met quite a few people. We're trying to figure out how to promote ourselves." Jones said to Eyd. "Tell me later," Eyd replied as they drank more whiskey. Ottie stepped up to the DJ decks next and put in his song. Meanwhile, Jones felt as if the world was spinning. "This world is kinda crazy, yeah?" Jones said to Brenger as Brenger sat down. Jones had no idea what to say but tried to keep the conversation going. "What's that song?" Eyd asked as Ottie took over the decks. "My own," Ottie replied. "You know, that's really good, Bro. Hit me up sometime."

Jones pulled out his phone at the ready, taking down Eyd's number and Facebook information. Meanwhile, everyone was up and moving around at this point. Jones downed another whiskey as he blinked, wondering how a fish tank filled with whiskey would taste. "What if a pool was filled with Jell-O?" Jones brought up the thought aloud. "Sounds horrible." Eyd replied, "Imagine trying to swim in that. What if you got stuck?" Jones wrote it off as a poor idea. Who would want to eat out of a pool anyway? Ottie took a single sip of orange juice and rum as the private party carried on. This had become Jones and Ottie's first solid connection in Los Angeles as they searched for the music celebrity, Idol. Eyd received a call and picked up his phone. Slowly his smile faded. "We have to turn it down, everyone. The neighbors aren't too happy about the volume." Eyd shouted over the song.

Garne went off to fade out the two vinyl decks and CDJ's that sat near

CHAPTER NINE – DEPRESSION TRIP

the fish tank. "Alright, man," Garne said, agreeing as the rest of the crew chattered on. "Let's get back," Garne suggested to Ottie and Jones. "I'll take you guys upstairs," Eyd said, reaching out to grab the last whiskey as he tipped his hat. "Let's get you three out of here." Jones shook Eyd's hand as they all went out the front door. Standing outside near the cars, the sun faded behind the mountains. Ottie got back into the car as Jones walked over to the Jetta. "Yo guys! Come over to my place. It's close by!" Garne said, welcoming them to stay for a bit longer. In Jones' drunken state, he didn't care, "Yeah man, I'm all about it!" Ottie shrugged his shoulders agreeing. He waited for Jones to get in the car, then reached out and turned the key. "You know Ottie, people just judge to inflate their ego. The world is pretty fucked up like this. We have the big boys selling oil and a need for validation over the internet.

When's the last time we even said hi to one another in person before making a match on those good ol' dating apps? I mean, we say the same old shit over and over. Sometimes applications are updated every so often and then marketed out to us as something brand new. We're just regurgitating information to each other, the same information over and over. Ottie, what in the fuck are we doing?" Jones hesitated as the two of them were sitting in the car. Ottie replied with a simple sentence, "Just trying to live like everyone else. Some form of comfort and laughter." he said, converging with the state of the world. By questioning their position, was this how he was going to spread ideas? Jones questioned himself. The galaxy wouldn't listen to logic and reason in the form of a complaint. After all, the galaxy itself was run based on the war on imagination following Nepharius' control. "Let's get back to Garne's house, Jones. You're drunk. Just say hello and try to chill." Ottie said, trying to lighten the situation. Jones clapped his head, "See this is the problem. We refuse to acknowledge ourselves and question our actions." Jones stopped his statement waiting for a rebuttal but there was none.

"Alright, you win," Ottie said as he pointed towards Garne getting into his car. Ottie smashed the pedal down to the floor, "Let's gooo!" he shouted, taking the parking brake off. Jones didn't understand if speeding in Los Angeles was simply because no one cared, or if the road warriors were watching over him. Regardless of what Jones had in his mind, he laid back in the seat as his head spun. Garne tailed behind them at first signaling that he needed to lead. Ottie and Jones had no idea where his house was so Ottie slowed down to let Garne pass. Ottie turned up the music for the ride. As a stoplight came up, they stopped next to one another. "Hey, we're almost there!" Garne shouted honking his horn jokingly. "Jones! This place is awesome!" Ottie shouted as he put his hand up through the sunroof of the car. Jones's head was still spinning from the alcohol. He smiled and gave Ottie a high five as Jones had no idea what else to say. "Almost there," Ottie said as the light turned green. He floored the car again. Following Garne, Ottie started to speed around the next corner.

Dodging traffic, they entered Garne's neighborhood. "Hey, we're here. Park anywhere in the driveway." Garne said reassuring Ottie and Jones so that their car wouldn't be towed. The front door swung wide open, "Oh Garne! You are home!" a blonde-haired woman stood in the door, tall with a classy look in her eyes. "Who are these friends?" she said, giving him a hug and a noogie. "These are my buddies from San Francisco," Garne said trying not to break composure. "Come on in, it's cold." she signaled for them to walk into the house. Furnished wood and lavish marble stood out as Jones first walked into the house through the doorway. The kitchen felt extraordinarily clean. Jones put his finger down swiping across the countertop hoping to pick up a speck of dust to give himself a sense of being at home. "Garne, show your friends around." his mother ordered as she pointed towards his room. "Well, there's not much to see, but we can go into my room for a moment," Garne said. Jones and Ottie agreed as they went into the light blue room where CDJ's and decks were displayed "We can use these for practice later." Garne mentioned. Ottie yelled out, "Yo! Dope!" impressed by the setup. "Are any of you hungry?" Garne's mother asked from the other room.

CHAPTER NINE – DEPRESSION TRIP

As the night slowly fell, the three of them had come to an agreement. They agreed that a few of them could meet up at Idol's place once Ottie and Jones found it. Jones' feelings didn't hit him until he realized he was sitting in Ottie's friend's house in Los Angeles. It was the first step. "Hey, when we find this guy Idol, we'll contact you to come down," Jones said. Garne looked back at them, his face turning serious, "You two have a lot of talent, but I'm telling you if you don't focus, and instead follow grandiose ideas, you'll never make it. Saying you want to throw a giant festival takes a lot of work." Garne eyed them. "If you guys can get something reasonable going, I'll bring the big crews." This to Jones was an opportunity and a challenge. Ottie also felt intrigued by the idea. "Let's do some searching around first and then we'll talk later," Ottie said, trying to diffuse the seriousness in Garne's vision. Jones kept quiet; would a space pirate be interested in a giant event? Would the people that Ottie and Jones met already even partake? Regardless, Jones pointed towards the decks, "We best practice at least and enjoy our time." Jones mentioned. As the three of them crowded in the room waiting for dinner to be ready, Garne put on the decks. Jones wandered out to the living room where the couch sat along with the television.

"What part of Los Angeles are you planning on going to?" Garne's mother asked as she prepared a few small plates. "Oh, maybe the Arts District," Jones replied, brushing off the question not knowing where Ottie and Jones were going to go. Garne's mom stopped for a moment, "The Arts District is an alright place. But be careful not to stay out too late." she warned. Jones sat there wondering what she meant. In this gentrified part of town, it didn't make much of a difference to Jones as he hadn't much to lose. Garne's mother jumped back into action as the buzzer went off for the fries in the oven. "Oh! That's it!" she said happily as she had been waiting for the fries to be completed. She put them on a plate and handed them to Jones as if he were going to be the delivery boy into the next room. "Carry these to everyone won't you?" she politely asked. Jones agreed, "Alright!" he smiled. Heading towards the room where music was blaring, Jones called out, "Dinner guys!" hoping to grab Garne and Ottie's attention. Garne and Ottie turned towards Jones taking the plate out of his hand.

"Nothing better than some fries!" Garne said excitedly as he bit into the cooked potato. Garne reiterated. As Jones and Ottie finished their plate of ketchup and fries shortly after, Garne reiterated, "Call me when you two have it figured out." Jones and Ottie headed for the front door as Garne's mom waved them goodbye from the living room. Jones was ready to venture out further into LA. Now back at the hotel, the front desk lady smiled at them as they walked towards their room. "No point in that USB yet, huh?" Jones queried. Ottie waved him off considering what had happened earlier in the day. "You know that old broken-down factory that used to make toys? We should head there." Ottie said, thinking ahead. "Tomorrow let's go to Staples too. See if we can make something worthwhile, print out our EPK's and such." With that plan stated aloud, Ottie hopped into bed and pulled the covers over himself. Jones lay in the other bed thinking to himself about how to find this place. He slowly drifted off to sleep as for the first time in a while, there were no dreams or noise in his head.

Chapter Ten – District Nothing

The next morning came bright and early. Ottie had just gotten out of the shower and got dressed after brushing his teeth. "Let's go, Bro!" Ottie said to Jones as he shook him awake. Jones woke up, rolling off the side of the bed disoriented, forgetting he was in a hotel. He caught himself from falling onto the floor. Saying nothing, Jones picked up his clothing and headed to the restroom. He went inside and closed the door, turning the water too hot as the shower slowly calmed his nerves. After fifteen minutes Jones was ready to go. Ottie waved Jones towards the door, "C'mon, Bro. Let's get an early start." Jones rubbed his eyes as he tossed Ottie the car keys. They walked out the door and down to the car again. Jones noticed that the floor of the car started collecting dirt as if the car felt like it had an old touch to it. Ottie turned up the music to max volume as Jones laid back in his seat. With all four windows rolled fully down, they ended up in stop-and-go traffic as they approached downtown LA. Passing through the mundane of Pasadena, the place felt no more than an urban stop. Jones pointed towards an exit, "There! That's where we want to get off!"

A bridge struck over towards an area that looked industrial. Ottie turned into the street where a three-way stop sign was and parked by the old factory that had once made toys. The windows had been blown out. There was glass all over the vacant factory floor. "There doesn't seem to be much here, man. It's a good start, but I think we're off the mark." Jones stated.

Ottie waved the idea away, "There's a giant psychedelic eye painted on the wall over there. This must be right. Let's go exploring." Ottie was right, Jones could feel the Art District's energy in his mind. The galaxy of interesting people was calling out to him as his ears picked up music coming from close by. "Yes, there's a lot of weird paintings around here. Let's follow it through." Jones said. They walked down the streets towards Sixth, stopping right by the bridge, Ottie spotted a warehouse that had boutiques with clothing and antiques. Two black gentlemen dressed in tuxedos welcomed them in. "Hey, guys! How can we help you?" one man asked. He held a notebook along with a fancy black pen. The inside pages were golden showing from the side of the black notebook. A fan lay on the ground pointing in one direction as jazzy music played in the background.

Ottie replied, "Well actually, we're looking for a few music artists around here." Ottie was cut off by the gentleman, "Oh, you mean the Arts District. It's down that way." pointing the same way as the fan was pointing. Jones, feeling a no-holds-barred attitude, blurted out, "My friend here creates original music. Mind if we play it on the system?" he asked the gentleman. The man thought for a second, "Go ahead." Jones loaded up Soundcloud and plugged it in. The song blared through the warehouse as they window-shopped picking up small antiques to look at them. "That's pretty good!" the man smiled, "Let me show you something." Two big red curtains hung down around the corner of the warehouse. Behind were paintings of many great jazz artists that stood over Jones' head. "Wow! This is something." Jones said as he admired the paintings drowned in color, that was framed in gold and hung down around the wall.

"Many of the platinum artists you've heard of have visited here at one point or another. You see, the Arts District has a love for music, no matter where you come from." the man exclaimed. "Why don't you guys put your email down in our special guest book? Come back some time. It could be a good way to meet someone who you're looking for." Ottie and Jones wrote their names and emails down as the man handed them the

CHAPTER TEN – DISTRICT NOTHING

fancy black pen and the book woven in gold. As they left the warehouse Jones turned to Ottie, "We probably won't do that you know, but that place was really cool. I think we're in the right place." Jones smiled, feeling like the two had made the right choice going on this journey. As they walked further down the streets, Jones and Ottie noticed shops hidden away. These weren't normal urban shops sporting glass windows with bright displays. The windows were all covered up as if the area had been run down and forgotten. However, once inside, each shop was clean and extravagant, showcasing the best items. "Maybe we should ask around for more details in one of these shops," Jones said to Ottie, reminding him of the goal they had set up. A man walked up to them as Ottie and Jones were talking.

"Please sir, can I get a dollar for some food? I sing a lot, you see, but it's been hard lately." In the bag that he was holding were two broken-down shoes. The man seemed distressed as if he had just been chased. "Alright. Here you go" Ottie said, handing him a dollar bill. The man started to sing in front of them. Not expecting much, Ottie and Jones were impressed. He had the deep voice of a well-trained jazz vocalist. "Thank you, guys. I will sing over tracks for food if I can find work," he said. Otter smiled, "Your voice is really good. I make music too, my guy." So Ottie played his song for the gentleman in return. The gentleman complimented them back and headed on his way down the street. "We are certainly in the right place now," Jones said, agreeing with Ottie. The two of them saw the graffiti of the eye a little closer. "Hey Jones, if you were going to get a tattoo what would it be?" Ottie asked. Jones replied laughing, not knowing why he asked that question. "Well, it'd have an image of an eye with music notes saying that 'music is my religion." On the other side of my arm, it'd say that 'water flows through you' with an image of a river."

Ottie laughed, "That would be pretty tight actually." he said looking at the wall that inspired the idea. The red bricks stuck out as they kept walking towards the main street. "I'm getting pretty hungry," Ottie said as the two of them walked around town. "Time to go!" a man shouted, dressed in a silver suit. Jones looked behind him, noticing a rush of people all dressed in grey with prominent watches walking quickly up and down the street. A rugged man complained, "Damn galaxy loan sharks are trying to steal all our land!" His one eye stuck out in yellow and the other one was a fake eye. He stared at the two of them. Jones pointed to this odd man while tugging on Ottie's shirt, "Yo, this guy is looking at you, we should really go." Ottie turned around and acknowledged the man, "Hey do you know where the Arts District is?" Ottie asked, without questioning, that the man was weird. The man turned his good yellow eye and pointed to the left, "That way." The rugged man noticed Jones in the back trying to keep his distance.

He smiled, "Soon these galactic rats will be gone!" Turning away from Ottie and Jones as he walked off laughing. "That guy was pretty strange, huh?" Ottie commented, oblivious to what just happened. "Yeah," Jones replied, not wanting to get into detail. Jones turned away from Ottie for a moment eyeballing the cafe that was across the street. The smell of sausages and croissants hit him as hunger struck. "Do you want a sandwich?" Jones turned around to ask Ottie and found Ottie focused on his phone. "No, I think sausage would be good. A place that our musician Idol goes to a lot is around this area. We might find him here if we're lucky." Ottie scoped out the area walking past the men in grey suits. The smell of sausage grew stronger as they came across two glass doors with a sign that read "Closed until further notice for the day". Ottie and Jones looked at one another. "Well, it looks like we'll have to come back another time, Bro. It's not so easy here." Ottie said shrugging. A man with blonde hair and tattoos who seemed to be moving into the apartments continued loading his furniture into his house.

"Yeah, this place is nice," Jones commented as they walked down the sidewalk. Not a single crack was in the sidewalk they walked down. Every road looked fully paved as if it were brand new. A gate across the street

CHAPTER TEN – DISTRICT NOTHING

popped out at Jones and Ottie. "Yo, this looks interesting," Jones remarked, pointing towards the colorful graffiti on the long gate. Music could be heard playing from inside the gate as Jones and Ottie were drawn in by the action. "You go first." Ottie dared, egging Jones ahead. Jones's feet didn't want to move forward. An overwhelming sense of embarrassment overcame him as his confidence left him. Suddenly he didn't feel right exploring the Arts District unannounced. "Hey Ottie, it's getting late. We should come back to this. Like really." Jones mentioned trying to hide the shame in his voice. Ottie became more curious by the moment. He didn't want to let up the exploration opportunity that fell before them. However, Ottie also didn't want to stay out too late regardless of if the two of them came back empty-handed from the first day.

"It's alright," Ottie said, calming Jones down. "We can always come back across this bridge. I'm sure something will be going on as it's the weekend." Ottie pointed back towards the car. "For now, let's get back to the hotel. We'll come down here tomorrow." Feeling defeated, they walked back towards Jones's silver Jetta that was parked under the two-hour sign. Jones blinked as a sign showed a sad face lit up in lights to tell them that it was time to move from the spot. "Clever," Jones said to himself, as he mocked the sad face. "Time to go I suppose." Jones laughed aloud as they got into the car. "I need some fresh air to cool off!" exclaiming, as he rolled down his window to clear his head. Lights guided the two of them across the bridge onto the other side where the town was quiet. A beautiful overhang lit up the way above each building as a Chinese restaurant stood out to Ottie. The sign read 'Warped Door' on the glass door written in red. "Sounds like an interesting place," Ottie commented as his stomach rumbled again. The two of them hadn't eaten since they left the cafe and sausage place. "Do you want to stop here?" Jones asked, wondering what was on Ottie's mind. "Let's just grab a bite to eat and then head home. I don't care where at this point." Ottie said, with his hand on his cheek and arm on the window.

Jones, eying the Chinese place said, "Alright then, Chinese cuisine it is." Jones sealed the deal for their food for the night and drove around the block to find parking close by the restaurant. A light flickered almost as if a strobe party light went on under the Warped Door's restaurant awning. There was an open parking spot. Jones was intrigued by the busy, but quieter town across from the Arts District into which the two had just tread. Ottie walked over to Jones smiling, "Finally, we can get some food around this place!" Two glass doors popped out at them. Jones went over to the door and opened one, "After you," Jones said, making a joke. The restaurant had a stairwell going upward, almost as if the small entry had welcomed them to the expansive two-story building above. Jones and Ottie already felt at home. A beautiful woman dressed in red and gold came out to welcome them. "What can I get you two tonight?" she said politely. She led them to a table and put fancy plates in front of each of them. "Got any spring rolls?" Ottie said, asking for something simple. "I'll have chicken fried rice," Jones replied.

The both of them weren't too keen on spending what little money they had left. Ottie reached over and downed a glass of water. "Pretty intense day, huh?" Ottie said wondering what type of response he would get from Jones. "I suppose," Jones said lackadaisically as his mind drifted elsewhere. The lady in red and gold listened in on their conversation. "Do you know Sao?" she asked Jones through his mind. Jones looked behind. He thought he heard her mention the guy who was running from the CIA that Jones had met at Club Temple. Jones shook his head trying to keep it focused. The lady in red receiving no response bumped his chair and walked away to grab the first dish. "Jones, you alright?" Ottie asked as he rubbed his eyes. "I'm feeling a little sick." Ottie sighed. "Well, we haven't had any decent rest or food in a while," Jones replied. "Let's just eat something simple and get out of this place. I don't like it here." The beautiful lady came back and put the spring rolls on the table.

"Thank you," Ottie said, feeling he had been served with premium service.

CHAPTER TEN – DISTRICT NOTHING

Jones also nodded politely to the server as she put the fried rice in front of Jones and smiled. To Ottie Jones said, "We need to find a connection now that we know the area. That sausage place next to the cafe will be great to go back to tomorrow. Still, this is pretty fun, huh?" Jones reiterated as he twirled his fork around. Ottie scarfed down his spring rolls and chugged his water. Jones did the same as the server came back around the corner. "Here's your check." The beautiful lady put the check down slowly on the table as Jones noticed the discount. A small amount shown in the payment total line as Ottie put down the cash. Feeling uneasy again, Jones got up and started walking down the stairs. He needed fresh air, away from all of the noise and commotion going on inside of his head while in the quiet restaurant. He proceeded to take out his chewing gum as Ottie rushed down the stairs behind him.

"What the hell man? You didn't even tell me you were going outside?" Ottie complained to Jones. "We need to get back to the hotel," Jones said as his phone read "low percentage battery". "There's nothing for us left here," he said with urgency, giving Ottie a hint that the place felt unsafe. Ottie went to the car with Jones not questioning the rush. Although Ottie was angry at Jones for taking him away from a good dinner and a beautiful woman, he quickly forgave him. They pulled out of the parking spot and headed back down towards the hotel. Jones's mind was now focused on how to promote Ottie rather than how to party hard. After an hour's drive, they arrived back at the motel. Feeling accomplished, Ottie sat down on the bed to play Fortnite. Jones lay on the other bed thinking things through, wondering when he would be able to return to the mission of the galaxy, the mission of the war on ideas. He started to get lost in himself, was he an arbiter? A musical warrior? Or was he simply Jones? Jones took another look at his hands to double-check although he felt human. "Yup, perfectly human," Jones said to himself.

Drifting off to sleep he thought, "How lonely this world is. Take away someone's hope and you've mentally killed a human. It's all most people have left, it's all anyone has." Jones shook his head. "Hope though, hope is a part of having the drive. It's a chance and we strive for chances." He spoke to both sides within himself, his dark thoughts and the light within him. Jones clenched his fist driving the negative thought away, "I will not be a slave to hope, however, I will see everything for what it is." Ottie kept on watching movies and different anime in the background. "Man, there's nothing good on TV right now," Ottie said quietly. Jones rolled over to stare at the blank wall. "Alright, let's try to get some sleep. Tomorrow we'll go back and contact more people." As Jones said those words he stared at his phone. The cursor lay in writing but nothing came to mind. Then words started appearing ahead of the yellow line in Notes as if it were telling him what to do and where to go. Jones shook his iPhone briefly and blinked. "Nah can't be real," he said to himself as the words on the screen continued to write ahead of him. He drifted off.

Jones woke up briefly and looked at his screen. He felt almost as if he could see every pixelated piece mixed with the grease and oil of everything he had ever touched. The pixels on the screen stuck out at him almost as if in a wavy trance. The light broke apart as if his mind understood how an iPhone was made piece by piece. Jones felt that the lack of sleep continued to affect his body on the trip. His mind had already been taken so what would be next? Jones drifted off back to sleep, back into the darkness that he so enjoyed. The next day Ottie turned around with the laptop still playing anime in the background. Jones was deep in his sleep though Ottie could still see the bags under his eyes. "I'll wait and let him sleep." Ottie quietly said to himself as he got ready for the next discovery. "Another sunny day in good ol' California," Ottie said to himself semi-jokingly. Then laughing, "Oh! I know, I can make those EPK's!" Slowly rolling out of bed, Jones went over to get changed and get ready for the day in LA. "Okay, so where are we going next?" Jones asked Ottie.

"What do you mean next? We go back to the sausage place and try again like we agreed last night." Ottie said. As if his eyes started working faster,

CHAPTER TEN – DISTRICT NOTHING

it seemed as if Jones could see every letter pop up as he typed onto his tiny phone. Jones started to make notes to himself. "Ready?" Ottie asked in an annoyed tone as he sat by the door waiting to go. He sneezed as Jones got up and headed towards the door. "Yeah, I'm ready," Jones replied in a tired voice. They proceeded down the hallway back out towards the garage. "You know, music really is the galactic vibration of communication," Jones said as a conversation starter. "I mean we don't even need to understand the lyrics to understand the feeling or the beat. Isn't that worth something?" Jones exclaimed. Ottie smiled, "Bro, most people understand this by now, I hope. I mean from a musician to a musician, that's where titles come from too. The music is that emotion, captured at that exact time. It's a history piece that lasts forever, just like the stars." Jones replied, "So much music is made every day so people will try to reach us that way too." Ottie stopped for a moment and put his hands on the wheel. "Let's go."

They started driving back towards the bridge in the Arts District. It was already day three in LA. "I need some paper," Ottie said as he pulled into the parking lot of an office supply store that was nearby. "Paper for the EPK?" Jones questioned as the building seemed to stick out at him. "Yeah man, but let's get some coffee too," Ottie said, trying to convince Jones that he needed a morning boost. It seemed that Ottie wasn't going to let up that he needed his coffee. They walked towards the coffee shop door where a man rode around in circles with a hat on. "L.A. Woot!" he shouted out loud, mockingly. "You're the best!" The man seemed troubled by the place. As Ottie ordered his latte, Jones walked over to the man. "Bro, LA isn't all that bad, right? There's music at least." Jones asked. Ohs stood there for a moment. He stopped riding around on his bicycle contemplating what Jones had just said. "Say that again?" Ohs asked. "I said there's music at least in L.A.," Jones replied.

Ohs's eyes lit up for a moment as he looked towards the sky. "People with some common sense!" he shouted. "What's your name?" Jones asked Ohs curiously. After all, the only friends they had in LA were Garne and his acquaintances. "It's Ohs and you are?" Jones shook his hand briefly and then gave him a fist pound. "Jones man," he replied. Jones dropped his tone and relaxed himself feeling the positive energy around the man. There was no need to be on guard. "What are you doing out here in LA, anyway. Do you live here?" Ohs asked him. Jones replied quickly, not leaving any room for speculation, "No, we're searching for a musician named Idol. They are around here." Jones said. Ohs smiled, "You mean the guy I live right next to? Yeah man, I know all about him!" he shouted. "I'll take you to him. Add me on Facebook and we can contact you there. I have my bike so I can't roll in your car at the moment." Jones and Ohs exchanged numbers as Ottie introduced himself holding the coffee in his hands. Jones explained what he had heard catching Ottie up to speed. "My guy! That's pretty cool!" Ottie exclaimed. He was excited now that they had found their lead.

"We need some paper first. We're going to make some EPK's before we leave for the Arts District." Ottie said excitedly. Ohs and Jones sat around the parking lot together chatting for a moment as Ottie walked in to buy paper and laminate his profiling. "Yeah man, I do the art show thingamajig in the Arts District," Ohs said to Jones. "You two should come by at the Majig. I'll take you to all the music shows around there. You know, whatever man." Ohs pulled out a pipe to smoke some weed. "So, what's your story?" Jones asked Ohs. "I used to live on the sixth row for a while out here," Ohs mentioned how I've met a lot of people, but I live in a small spot now." Jones nodded his head paying attention to every word. The man did seem to know what he was talking about regarding the general area. Ottie came out finishing his coffee holding a few laminated printouts of his artist name 'Allorium'.

"We're also here to hand this USB to Idol with our music on it," Jones said, trying to explain the situation to Ohs, hoping he would invite them in. "Totally, man. Come by the show." Ohs repeated. Jones asked in return, "What show?" wondering what show he was talking about. Ohs stuttered

CHAPTER TEN – DISTRICT NOTHING

a little bit, seeming to be not all there, "Just a show up here. It'll be fun and stuff. Later tonight. I'll take you there." he said. Jones did have his number so sent a text just to be positive that it went through. Ohs' phone responded in confirmation. "Alright, we'll see you a bit later today," Jones confirmed as he and Ottie went into the car. Jones and Ottie gave one another a high five. "Bro, we got it," Ottie said with a huge grin on his face. Jones laughed back, "Yeah we did! He seems okay, a little off though." Jones said, trying to downplay their interaction. "Where to next?" Jones asked. "Well since we're headed back over the bridge, we should go to that sausage place that Idol frequents. I don't know why, but I feel it." Ottie said.

Ottie and Jones headed to the same place where they had parked last time, near the building with the giant psychedelic eye painted on it. The whole District was starting to come to light as it opened up to the two of them. Jones and Ottie went up to the sausage place door and opened it as the strong smell wafted over to them. "One sausage each coming right up!" the front desk man shouted. Jones went over to the right side of the brown desk as the man pointed over to a soda cooler. Ottie took the soda as well. "Are you staying to eat or walk-on-out?" the man asked with curiosity. "We're staying to eat," Ottie replied. Jones looked off to the left towards the music that came from the background. "This is it!" Jones said. Ottie looked at Jones as if he had three heads. "What is it?" Ottie questioned. They walked around the corner with hot dogs in their hands. Ottie almost dropped his plate as a vinyl record player encased in wood with balloons rising from the helium caught their attention. Their Idol's spot confirmed it.

"This is the same place we saw in the documentary!" Ottie said excitedly. Musicians were dancing around the vinyl laughing, conversing about how their next big shows were coming up. A man passed Jones as he picked up another record and headed to the vinyl to put on a new song. People were congratulating someone on their birthday. Jones and Ottie picked a table and sat down to watch. Ottie took out a little marker and drew his name on the table. "Ottie! What are you doing?" Jones shouted. "Bro, just draw something. It doesn't matter." Ottie said encouraging him. Jones took the pen and drew a smiley face next to 'Allorium'. "See? That wasn't so bad." Ottie said smiling. Jones took in the smell of the wood, the laughter, the music playing on the vinyl, and the rest of the scenery. Due to the aroma, Jones felt sentimental as if he had finally started on a purposeful journey. The electronic music blared as Jones slowly chewed on the sausage and bun. "You know Ottie, this should be us," Jones said, suggesting that their music could be heard throughout the area.

Ottie contemplated the idea for a moment, "Yeah, that's what we came down here for. We have to find him." Ottie said agreeing. With that said, they finished the last bit of the sausage. Getting up from the table they smiled. Their pen drawings would be there for a very long time. Jones and Ottie proceeded to head for the door as the happy birthday sign with balloons sat by the vinyl encased away in the back of the room. Feeling fully accomplished that they had found one of the hotspots, Ottie and Jones walked out the way they came in, giving the front desk gentleman their thanks. The man waved back and told them to come back anytime. As Jones exited the building, he looked up at the sky wondering how the universe would pull them further towards their goals. Ottie slapped him on the back. "Yo, we still got some time! We should check out around town more." Ottie said. Both were more excited than when first arriving in LA. "I'm all for it." Jones agreed. They walked back towards where they originally saw the warehouse places. The District was bustling with more people today, as the two of them walked in and out of the stores.

"$300 for a shirt?" Ottie wondered aloud as Jones questioned it as well. "Yeah, $300 for a shirt that will probably be recycled in a week." Jones laughed. As the two of them shopped through more stores, one stood out. "Yo, that's the shop from the documentary!" said Ottie just as Odu's showed up on the front of the place. Jones and Ottie went in to look at

CHAPTER TEN – DISTRICT NOTHING

the shirts. "Whoa, Bro! $500 for a shirt?" Jones said this time. "Yeah, man! Come by later. We're having an open house party." a man said to them from behind. He wore a white blazer sporting long blonde hair. "A house warming event?" Jones asked out of curiosity. "Yeah! It's going to be huge. Where are you from? My name is Gemmy." he said. Gemmy didn't seem as if he was the average, run-of-the-mill, sales clerk. Jones felt as if he knew where this was headed.

"Well, this is Ottie and I'm Jones. We're looking for the musician Idol. Know this guy?" Jones asked on a whim. "Oh yeah, Bro!" Gemmy said in return, "One of our staff here at Odu's can take you right to him!" Jones and Ottie gave each other a cautious look, taking a small step back. "Isn't he on tour?" Ottie asked. Jones gave Ottie a nudge. Gemmy replied quickly, "Yeah well." Jones piped up, "Well! All good. We have no idea, but we'll be glad to come along." Gemmy smiled briefly, "See you there!" Jones and Ottie shopped around in Odu's to remember the storefront then left down the road. The Arts District felt more like home each time the two visited."Just follow the music, right?" Jones said to Ottie, lighting up the mood. Ottie smiled back, "If it's bumpin', Bro, then that's where we go." The white store and blank space still crept into Jones's mind. "So, this is what a blank space to create something new feels like." he thought quietly to himself. As the day passed towards evening, Jones couldn't stop the thought now. Every waking moment that passed by was another musical warrior's fight lost. Another war failure on people's imagination within the world.

"We're supposed to meet Ohs, right?" Jones asked Ottie. "Oh yeah, dude. Text that guy." Ottie replied. Jones opened up his phone and sent a text directly to Ohs, "Hey man, where are we meeting?" A few minutes went by as Ottie and Jones walked back towards the car. Ohs hadn't responded. "He's not texting back," Jones said worried as the night was starting to fall upon them. "Call him then," Ottie suggested. Jones attempted to give him a phone call. This time it went through. Ohs picked up the phone. "Hey!

Cool! Music and stuff, right?" Ohs replied. "Yeah, man. Where should we meet you?" Jones said, trying to hide the realization that Ohs' ability to function in conversation was problematic. "There's this rock showplace. It's going to be cool, free and all. I mean come on down. Free, right?" Ohs said again. Jones hadn't checked his spam email in almost a week now. Ever since Nepharius had told him to go on his own journey. For a while the emails read, 'Where is he?' and 'Come back to us.' Jones didn't reply to their calls. "Yeah, got an address?" Jones asked as Ottie listened in. "Type in the Webut," Ohs answered. Jones loaded up Waze on his iPhone. Jones tapped a hidden box in a section that hadn't existed before. The 'Road Warriors at Your Service' link came up on his phone. The Webut was a short walk from where Ottie and Jones had been. "Alright, we're on our way," Jones said as the two of them started walking. "It's kinda cold, Bro," Ottie complained.

"Yeah, it'll be warmer inside," Jones said, thinking about the show. After a few minutes of trudging through the nooks and crannies of the District, Ottie, and Jones arrived. Ohs was standing outside Club Webut waving at the two. His white cap was put on backward as the bike lay on its side. "You made it!" Ohs exclaimed, holding out his hand to give them a fist bump. Jones gave him one back as they walked inside. The building had a two-story patio with a bar out front. In the back, rock speakers were set up with a microphone. At first, the place was semi-filled almost as if it was pre-party time to talk. "Bro! This place is popping!" Ottie said as he looked at the beer options listed on the wall. 'Webut the drink –we serve well' was written on the blackboard. Ohs started talking to a woman he seemed to know about radio talk show hosting. "Yeah, beer and stuff are around. Grab one!" Ohs said, "Party woo!"

Jones and Ottie went around to the front side where the two stories were. Just as Ottie held a beer in his hand, Ohs went up to the front where people with guitars sang on the microphones. The world began to spin for Jones. He could feel the energy of the people. Each person started to speed to

CHAPTER TEN – DISTRICT NOTHING

where they wanted to get to as if they were teleporting. Jones couldn't keep up and retreated to where Ottie was standing. "Yo, look at Ohs!" Ottie said. Ohs was standing towards the front, high-fiving his friend who was playing the guitar on stage as the rest of the people jumped around. Ottie wandered off towards the front to grab another beer as a woman stood behind Jones. "Cool show. You make music I hear." the woman said, not giving Jones any time to think. "How did you know?" Jones asked, turning around. "Alexa," she said, holding out her hand with a smile. "I'm with the Galactica Musicians Company and we'd like to promote you and your buddy. Right now, it is a bit soon, but hold this contact." Jones looked at her finger as she put it on his iPhone. Her contact information appeared there as Soundcloud loaded up. "See here? Now you can see all the Galactica Musicians and their feelings." Alexa said.

Jones blinked his eyes again, Alexa disappeared from view as all he saw was an older lady drinking a beer. "What?" Jones said to himself, half ignoring what had happened. He started walking upfront as Ohs retreated towards Jones. "Bro, sick party, right? I mean, whoa!" Ohs said again, loading up a pipe full of weed. "Don't smoke kids." He laughed to himself as he smoked, laughing with the rest of the crowd that was dancing to the live music. This time there were no costumes as before. All the people within the crowd dressed up beautifully, but casually. Ottie came back towards them with another beer. "Where do you live, anyway Ohs?" Ottie asked with curiosity. Ohs turned to him smiling, "Right across from your Idol in the Galaxy Apartments." Jones, taken aback by this information, jumped into the conversation. "That sounds awesome. Will you show us?" Jones asked politely. Ohs agreed, "You know your Idol used to live above here on the second story. We used to rent it out to him." he said smiling. "Awesome," Ottie replied.

As the night went on, the three of them stumbled out towards the main entrance. "Alright, Ohs. We'll see you tomorrow!" Ottie said gleefully as Ohs went off on his bicycle waving as he rode away. Jones thought for a moment. He decided to keep the interaction between him and Alexa a secret as he didn't want to startle Ottie. "We better get going. It's almost past time." Jones said, realizing that night was ending as his phone's battery was drained. They walked back to where the car was parked. The sign showed a sad face. "Where's my car?" Jones said at first. "Oh no... No, no, no! It's not here!" he cried. The realization that his car had been towed in LA hit him fast. "If only my car had a sensor that someone could press and call me, I'd move!" Jones said, complaining as Ottie sat there silently. "I guess we'll have to walk to the towing place..." Ottie trailed off with his voice trying to calm Jones down.

Jones continued his rant, "I mean, a sensor that called my phone through an app. So simple. I would've just moved my car. What is this bull crap!" Jones yelled louder, almost losing it. Ottie loaded up the towing place on the mini-map. "Let's start walking I guess," Ottie said calmly as Jones followed behind him. The grated fence with rust was strewn along the walkway. A man in a tattered sweater slowly walked past Jones and Ottie as they trod towards the towing lot. The man mumbled to himself as he went by, not noticing the presence of Jones or Ottie. "Yo dude, it's kinda harsh out here, huh?" the man mumbled. Jones sensed the zombie from the galaxy inside of the man that walked by them. "I guess," Jones said, ignoring that he knew what this man really was. Another tattered woman walked by the two of them as few people seemed to be out at night. They saw more of them going left and right as

Jones and Ottie grew closer to the towing center. "You really should have read that sign," Ottie said. Jones retorted, "Shut up!" as they continued forward. A security guard drove with its lights blinking yellow towards them. "Excuse me! Do you know which way the tow place is?" Jones yelled towards the security. The security guard stopped for a moment as Ottie tried to bring up the GPS on his phone. Not able to get the exact location, the security guard pointed north. "Yeah, it's about two blocks that way. You guys are pretty close but be careful out here at this time." the security

CHAPTER TEN – DISTRICT NOTHING

guard warned. Jones thanked the man, but grumbling to himself. He was going to have to pay money for this blunder.

Jones' phone beeped at him in his spam email.'Now serving Roudites. 20 of these in Galactica currency could buy you anything in the worldwide universe!' Jones deleted the email. Ottie saw this as the two were a block away from the station. "Why are you looking at your spam email?" Ottie asked. Jones replied, "Just deleting some spam so I can see what's going on." Ottie's curiosity died with the spam. Arriving at the building, Jones and Ottie went over to the lady in the window. "Do you have a silver Jetta in your lot?" Jones asked. The entire building was empty except for a few people. "Let me check." she sighed, rolling her eyes. After a few minutes, she pulled it up on the computer. "Yes, that will be $430." Jones wide-eyed, raised his voice, "$430!? That's basically robbery, lady. We're just visiting LA. This is complete bullshit!" Jones felt at the end of his rope. Ottie patted his back, "Chill, or we won't get help." "Hm. You'd better listen to your little friend there. You'll get a mailing when you get back to your address attached to the car." the lady replied, trying to get them out of there as quickly as possible. Jones sighed, paying the credit card fee, "Okay, fine whatever, just give me my keys." A few minutes later the car came out of the lot. Jones and Ottie got in driving out to street level from the underside.

"Let's get back to the hotel. We have a lot to do tomorrow." Jones said to Ottie. They drove back to Motel 6 to get some rest. However, Jones couldn't sleep that night. His head was spinning with all the potential and opportunities of what had happened so far. But they also had less money to stay in LA now. Four days had passed.

Chapter Eleven - Unclear Discovery

The problem with things that happen to you in life is that once they happen, they cannot be changed unless they're still there.' Jones thought to himself. He didn't want to take any more losses but knew he would follow this path. And it was too late to change this path. Ottie and Jones would see this trip through. Ohs texted Jones, "What are you going to do today? Let's meet up!" Jones replied quickly, "Yeah man. We would like to see your place." Feeling sore from yesterday's losses, Jones got in the shower making it hot to clear his head. "Ottie, you ready bro?" Jones asked. Ottie coughed a couple of times, "Yeah man. But I think I'm starting to get sick." Jones replied, "That sucks man. Let's take it slow. Just drink lots of OJ. We'll buy some at the store on the way to Ohs'."

After an hour of sitting in stop-and-go traffic, they arrived at the apartments. Ohs waited outside wearing a white cap and bomber jacket. "Yo! Come on inside!" Ohs greeted them. Jones and Ottie walked up the small steps that led to multiple rooms. "This is my friend Andy over here. He paints a lot." Ohs said. A man sat painting in a small wood-floored room. A small bed sat in the corner as a door was painted over the window. He waved at them as Jones and Ottie waved back. "And here's my room." Ohs continued. Music and murals were plastered on his wall. He had his computer set up with a microphone. A giant American flag sat in the back along with a chandelier that changed colors. Ableton Music Production software was showing in the background with attached speakers. Ohs

CHAPTER ELEVEN - UNCLEAR DISCOVERY

also had an iPad with multiple programs on it. "Woah, this small place is dope!" remarked Ottie, taking it all in.

A little oven pot sat in the corner with kale and carrots cooking. Next to that was the fridge. A couch sat squished right behind the computer. "It's not great and sucks to eat like this, but it's my pad," Ohs replied. Ohs took his weed pipe and smoked it. "Do you want to smoke too?" offering it to Jones and Ottie. They both nodded yes.

"You guys should make something here, like, right? It's fun stuff, right?" Ohs suggested. Jones sat down in front of the Ableton screen as he went through the programs messing with the oscillators. Ottie asked Ohs, "Yo, can we play our tune through the speakers?" Ohs replied, "Yeah man, whatever. Like, let's do it." as the speakers blared Ottie's song. Ohs got up and danced in his chair, bumping to the beat. "Man, you guys are living the dream, songs and all. I'll let you play at the small gig I got. I play for the museum and stuff." Ohs suggested. Ottie replied excitedly looking at Jones, "Bro, let's do it!" The three of them sat for a moment thinking of the possibilities. Then Ohs asked, "Hey didn't you want to find your musician guy, Idol?" "Yeah, I do," exclaimed Ottie. They got up off the couch after crunching some kale and carrots. Then, taking their time, they meandered down the apartment hallway to the set of small steps they entered from. They walked outside towards the river through a small entryway leading towards a gutter.

"See that guy on the road? He's a friend of mine." Ohs said, pointing to a man sitting with a guitar on the streets dressed in all red, white, and blue smoking a cigarette. They walked further towards the dam where an entryway sat. You could walk down the hallway to the very end and back. "I don't think anyone's here, but this place is nice," Ottie said as they strolled. Jones agreed with Ottie, understanding that the mission was a failure. They looked up as luxurious red and black cars rushed up from behind them. One of them turned around and set up to drive down the small square tunnel in which they had just walked. "What's this all about?"

Jones inquired. Ohs saw the cars, "Oh, they are always shooting movies and whatnot around here. Just movie stuff you know. Hey, I can't be out too long cause I'm kinda hot right now. You know?" Jones wondered what Ohs meant, "Hot as in tired from the sun?" Jones asked, making a poor joke. "No man, hot as in things are kinda rough right now. Lots of eyes you know." Ohs replied while looking around him. "Oh, I see," Jones said as the cars and cameras drove away after an action scene was shot.

Ottie looked across the way, "Bro, I think that's him sitting on the other side, on the grass. There." Ottie said pointing, "Should we go over there?" Jones replied quickly, "No, let's catch him another time. This could totally be someone else." Jones made sure that Ottie didn't run off after him, "I have to promote you, right?" Ohs overheard them, "I could make the QR scanning work for you and make it spin or something. You know, to promote yourself or something." Ottie went over to Ohs, "Bro, I would really appreciate that." They walked back to town towards the grocery store as they continued chatting. "I can introduce you to some teachers, too," Ohs said, offering up the rest of his day. "Yeah! I'm all ears." Jones said. "Alright, tomorrow I have class. Just pick me up from here." Ohs mentioned as Ottie trailed slowly behind sniffling from his nose. "Yo, we should meet up with Garne." Ottie said to Jones, realizing that Garne was waiting for their call.

"Yeah, we found it. Now we can hunt together to say hello. Everything's in place. We know where to go." Jones said looking at his iPhone. "Oh shit! The party at the clothing shop!" Jones reminded Ottie. "Hey Ohs, can we meet up later? We have somewhere to be," asked Jones. Ohs finished up his grocery shopping as they all headed out towards the front of the store. "This is our shot, Bro," Jones said to Ottie as they walked towards the car to the silver Jetta. Not wasting any time, Jones stepped on the gas and headed out towards the warehouse section. They understood the area well after searching around for several days. A table was being set up as they arrived at Odu's clothing shop. A man with a hat along with twenty

CHAPTER ELEVEN - UNCLEAR DISCOVERY

or so other people sat around on the benches. Alcohol was set up on the table. Jones felt stressed. The members of the clothing shop came up to them. "Hey, glad you could make it!" One of them said as Jones and Ottie sat around the table. A well-dressed lady showed up, as a man wearing the store's clothing DJ'd in the back of the shop. Night had fallen upon the warehouse as the people started throwing their promotional block party. Jones sat there talking to the server, dressed in a black tuxedo, who seemed to be serving at a fast speed. "Oh man, how long have you been doing this?" Jones asked.

"About ten years, man. Who here wants a beer? Relax! It's a party. You're too tense." the server, smiling, handed beers to both Jones and Ottie. Walking around the shop, the lady dressed in all white came up to them to have a conversation. "I'm an entertainment lawyer. You'll need me someday, but not yet," she said, handing her card over to Jones. All of the pieces seemed to be coming together. Jones tried talking to Ottie. "Hey man?" Jones started. Ottie wasn't paying attention so Jones tapped Ottie on the shoulder. "Look man, let's go to the car for a moment." Jones requested. When they got to the car, Jones said to Ottie, "Get in!" Ottie reluctantly came over to the car and got in. Then they began arguing in earnest, "Don't ruin this!" Jones yelled. Ottie started replying with an attitude, "Ruin what?" "Bro, you're not listening to me, or networking; You're just messing around! What did we come to LA for?" Jones yelled even louder. Ottie started tearing up as he sat there silently.

"Alright, sorry," Ottie said. Jones calmed down, "I'm sorry too. It's just this whole LA problem. Let's go back to the party." They got out of the car and headed back to the party. They sat back down at their former table. "Sorry about that, man. Hey, you know the musician Idol, right?" Jones asked the server. The man from the clothing shop team said, "Yeah, we know him. Stop by tomorrow." Ottie and Jones both shook his hand as the party dwindled to nothing. "You know, despite this LA trip being a complete failure so far, we can still have fun with it, right?" Jones said to Ottie. Ottie smiled, "Call Garne? Let's invite him to go through the District with us tomorrow."

"Let's plan on giving them fliers of you and promoting you. Come up with cool ideas." Jones said, getting excited. They looked over towards the old factory where giant letters hung. "Hey, what if we bought materials to hang a giant poster down from over there? Throw some confetti off the top of the roof or something? Or we could put confetti in a balloon and pop it over the city." Jones suggested. "Bro, that sounds amazing, but we should ask first. Sounds like trouble for us." Ottie cautioned. "Well, for now, we got this." Jones showed Ottie the QR scan code spinning link on his phone that Ohs had provided. Even though it had all of ten views on it, every time Jones clicked, 100,000 views flashed towards the Galactic. Ohs must have been a Musical Warrior. "So?" Ottie wondered.

"Well, at least it's something. Ten views are a start," replied Jones. They got back in the car and started heading back down the road towards the Motel 6 hotel in Buena Park, Orange County. Tomorrow Ohs will show them to the music teachers in the afternoon. Before then, Ottie and Jones would have time to waste. "Hey, Ottie," Jones said, tapping him on the shoulder as they arrived at the hotel. Jones poked him again, "Ottie, we're here." Ottie mumbled as he drunkenly opened the door, "Bro give me a moment. I'm feeling so sick right now." he said. Jones replied, "Need something? We can get some ibuprofen or vitamin C at the front desk." Ottie didn't want anything as he waved his hand towards Jones, "No, I'll be all good. Just let me just rest a while." Jones replied in return, "Alright, for sure."

Jones walked into the hotel lobby, closing the door behind him. Emotions flowed through his head as to what happened. Up in their room, as Jones lay on the bed recuperating, he slowly recapped the day. He wondered if this experience would be a waste of their time. Drifting further into the galactic space, he lay there for a moment quietly. Alexa and the Entertainment Lawyer he had met, seemed to be connected. He felt he

CHAPTER ELEVEN - UNCLEAR DISCOVERY

could use their help later down the road. Odu's clothing shop had taken a liking to them both, but that wasn't enough yet to support them. Jones felt he was still missing a piece, but what was it? Jones sat there contemplating this for a while. Startled by the bathroom door opening, Ottie walked in flipping onto the bed and passing out. His sickness had become worse due to the long day of traveling and lack of rest. Jones woke up hearing his coughing as he was brought back to reality. "Yo, I need some rest," Ottie said as he promptly passed out cold. "Tomorrow we'll get you some medicine right quick," Jones said as he shut down the computer.

The next day, Jones woke up while Ottie was still fast asleep. Although Jones had not yet bought the medicine, Ottie was able to rest throughout the night without waking up. Jones meandered down the hallway taking in the marble on the ground floor of the hotel. Ohs had sent him three texts wondering where he was. "Hey man. Trying to reach you and stuff. It's already 1:00 PM and whatnot." read the texts from Ohs. Jones replied, "We'll be there a little later. Sorry man, my friend's a bit under the weather." Jones sat around the room for a moment thinking of what to do as Ottie slowly woke up. "Yo, let's do this," Ottie said. Jones and Ottie headed out while texting Garne, "You ready?" Garne quickly replied, "I'm always ready, my dude!" They met up shortly afterward at Garne's house as Garne got in his car. Jones felt that it would be a long day of discovery as Ottie and Jones drove back over the bridge towards the Arts District.

Garne veered off left, "Yo! I got a text. And I've got something to take care of. I'll be back." Garne texted. Ottie and Jones parked in a safer area around the Starbucks near the apartments. "Let's go for a short walk. You might feel better." Jones said, encouraging Ottie to get up and about. They walked down the sidewalk where not a single bad crack was showing - all newly paved. 'Bit apartments' was written right above the entry door. "Bit Apartments?" Jones said aloud, questioning the odd name. The door was left slightly ajar as Jones and Ottie walked in. A man was walking towards the door. "Do you guys want to see the apartments? " he asked, " Name's

Dane." He was quick to notice the USB, held in Jones' hand. "Yeah, man! There are paintings on the wall and everything. What is this place?" Jones asked curiously. Jones realized that they had pretty much snuck into a residence place where they weren't supposed to be. The only way out was to talk to the gentleman. Dane laughed, "Follow me."

He waved the two of them further inside the building as the hallway and rooms were built and almost fit for kings and queens. Opening the door to his apartment a woman stood there. She was practicing on an S4 Tractor. "You DJ?" Ottie asked out of curiosity. Jones sat by and watched, surveying the situation. "No, but my girlfriend does!" Dane said proudly as his girlfriend was standing over to the side, enjoying the time. "For whom?" Ottie asked again, pushing a little out of curiosity.

Dane took a step back, "For Idol." Ottie's excitement went through the roof. "Wait, what?" Ottie said putting two and two together. By chance, they had stumbled across their biggest 'in' besides meeting Ohs who lived down the street. Jones realized how everything was starting to connect. As they meandered around the apartment, Ottie and Jones thanked Dane. "So that USB?" Dane asked with a question. Jones immediately handed it over to Dane. "It's some music he made," Jones said, pointing over to Ottie. Dane eyed the USB up and down, "Pass me a number. Let's grab a beer." Dane said kindly, offering Ottie a time slot to talk.

"Sure!" Ottie said. Another opportunity had arisen in reality. Jones started to feel as if the two of them finally got somewhere. Ottie and Jones then left the apartments moving towards the Café where they would wait until they heard from Garne. Garne eventually texted them, "Alright, errands done! I have some medicine for Ottie too. Where are you guys?" Ottie and Jones sat down at the Cafe as people dressed in beautiful clothing walked in and out. "$10 for an avocado sandwich!" Jones said to Ottie aghast, "Let's grab a coffee instead. This place is pricey!" Ottie laughed for the first time during the day, "We're at the Cafe." Ottie texted Garne. In a couple of minutes, Garne showed up. "Okay, what did you two find?"

CHAPTER ELEVEN - UNCLEAR DISCOVERY

Garne asked, questioning Ottie and Jones' big grins and antics. "Yo, we found Idol's secondary place, among other things. Come with us." Jones said. As they left the Café and started to walk downtown, Garne got a text from Aps. "Bro! Aps wants to come too!" exclaimed Garne. Jones and Ottie were surprised. They had met Aps prior and remembered that he was living close by in LA. "Alright, why not?" Jones said.

They started walking the same trail that Ottie and Jones had explored earlier, showing Garne all of the interesting spots. Then Aps came down, showing up with one of his friends and ten other people. Jones's eyes went wide, "Woah! What is this, a film crew?" Aps had a love for filming and running around places. "Bring in the cavalry." Ottie joked as the fifteen of them began trudging through the town. Walking past the red warehouses, the group stumbled upon the Odu's clothing store again. A small crew of Odu's servers sat outside at a table eating chips as they waved them over. "Yo!" a lot of them said, "How are you?" Jones felt flustered as the night didn't go over as well as he wanted at the block party the night before. "Good! These are my friends." Jones said introducing them, but trying to hide his emotion. The clothing shop group politely welcomed them as a man in a white suit with blonde hair sat at the table. Jones didn't know what to say, flustered he asked the man for help but was turned down.

"Help with what?" the man said, questioning Jones. "Help with promotion? I'm not sure yet." Jones replied. The man sat Jones down, "Listen, kid. I like your vibe, but remember this in LA. Don't waste time." Consoling Jones, he offered him a few cheese chips. "Here man, sit down and converse. But I can't help you. Sorry." Jones had a feeling that it was coming. Everyone in the group mingled and talked as they enjoyed the sunny day beating down on the table. Jones pointed to the factory across the street, "We'd really like to make a statement by covering up that damn broken down place with art." Two people out of the group laughed and agreed, "Yeah, too bad it's owned but not fixed up. We would like that too." sighing as the closed down factory felt like a stain on the entire District. "Let's move on," Jones said, waving Garne and everyone forward. Walking further down towards the red brick warehouse, Aps started plotting with Garne and Ottie. "Listen, guys, let's go find all of the Idols' in the buildings! If we can get a chance to meet him, that's good enough!" suggested Aps. The musicians walked around as a party went on in one of the warehouse buildings. "Yo, the back door is open, Ottie said as he wandered in with Jones.

What is this place?" They saw many people dressed up in tuxedos and luxurious dresses. Walking in further, Ottie started eating some of the food after taking the medicine Garne had given him. A man quickly shouted at them, "What are you guys doing here? You can't be in here! How did you get in?" The man seemed flustered. Ottie replied, "We're looking for the musician Idol." The man pointed Ottie out of the door. "Not here! You guys broke into a wedding." the man said angrily. Ottie apologized as Jones left back out the door. The man shut the door to the warehouse after escorting Ottie out. "Yeah, maybe that helicopter flying by up there is Idol with his buddy." Jones joked, trying to lighten up the mood. Aps came over with Garne, "Let's start heading back. It's getting late. We will come back tomorrow." he said. As the crew started walking back through the District, there were loads of people partying in the streets. A Korean woman was sitting in a souped-up car. Many people dressed in suits or weird clothing were making noise as another group was walking out. "Whoa!" a man said in a leopard hat. Jones went up to him as Ottie and Aps went towards the back of the place. "What's going on here?" Jones asked. "Grab a drink!" he said, "Free drinks for everyone. Come on in and check it out."

Inside, the place was fully crowded as art hung off the walls. EDM music played in the background as artists from everywhere talked and smiled together. Jones looked back over at the Korean woman sitting in the car out front staring at her phone. He assumed she must have been a popular singer from the band. "Alright," Jones said, accepting entry into the place. Plaid walls with many paintings and a little cutout for the DJ

CHAPTER ELEVEN - UNCLEAR DISCOVERY

to play through had been set up. "So why are you here?" the man in the leopard hat asked Jones. "Well, you see, we're trying to find Idol. A lot of us are musicians." Jones replied. The man offered to let them to come by another time, but Jones turned it down. "My friend is sick, unfortunately. We'll see if we can make it." Jones said.

The man didn't seem bothered by this. He backed off to enjoy the party. A moment later Aps and Ottie came running out of the back end of the gated area. "Yo! We have to go now!" Aps said with Ottie in tow. Garne ended up running as well. "What happened?" Jones asked as he walked outside with a drink in his hand. "We'll come back tomorrow and explain later. We have to get out of here." Ottie said. Ottie gave Jones the car keys as they all briskly walked away from the party. "Bro, that was dope," Ottie said, hinting at what had happened. Aps laughed as well, "Who thought we would've got kicked out. Listen Jones; the security guard hinted at Idol's place. He uh, well, he said yes, but not really."

Jones questioned their antics, "So, he said he's there basically?" replying calmly, as the four of them took a breather from walking away fast. "Yeah, he's here," they said, High Fiving one another. "We will be back in a couple of days," Aps said, calling his crew over. Each group departed their separate ways. As Jones and Ottie headed towards the car Jones said, "What a good day!" Ottie walked slowly, battling the onset fever that had come, "Yeah man, we really found what we were looking for." Ohs texted Jones, "I'll take you to the teacher's spot tomorrow instead. Okay?" Jones texted back, "Yeah, that sounds fun. Sorry, we missed it today." Both Jones and Ottie had fun for the second time this trip. As night fell Jones imagined himself on stage briefly, "What you imagine is what you create." repeating through his head as he looked out the window. This time Jones drove for the third time during the trip. "I guess so many souls listen to music to drown out the noise of everyone else," he thought. Voices responded through his head, "It's how we communicate easily."

Jones tried to tune it out by listening to music. But words sprung about,

"You get yours and I'll get mine." Ottie fell asleep in the passenger side of the car trying to rest on the way back to the hotel. Once in the garage, Ottie went straight to the room while Jones tapped the Caution 'energy' sign hoping to get power. However, nothing happened. Jones tried to press his hand on the sign again as the lady from the front desk tapped his shoulder. "Can I help you with something sir?" the lady asked. Jones didn't have an answer, but thinking quickly he replied, "Just looking at the sticker on the sign." She looked at him oddly. "Do you have a room here?" Jones pulled out the keys from his pocket, "I do Miss. Roomin' away." trying to make a joke to diffuse the situation. "Please step away from the lobby door, sir. You've been staring at the sign for twenty minutes." the front desk lady politely asked as she laughed, "You should get some rest, sir. Do you need help finding your room?" Jones declined. He thanked the woman from the front desk and started walking towards his room. "I warned you kid, Nepharius is trouble." the voice rang out through his head. "Now you're following the same footsteps as his, even with distance in between."

Jones realized by the sound of the voice who it was, "Mira, you've been trying to trace me all this time, haven't you?" Jones answered, fearing the worst. "I told you to stay in your lane, kid. You're discovering too much. I'm on your side, but if you keep digging, then Nepharius might be your only friend left. That's not something you want." Mira warned him again. "Life is about balance. Why do you think so many people sing about this stuff?" She continued trying to convince Jones to fix his newfound self, "You're out of balance right now. Even the CIA is going to come for you soon." Mira continued her lecture as Jones tried to wave away her voice, feeling cold inside with a mixture of warmth in her breath. "Alright, alright!" Jones replied, "Mira, I don't understand a thing you're talking about." She hinted at his past again, "Humans are made of stars, you're an…" she stopped. "Stop Mira, you're messing with my crew!" Nepharius shouted, the sound echoing through Jones' head.

CHAPTER ELEVEN - UNCLEAR DISCOVERY

Suddenly Jones felt tired. He didn't hear the woman from the front desk call his name from down the hallway, asking if he was okay. Stumbling to his room, he passed out on the bed in full clothing. Jones was too in his head to understand reality. Mira disappeared as her voice was gone. Nepharius also stopped talking. "Keep your head clear." were the words echoing in Jones' mind. The next morning Jones woke up hearing Ottie throwing up in the toilet. Still refusing to stay in and get rest, Ottie fought briefly with Jones. "Ohs is showing us around today. I have to see." Ottie insisted. Jones eventually gave in feeling tired, "Alright bro, but you're sitting in the very back." Laughing, trying to make light of the situation. Ottie fell asleep as soon as he curled up in the back seat. An hour later Jones and Ottie arrived at Ohs' house. Jones shot Ohs a text. "Hey man, is today a good day to show us? We're here."

Ohs replied right away, "Right on, like, awesome Bro. Be right out." Jones felt tired but hid that feeling away under his excitement. "Are you guys hungry?" Ohs asked. Ottie nodded lightly as Jones agreed. After an hour of driving towards the spiral building known as Star World Records, Ohs sat down staring out. "See this? This is real LA." Ohs said. Cracks and dirt lie everywhere as homeless and beat-down people dined at the burger spot. "It used to be so different. Times have really changed." lamented Ohs. Jones sighed, relating again, "I'll inspire people. Let's change this!" he thought in his head, as heads around him perked up almost as if they could hear him. Dogs looked at Jones without him saying a word and stopped barking. He calmed his mind realizing he hadn't said anything at all. Ohs stared at him waiting for a reply. "What do you think man?" Jones played it off as if nothing had happened within those few seconds. Ottie and Ohs hadn't seemed to notice.

"I think I'm excited to meet these music teachers!" Jones replied excitedly. Ohs threw away his burger wrapper into the trash. "If people would simply eat their own packaging and waste, we wouldn't have this problem," Ohs said as Jones nodded in agreement. "Huh?" Ottie perked up, feeling better after he ate. "Bro, so where is this place?" Ohs gave them the address as they all hopped into the car driving a short distance to a parking garage that gave a hole-in-the-wall feel. They walked up the steps as Ohs waved to the students. "Hey man, this is my thing. Where I do radio and stuff." Ohs said. Ottie and Jones could hear a teacher giving a lesson to a class. Three students sat in the leather black chairs moving their mouse's around as a digital audio workspace loaded up on the computer. Ohs waved to one of the students. "Woah!" Ottie exclaimed as he went up the stairs towards multiple pieces of vinyl that sat over in the back. This is pretty awesome!" he said, seeing the vinyl all in a line with the microphone.

"Want to take classes?" Jones joked as the view showed a beautiful overlook of the city. A student walked down the hallway to where Ohs stood and waved. "This is one of the talented students here. He's a friend of mine." Ohs exclaimed as he was happy to be in a place that accepted him. The teacher invited Ottie and Jones to sit in the leather seats as Ohs stood behind them watching from the sidelines as students worked away at their songs. After watching a while, Jones asked, "So, Ohs, who else is around here?" wondering if there were other teachers off duty. "Oh, Miss K, one of our teachers is pretty sweet," Ohs said, leading them forward towards the front desk that sat with gold-plated names. 'Team Kull' was written on the plate plastered on the wall of an office that Jones had noticed. An award stood on the desk as Ottie and Jones went over. Ottie seemed to know more about the Team than Jones did. Jones wandered towards the other side of the building not knowing what to say. He zoned out in his headspace again, taking all of the scenery in, not wanting to think at the high rate of speed he had been thinking. Ottie finished talking with the Team and Ms. K. Ottie's body had begun feeling sicker. He was grateful for the connection, but it was time to go.

So, they said their goodbyes and walked out of the building. "It's 4:00 PM. What do you guys want to do?" Ohs asked. Ottie said he wanted to grab a haircut. "Bro, what? You want a forty-dollar haircut?" Jones asked jokingly, knowing that prices were a lot higher than usual in this area. "Yeah, man. Layers and everything." Ottie joked back. Ohs whispered to Jones, "Yo, your vibe is cool, but your friend's vibe is kind of crazy. Drop me off first." Jones went over to the car and got in. "Alright, but after the convenience store." Jones said to Ottie, "Remember how we talked about popping a balloon off the roof and hanging a sheet? Let's do that." Ottie agreed as Ohs followed along with the plan. After walking around the store, they bought paper and cutouts along with spray paint. Then they picked up balloons. "Are we really going through with this?" Ottie asked. "Well at worst, if we don't do it, we can always return the stuff we don't use," Jones said. Jones dropped off Ohs back at his house. Before closing the car door, Ohs said, "Hey, meet me later at the Bunny Club."

Jones figured this would be the last time Ottie and Jones saw him for a while, "Alright Ohs, we will text you." And they drove back towards the haircut place. "This place is owned by Idol; it must be somewhere here." Ottie shook his head as they walked through an alleyway where artsy graffiti ran rampant. The both of them stumbled upon the glass doors as they walked through the alleyway. The glass doors swung open to the haircut building. Merchandise and branded clothing were displayed around the store all priced above $199. Ottie waved to the front desk lady who called him over. Without a further word needed between him and the front desk, he went over to the chair to sit down for a haircut. "Name's T-man!" A tall man with brown eyes came up to them and shook their hands. "I'll be cutting your hair today, dawg". he said with scissors held in his left hand. Black leather seats and marble filled the room. "Pretty fancy for a haircut parlor," Jones remarked, complimenting the place.

"So, what brings you out to this place?" T-man asked. "I don't recognize you guys." Ottie looked back at Jones, "Well, I make music." Ottie said. "Oh, music? Hey, that's pretty cool, man. You know we have a DJ set back there. Let me show you." T-man escorted Ottie and Jones over to white curtains which cut off a back room that was much darker. Lights and music played softly as there was no one in the room. "You should come by! Play a set for us while we work!" T-man offered. Ottie networked again, "Yeah I'll give you my email!" Jones blinked for a moment; many people started dancing on the dance floor. He blinked again and they disappeared as if traveling at hyper-speed.

T-man sat Ottie back down in one of the black leather seats as he layered his hair. "We'd be excited to hear you play sometime." T-man reiterated. Ottie shook T-man's hand as he finished up the cut. "Yo, how does it look?" Ottie asked Jones. "Pretty sick!" Jones said in return. After paying for the haircut and a few minutes of window shopping they went out of the place. "That's our next connection," Ottie said excitedly about the possibilities. "Yeah man, hope you got his email," Jones replied.

The clock struck 6:00 PM. It was time to pick up Ohs. Jones put on the gas to the car and raced as fast as he could down the highway Every eight seconds a hole appeared in the highway lanes that allowed Jones to go as fast as he could weaving in and out of the cars. "Jones! Slow down." Ottie shouted from the passenger's side as the music blasted loudly in the car. Jones slowed the car down and stated, "We're already here." as the night fell. Ohs rushed out of his house with his hat on, taking a small weed hit before getting in the car. "Heyyy! We're going to a friend of mine's show. To go talk a bit. Artists and stuff." Ohs chatted excitedly. Jones and Ottie looked at one another and shrugged as they headed downtown. As they arrived outside of the building, a circle of people stood in front of two big red doors with black handles. The word 'Bunny' was written in large letters at the top of the place as people smoked cigarettes outside. Jones parked on the other side of the street. They got out to walk towards the door. "Hey! Ohs!" a man said from the circle of smokers, he was dressed in all blue with a blue cap, "I'm tryin' a rap still!" Ohs looked over at Ottie and Jones, "For sure man, these are my friends." Ohs said smiling.

"Yeah! Yeah, got Soundcloud? Let's get some studio space." the man in

CHAPTER ELEVEN - UNCLEAR DISCOVERY

the blue cap said happily. Jones took a step back, feeling crowded by the invitation, "I'm going to stand over here." Jones stepped over towards another man in the circle. This man wore a jacket with musical pins on it. "Hey, I'm also Ohs' friend," he said to Jones. Talking to the faces felt more as if Jones were talking to shadows. He felt cold, isolated, and alone stuck in between the world he was trying to inspire and the world he was watching. "Awesome, man. You rap too?" Jones asked. The man loaded up his Soundcloud as the man in the blue cap overheard. Ottie saw it on Jones' phone, "Dude's only got 10 followers, Bro." Ottie warned Jones. The man in the blue cap kept talking loudly about his abilities to Ohs. Jones blinked, this time there was no crowd behind the man. All Jones could see was emptiness. Ohs and the rest of the crew went inside. The guards welcomed in Ohs as more people flooded in.

"This is another spot tied to everyone," Ohs said. Ottie overheard some of the names thrown around in the club. He picked up the fact that this place was no ordinary place. "Ohs, who rolls through here?" Ottie asked out of curiosity. "One of your Idol's musicians who is under his label," he replied. Ottie went upfront as the musician sat there playing. The crowd, rather than cheering, danced more slowly to the bass playing out in the room. After an hour, Jones felt the emotion and wanted to leave. He couldn't accept that he could read what everyone else was feeling by simply standing there. As Ohs lit up some weed, he watched Jones walk out the door. He went out after him while Ottie stayed inside. "Where ya going?" Ohs asked out of curiosity catching up with Jones. "Outside here to catch some air. We should leave." Jones said. Ohs understood and went in to grab Ottie. The circle of laughter faded outside as the rappers and musicians said goodbye to one another. Ottie came out. "What's this about Jones?" he asked, questioning him. "Let's go back. The show's finishing up, replied Jones. Ottie sighed, "Yeah, alright."

They all walked back towards Jones' car. After a short drive, Jones dropped off Ohs and headed back towards the hotel. "We've got about two days left here. Ottie said to Jones. I want to send out some of my pictures and drop them off under doors in the area." Jones agreed. "Call Aps and Garne. We'll say goodbye to Ohs tomorrow and prepare to pack up." Jones felt good about the connections the two of them had made. After driving through the night and arriving at the hotel, Jones went straight to the room. Both Ottie's and Jones' clothing scattered the floor. They had been so busy going out and exploring every day that they hadn't taken time off for themselves. Realizing that the trip had been more than the two of them expected, Jones fell right on the bed. His head swirled with thoughts as he tried to gather up his thoughts about the connections he had made in LA. Ottie started snoring as the sickness slowly went away. Still feeling slightly under the weather; he had trudged through. Jones and Ottie were to wrap things up. However, both of them didn't know that after this trip it would be a long time before they saw one another again. The next morning Jones rubbed his eyes. He stared at the ceiling as if the highs of the trip had already passed. "Are you enjoying your journey?" a voice rang through his head. "You have a lot to do when you get back, as you've promised us." Thousands of voices echoed as Jones tried to calm them down.

"Yeah, I will get to it. Let me enjoy the last part of this trip." Jones said to himself, understanding what he had promised and the consequences that would follow. Ottie got out of bed, "Hey man, I'm going to shower first this time." Jones replied right away, shaking the voices out of his head, "Yeah, it's going to be a big day!" Ottie got dressed as Jones was already packed with his clothing. He reached for the door as he looked back at the room one last time. "Yo! Where are you at this time?" Garne texted. "Aps and I want another shot at this place." Jones texted back. "Yeah, follow us! We have this all figured out," replied Garne. Ottie and Jones got into the car as Ottie reached for the tissues. "Yo, I'm feeling a little better after all of this," Ottie said sniffling. Jones crossed the bridge, soaking in the trees planted along with the Arts District community along with the feelings of experiencing Los Angeles. It would be some time until he felt like he

CHAPTER ELEVEN - UNCLEAR DISCOVERY

should go back to the Arts District.

Garne and Aps came with their full crew again. "I have a plan this time for the apartments. The guard kind of told me all about it." Garne said. Ottie and Jones sat there with Garne as the three of them planned. "You know first though guys, I want to throw a giant festival!" Jones exclaimed. "Yo, Jones! Focus on the music first, before a festival, man." Ottie sighed. Jones looked around towards the warehouse that Ottie had spotted on their first visit. It had a large gate and a 'Beware of Dogs' sign. "You know, I wonder what's in there?" Jones pointed towards the warehouse building. The sign showed a happy face on it as the crew walked towards it. By coincidence the warehouse door opened. "What's this place about?" Jones asked as a bald, tall man walked out with a glass of wine and put it down on the table. "Oh, what are you all doing?" the man asked with curiosity. "I'm promoting these artists. And I'm kind of interested in throwing a festival, like the big ones we always hear about!" Jones said happily. "Come inside then, I've got something to show you." the man welcomed the entire crew in. "I've played at that festival you're talking about."

The crew gathered around to listen to the man's story about his drumming experience. "It's getting expensive to live here though," he exclaimed. Wooden furnishings and metal designs filled the house along with a cherry wood separator. The man was living comfortably. Jones couldn't say anything as he felt like he had mistakenly accomplished one of the missions. Ottie and the rest of the crew meandered through the place as time passed. The man thanked them for the conversation as the crew waved goodbye. "Well, now we know what's in there." Ottie said, "Would have never guessed that." Garne and Aps, feeling fired up, decided to head in towards the town. "Let's go find your Idol!" all of them shouted as they waved to Ottie and Jones. Ohs texted Jones, "Yo! I spotted your Idol!" Jones texted back, "What do you mean?" Ohs replied, "He's in his home across the street." Ottie grew excited, "Alright, we'll be right there."

The entire crew walked in and out of the buildings as Ottie left fliers of himself across every house that the crew had visited before. Each flier, with a picture of him sporting his new haircut along with his stage name 'Allorium', was passed out. Some of the fliers even slid through the door. "Well, that's one way to do it," Garne said from the side. The crew fully showed up at Ohs' house as Ohs pointed towards Idol and smiled. "Oh man, he's working away, huh?" Ottie said. "Well damn, alright!" But Ottie didn't want to disturb Idol or be seen as someone who just came across the situation; a sort of respect for a fellow artist making music. "Well, we saw him. Let's go over there." Jones said. The rest of the crew agreed, giving high fives. Ottie and Jones said their goodbyes to Ohs. "Come by anytime. I'll miss you, Bros!" Ohs said as the rest of them waved as they walked out the door. As a tribute to the mission of finding Idol all of them went into the apartments where the security guard was at the front desk. "Is he in?" Ottie and Aps asked.

"You guys can see the place only if you're buying." the man said sternly. "I can't allow you forward." Ottie and Aps went out the front door and snuck around back. A few minutes later a shout came from the garage. "Hey, I thought I told you guys! You can't be in here!" Ottie shouted to Aps, "Let's get out of here." They ran from the apartments veering off right, taking the steps down towards the front of the elevator. Ottie and Aps accepted their fate as the two of them calmly walked out of the apartments. "Don't worry, Garne and I will make it to the scene down here now that we know," Aps said. Garne and Aps smiled. Jones and Ottie looked at one another, "Hey man we tried right?" Ottie said. Jones shrugged as they turned back towards the car. "I'll see you at the hotel!" Aps yelled loudly. Ottie nodded his head in confirmation and headed back to the car. Ottie and Jones drove back to the hotel where their clothing was already packed. Jones felt a sense of success on the trip as well as a sense of failure as he looked at the floor feeling depressed. "This can't be all there is to the world, right?" Jones asked Ottie, trying to get confirmation that the trip had not been a waste. Both Ottie and Jones had gone completely broke. They had spent

CHAPTER ELEVEN - UNCLEAR DISCOVERY

all of their money on shows and outings to meet the people in town.

"What do you mean?" Ottie questioned Jones' statement. "I think I'm a bit depressed, Bro," Jones responded. Ottie sat there quietly for a moment. He recalled all of the times that he and Jones had drunk together and this entire trip the two of them had. "Depressed? Are you sure, Bro?" Ottie asked very concernedly. Jones thought about it again, "I think so man. I feel like we've failed, you know? We put all this time and effort into our music, and spent money coming down here. We got connections now but haven't accomplished anything." Jones went off on a small rant feeling hopeless with all of the money spent on hotels and food. "Yeah, I get that feeling sometimes as well. We have to keep pushing." Ottie said, trying to relate to Jones and his expressed failures. Ottie thought for a moment, "Hey man, Aps will be here in a bit. Let's say our goodbyes properly." Ottie's voice shook as well and Jones could hear the slight off in his voice. "If you need anyone to talk to Jones, I'm always here for you, Bro," Ottie said. For a moment Jones sat there as thoughts raced through his head. Everyone he had previously met wanted a part in the potential future he was about to create. Jones sighed, "Alright, I guess it's not so bad." He gave a slight smile to Ottie as Aps came through the door.

"Hey man what's up!" Aps came into the hotel room to say goodbye. "I brought over my laptop. Ohs' house was pretty cool man. He had a lot of interesting DAW stuff on his system." Aps brought up one of the songs he was working on and got to it. "Yo! All about dat bass." Ottie said jokingly, following it with a fake laugh trying to lighten up the mood. Aps, feeling sentimental, loaded up his tracks as the two of them talked for a while about their past meetups. After a couple of hours, Aps packed up leaving the Motel 6 hotel feeling empty and quiet. "Yo, it's time to go soon." Jones hinted at Ottie as their stuff was nearly fully packed. Ottie contemplated the homeward trip as he reached for his stuff in the restroom, "Yeah, alright." As night fell, they went to bed early that night. Ottie and Jones had to leave the next morning after spending two weeks in LA. A part of Jones didn't want to leave yet, feeling there was much more to do. However, he knew that staying there was no longer plausible. Ottie flipped on the T.V. as he sniffled from the final parts of being sick. "Bro, when we get back, we'll go job hunting again," Ottie said. Jones nodded his head, "Yeah, we have to man."

Jones woke up the next morning as Ottie had already thrown his luggage in the car the night before. He shook Ottie, "Get up. It's already time to go." Jones realized he was late for check-out time as he went up to the front desk cashier, "Did you two enjoy your stay?" she said, smiling trying to forget what she had seen Jones doing a few days earlier. "Yeah, we enjoyed the stay just fine," Jones said as the credit card swiped on the counter. Jones headed towards the car throwing his luggage in the back seat. Ottie turned the music up too loud. "It's afternoon man. Turn it down. This music is hurting my ears!" Jones exclaimed, trying to gain back control of the situation. Ottie didn't complain this time. He turned the radio down as they sat silently driving out of LA. "Are you hungry?" Ottie asked, trying to gauge Jones' mood from before. "A little bit, but not much," Jones replied. "We can stop soon for a burger or something." Waze loaded up on his phone, 'The road warriors are prepared for you, Sir!' Jones hit the cancel button on the screen hiding it away as he didn't want to be disturbed by the world. Jones turned the music on so he could focus on driving as Ottie slept through most of the ride back to San Francisco.

Chapter Twelve – Scattered Infiltration

After five long hours of driving, they arrived home. Ms. P was standing at the door. "Jones, we need to talk about Ottie's stay," she said with a warning. Jones waved her off, "Can we talk about this tomorrow?" His mother turned away peeved. She didn't want to argue as she had other problems on her mind. "Tomorrow then, no later," she said in a scolding tone. Jones nodded his head knowing what was coming. Ottie had promised to move out within two weeks and it had already been almost two months since he had been living in the house. Despite Ottie being respectful and having a low presence, he had overstayed his welcome. Ottie had failed to get a stable job for himself which he could continuously work at. Jones had tried his best to promote and help Ottie. Jones turned towards Ottie, "Hey man, let's go for a walk and talk awhile." he said with a heavy sigh in his voice. Ottie looked out over his laptop back at Jones sensing it was bad news. They grabbed their skateboards and treaded outside towards town. "Yo, my mom doesn't want you to stay in the house anymore. Do you have a plan?" Jones said. "You can shower here but you can't live here anymore," Jones repeated himself as Ottie looked down for a moment. "Oh.... maybe I can sleep in your car for a while at night?" Ottie suggested this as his first solution.

"Well alright, but only temporarily while you talk to a friend. Do you have any others here?" Jones asked, trying to fish for a better solution. "Jones, I've got a few. I can stay at a hotel for a couple of nights in Berkeley with the extra money saved too." Ottie said, trying to be responsible. "The places like Starbucks won't hire me because of a theft found through my background check. This dates from when I was in high school when my friend forced me to steal. I have a warrant over my head." Jones's eyes went wide. All within a few moments he had told Jones something way too late. "Why didn't you tell me this sooner?" Jones shouted, almost losing it."Look, I'll find a place within the next day or two," Ottie replied. They walked around the town taking in the scenery, both downcast. Jones was becoming tired of this reality and wanted to go to the other galactic reality he had been forming in his mind. "When we get back, start asking your buddies," Jones mentioned. The time for Ottie and Jones to part ways had come. The feelings that Jones began to have when coming back from Los Angeles hit him like a rock. The sun felt hotter, as they walked.

Jones remembered Nepharius' words about finding the experts in the world. Jones wanted to go out exploring for them around town. Jones thought to himself, "Okay, I want to escape to my own reality, but how can one create his own reality while still living here?" He questioned and pondered it after everything that had happened. "I know, I'll test those theories I saw. I'll test all of them as I go find the experts in the world. I mean all these weird people from galactic space are talking to me. I've already experienced some. How bad can it be? I'm joining Nepharius' crew." Jones mentally spoke to himself as Ottie chattered about a woman he knew in Monterey Bay. As long as he could get dropped off down there, he would not have to stay at Jones' house. "Stop Jones. This is a dangerous game you're playing." Mira spoke. "Remember, I warned you about the CIA coming after you." Jones shook his head as Mira disappeared. At first, Jones didn't want to accept her back in. Ottie still needed a place to go for a day or two more. Jones couldn't give in — give in to the depression that had become the driving force of his world's parallelisms.

"Alright, let's head back. I'll deal with my mother and park my car a little out of sight so you can sleep at night. You can borrow my laptop

CHAPTER TWELVE – SCATTERED INFILTRATION

in the meantime to find the place." Jones said, reconfirming the plan. They walked back towards the house. This time Ottie got on the laptop messaging friends and talking to the people who lived around the area. Jones said he would talk to his mom but it couldn't wait. "Mom, tell you what," Jones said as his mother turned around. "Yes?" she replied. "Ottie is looking for a friend's house to stay at. He'll be leaving tomorrow." Ms. P. 's face lit up. "Alright." Jones went into the room as Ottie called another friend.

"Hey, yeah. Monterey Bay. Yeah, okay. Bye." as fast as Ottie called her, she hung up. "So, I found a place in Monterey Bay. I'll sleep in the car tonight and we'll leave tomorrow." Ottie grabbed his stuff and put it in the car. Jones gave him the keys. "Have a good rest," Jones said as Ottie went towards the front door. He waved as he closed the door. Jones sat there in silence as Nepharius called him. "Jones. Are you ready?" Nepharius asked. Jones obediently agreed, "Yes, I'm ready." Nepharius got closer to Jones, "Alright crew! First, I want you to travel the iron horse road. There's a Valkyries school there. I need to promote Retragrammatron, the show, and I'm looking for those experts who understand this." Jones listened in. Nepharius told him the exact location of the school by the Army Base on the Iron Trail. "Listen, Jones, you're an arbiter and keeper of time. Take video games for example. Most of them are based on real places and stories. Visit the library and read them from time to time." Nepharius advised.

Nepharius disappeared as his chair faded. Jones was now able to go wherever he needed to freely. Or so he thought. That night Jones slept like a rock as he had been sleep-deprived again. He twisted and turned within the bedsheets, unable to shake the guilty feeling of failure. The bushes shook again as Ottie spoke out inside his mind. "Who's there?" asked Jones. The bushes shook again as the footsteps sounded as if they had sped up to the roof. "You guys leave here!" Jones ordered, afraid after their last encounter. The sound of scurrying went down the house and out into the driveway. Morning came as Jones rubbed his eyes. He walked outside to see Ottie asleep in his car, all fogged up from the windows being closed. Jones opened his car to air it out. "Yo, why is the car so foggy?" Jones questioned Ottie not wanting to know the answer. "Shut up, dude," Ottie replied, seemingly annoyed that he did not get much sleep. After getting ready, Jones got in the car with Ottie. The drive would be three long hours to Monterey Bay, towards the beach end of town. They arrived at a little gas station close to their destination address. The gas station had hotdogs inside and a sign 'Brand New' written on the door. What was a Warrior that was part of a crew against the theft of imagination supposed to do in Monterey? Jones didn't have much thought of the place as the two walked in. The man silently watched and smiled at them waving happily. Jones and Ottie poured themselves an Icee as the two of them chatted about Ottie's moving situation. "I got it, bro. I'm going to try to live here and if I can't, I'm going back." Jones replied, "Back where?" Ottie looked up at the sky for a bit as the car filled with a tank of gas. "Back to Ohio, you know?" he said in deep words.

"Oh, alright," Jones said slowly as the two of them spoke. "Let's go down to the beach sometime," Ottie suggested. Jones nodded his head as he drove the car towards Ottie's new area. A woman with blue dyed hair came out as Ottie walked up the stairs dropping his luggage off. "I'll be fine here for a while," Ottie said. Jones turned around waving as he got back in his car loading up Waze. This time the Road Warrior icon loaded up on his phone. Jones hit 'Yes'. As Jones hit the gas picking up speed on the freeway. Police icons started to pick up on the map. The faster Jones pushed on the pedal, the faster the policemen popped up. "Stop messing with others' will," Mira shouted angrily in his head. Jones said to himself, "Protection shield." A white light in his mind expanded as if he felt he was floating. He pointed his fingers towards each car selecting which ones he would move out of his way into the other lanes. The cars cleared a space for him allowing Jones to speed up through the traffic that stood before him. Road Warrior icons popped up all over the map in defense as bikers sat there with a

CHAPTER TWELVE – SCATTERED INFILTRATION

policeman at every face on Jones' screen. "This is incredible," Jones said to himself, smiling like a man who had found his wildest dreams coming true. "All I need now is a hat and a cane!" Jones always had watched T.V. shows, particularly appreciative of the acting. He was starting to believe that actors were simply putting themselves in those worlds, making their characters and alter egos real as the actors disguised themselves in the world. Jones believed much of the same thing was happening to himself as he felt he could see into the future. After all, the people and events that had happened around him would change anyone's mind.

Driving faster down the road, the three hours Jones was driving felt more like one. A car stopped in front of him in traffic as Jones slammed on the breaks. He had almost hit the car in front of him but his car came to a dead stop almost as if on will. "I told you Jones, Karma! For every situation you mess with, the world will give it back to you in some other way. If you move traffic for time? Traffic will be there again to take that same amount of time back." warned Mira. Jones thought in his head again, "Shut up Mira, what do you want?" Mira smiled, "I want Nepharius. I want him out of leading his crew as he's supposed to follow regulations." Mira turned around, "If it weren't for the need to capture him, I would have turned you in already, but I like you kid. That right now is the only wall holding me back from putting you right in there with him." Traffic moved again as Jones blasted music moving his hands around in a rotation. Neither of his hands touched the wheel as the car drove straight, even around the turns. The car turned with turns by Jones' will alone. Jones arrived home and walked through the door. "Hey, mom. Ottie's gone to Monterey Bay as promised."

She smiled and went back to her indoor plants, "Well, it was good having him here." Jones walked into his room. After going through the drive his heart beat fast. He rolled in his bed almost as if he got back playing off the wills of others. As fast as Jones got back into the house, he decided to go out again. Jones spotted a cane near the front door, the same cane that he had seen woven in black with a metal top. The cane had an old feeling to it as if a Veteran with a dark past had owned it before him. Jones reached down and took the cane walking outside with it. He stared at the leaves as the leaves turned red. Thinking about the City and BART stopping for him, the doors opening, guiding him where to go every time he was walking. Jones smiled, going towards the sidewalk as the old Army Base ran by under the bridge. A sign that said, 'Land Traps Present, Proceed at Your Own Risk' stood out at him as the curled rusted barbed wire sat on top of the sign. "Walk through the place, Jones. You'll make it!" Jones could sense the energy coming from the spots, almost as if the wind told him where to go as he stepped over from place to place.

The deer stopped in their tracks to watch him. A cat that crossed over the street along with a dog stopped in their tracks too. The animals could almost sense the energy resonating from Jones' body as he kept jumping from space to space. At the very end, he made it through the path, spotting a dirty pipe that dumped sewage in the water close by. "Fix up the pipe so that water's cleaner around the area. Got it." Jones imagined it in the future creating the construction that would happen by his very own thoughts. He wrote it down on his phone to bring the idea into reality believing it would converge both spaces for instant creation. Jones walked further into town towards the Veteran's building. He wondered what other people would sense. Babies in carriages instantly smiled as he walked by almost as if they were old spirits in new bodies. The clarity of the universe in which many things came out of hiding, unnoticed had now become noticed in reality towards which he was living.

"You know, a compass over our heads would be awesome." Jones thought to himself. The wind pointed towards the E on the Earl's Groceries sign. The giant red letter stuck out more than the rest at Jones as it was tattered. "Go east huh?" Jones thought. He walked down the street towards a second grocery store as the building opened up. "Time to do some shopping in the future," Jones said, closing his eyes for a moment. He re-opened them as

CHAPTER TWELVE – SCATTERED INFILTRATION

he walked into the grocery store. A flower in yellow color with a pen sat at the side of the store. He picked it up as the green bottom was able to write. "I feel I've done this before." Jones thought to himself as he pulled the pen apart from the flower. Then he put it back, "Ah yes, separating pens you can plant. Great!" Jones joyfully cheered to himself walking towards the back of the store where bottled water was on the shelf. 'Eternal' the brand read. "So, if I drink this, I will have eternal life! Not now. I don't think I want that." Jones put it back on the shelf as a woman walked by and grabbed it almost at the same speed that Jones felt he was traveling at. Jones walked over to the men working the oven as a calzone piping hot was being served up. "What can I get for you?" the man asked.

"That looks good." Jones took the calzone in his hand as the man handed him a box that looked like a pizza slice in cardboard. "There are phone chargers on the walk-in here too." the man said, pointing them out to Jones as he gave the man the money for the calzone. Jones sat down charging his phone as he was conjuring up the idea of how to put a compass above people's heads so people could tell one another where they are headed. As the sun beat down on him, he threw away the cardboard box. The brown wood chips now were the bright color of red and smelled of cherries and soda. "Man, this place is great," Jones said to himself. "To keep it to myself, I will only take three items a day from this future," Jones said as if he were talking to the galaxy. All the meanwhile people from the outside were looking at Jones as he quietly mumbled to himself. Feeling insecure, Jones thought about it, "I need a disguise." Ottie texted his phone, "Hey come down tomorrow. Let's go to the beach. I'll show you inside." Jones calmed down after testing out his newfound self. "Alright," Jones said to Ottie while marching back towards his car. He got in and blasted EDM from it. "That's right; the Universal car design. That must be my ticket to that brown felt hat." Jones laughed at the thought of his insanity turning real. Jones came home as Ms. P stared at him. "Where did you go?" she asked with concern.

"You worry too much, Mom," Jones said, trying to keep her out of his business. "You alright?" she asked again, questioning Jones' actions. He had always mentioned where he went casually. Jones usually had nothing to hide, the changes were becoming obvious. "I'm going back out," Jones said again. He didn't want to stay home as he now felt a purpose to go out and explore his local areas. An In-Law Unit sat at the back of the house by their pool. Glasses with a funky hippy vibe, blue glass, and a squiggly steel outer casing lay in the room. Jones put them on. I'll call myself "Vextrous Fortunata, the Arbiter." Jones declared. Jones had a musical persona that Nepharius and he talked about. Vextrous coming from one of his favorite books as Fortunata coming from his other. "Yeah; this is the perfect disguise. A hat now, I must." Jones walked back into the house, "How do I look?" he asked his mom as her face turned more concerned. "Aren't those your step bro's?" she asked, questioning him.

"No, the wind showed me the back room. The wind pointed these to me." Jones replied. Jones' mother instantly knew there was something wrong with Jones. "Jones, what are you talking about? You should get some rest," she said, her voice rising with alarm. Jones felt attacked, "Never mind, I'm going out." Now wearing the blue-tinted hippie glasses that Jones had picked up within his stepbrothers' room, he was wearing them constantly. This allowed him to focus his mindset, to help him navigate and bring out the people from hiding, all playing on the same level as him. Jones walked further east as he came upon a large black rock, commemorating a deceased person with engravings on it. "Has Ah, I get it, for me to understand anything I first need to understand where it all came from right?" Jones asked himself. 'Hand of peace' was written on the black stone engraved in gold.'Donated to the City of Walnut Creek' it said with a plaque describing the history of a man. The wind blew again as Jones changed directions; a Watcher looked at him from afar. As Jones noticed him, he decided to avoid eye contact.

"So, you want me to find the history to help bring back some development

CHAPTER TWELVE – SCATTERED INFILTRATION

and imagination?" Jones said in his mind. "I will solve these problems as we get to them." The wind started up again blowing around him as the leaves pointed forward in a zigzag line. By reading through the tips of the leaves and the trash on the street Jones would know where to go next. Jones walked down the City of Walnut Creek streets turning the rest of the lights green. He sat on the corner of the pizza shop staring through the octagonal shape in the road. The yellow poles stuck out of the ground giving him a geometrical perspective on the world. Jones had all of the pieces of the theories he had been watching on T.V. working together in his realities. Feeling content with his newfound feelings and abilities he walked home preparing for tomorrow's journey. The next time Jones went out he would be trudging through the streets of the Iron Trail towards the school. Jones opened the door as his mom got on the phone. She locked herself in the bathroom calling upon friends for advice. Jones moved his head close to the room; he knew that without hiding he would get caught. His own family was ready to incite his insanity over to the very people Jones was trying to avoid. Jones quietly went into his room as bits and pieces of conversation flowed towards his ears.

"Yes Ms. P, yes when my son went through the same problem, we got him immediate therapy. Right away Ms. P, I understand." the voice on the other end of the phone said. His mom's voice and actions changed towards Jones that night. Jones knew, on this entire journey it wouldn't be over until he "Got the help he needed." Jones drifted off to sleep as he was too tired to continue using his mind. The next day would be filled with surprises, he thought. "I have to keep going." The next day came quickly. Jones looked up at the ceiling as Ottie texted him. "Yo! Let's go to the beach." the text read. After yesterday's experience, Jones' entire body felt completely drained. He slowly got out of bed lacking sleep from the night before. Feeling woozy, he went into the restroom to check himself. His mind was spinning with all of the ideas as he still felt on top of the world, but his body was not complying. His heart felt like it was giving out. He turned on the shower as the warm water went down his face, trying to slap himself awake to go meet Ottie. By now it didn't matter how much sleep he was getting, every day felt completely draining on his mind. "Okay." he texted Ottie.

Jones' mother turned silent and had gone out shopping. Her voice changed when around him and every time she saw him. She was trying to figure out what had happened to her son. Jones didn't want to get into more arguments. After wolfing down his food he began the process of heading for the door and getting in the car. But brushing his teeth even seemed like a hard task to accomplish as he forgot where he was putting items. "Keys?" he said to himself,"Check!" As soon as Jones patted his pocket, he realized he had forgotten his wallet on the nightstand. If it was one of the two items necessary, he had been missing the third, placing them down around the house and then leaving them behind. "I can't let my phone die," Jones said silently to himself thinking that the phone had been a big source of his power. So back into the house once more for the car charger.

Jones turned the car engine and the music up to full blast to keep himself awake. Bobbing his head back and forth he sped off down the road past the first stop sign. The entire road behind him left wheel marks deep in the gravel as the axel of the car bent. This time Jones drove as fast as he could towards Ottie, while not messing with people's will to try to let the world function at its own pace. Three hours later Jones showed up at Ottie's house in Monterey. This was the day the two wouldn't see one another again for a while. Jones knew it. He could feel Ottie's energy. "Hey, Jones!" Ottie waved, opening up the door. Jones waved back, "Hey Ottie!"

"Come inside," Ottie said welcomingly. Jones walked in holding the door open, "Yeah man, what's up. Let's go out and explore." Back inside, Ottie sat on the bed watching some T.V. as he went looking for some way to get hired. A laptop sat on his lap."How are you liking it down here?" Jones asked curiously. "Bro, I love it down here, my dude," Ottie replied quickly explaining the situation. "Let's go out to the beach for a walk, I'll show

CHAPTER TWELVE – SCATTERED INFILTRATION

you around." Jones didn't say much, "Alright." They went down to the beach where birds flew around. The wind blew harder as Jones and Ottie looked around tossing rocks across the sand. Upon the hillside, a sewer pipe protruded. It looked like it had been torn away from the land with time. Jones took a picture of the signboard that talked about 'Making fresh water'. "This could be useful for the world someday," Jones said to himself as he looked below the square wiring. Ottie sat on the cement wall staring out into the ocean. "So, I've been playing a lot of game cards lately," Ottie announced.

"Cards?" Jones asked. "So, how is the nightlife here? he said, questioning Ottie about his comment. "The nightlife is pretty fun, my guy. Let's go into town and get some coffee." Ottie replied. Jones and Ottie went into town as Jones thought back to the 'Making Fresh Water' instructions. "I bet a city lives down there under the sea," he said to himself. "But it's not a city I'd want to go to." The two of them walked to the Safeway. As Ottie ordered two coffees, Jones went over to a scruffy, beat down, homeless man who sat on the bench near the door they had entered. The scruffy man looked into Jones' eyes as he came over to him. Jones asked the homeless man, "Are you a billionaire?" The homeless man lost it and yelled at Jones. "I'm going to hit you!" Ottie looked over at the situation. It all happened fast and he got scared. Ottie grabbed the two coffees, "Dude, what are you doing? Let's go!" he warned Jones. "No, this man is important." Jones blinked his eyes twice again, completely sleep-deprived.

Ottie walked away outside after trying to calm the situation down. "Sorry about your friend." the homeless man said to Jones. "I had to scare him a little bit so we could speak privately." The old man winked at Jones as he went to sit back down."This town has a lot of aspects to it." the old man said. With that said, the old man got up and walked out the door. People nearby looked at the situation surveying what had happened as Jones went around the grocery store looking for Ottie. Eventually, Jones gave up walking towards the outside. Ottie was gone. A man with a hat walked through the parking lot! "Hey!" the man said. "Hi, there! "I haven't seen you in years!" Jones shouted to the man with a brown hat, a hat just like the ones that successful people had. Like the ones Jones had seen in all of the places, he had been. The man hugged him, "Oh it's so good to see you my friend!" he said. "What's your name in this day and age?" Jones asked out of curiosity.

"You can call me Anto by my earth name, but I am the Spirit of Music known to you, really a Blue Cargon from planet Garth. Don't worry, we are peaceful creatures" Anto surveyed the area. "Come with me I have a place to show you." The two of them walked back towards his apartment. Many kids were playing outside, throwing their toys up and down, and laughing together. An old lady with splotches over her face, who looked like she was disintegrating, waved over to Anto. He opened his door and invited Jones in. A piano sat in the corner of the kitchen. Everything was symmetrical, even the brightness over the shadows on the kitchen tiles. Jones's mouth fell open as he silently said 'wow' about this area of the house. They walked further into the apartment. "I've been watching you. Everything here is in perfect chi in my small room." Anto smiled. A single picture of an old red Jaguar car hung on the wall next to a single wooden table within an empty room that was crystal clear, cleaned beyond any normal floor that Jones had seen. Even the shadow in the corner of the room seemed to sparkle; as a peaceful but lonely feeling came over Jones like a wave. The shadows that were in the corner and the sun that shined through the window onto the floor were synced in perfection. Jones had been noticing this same symmetry before with doors that he had opened and closed during his previous travels with Ottie.

"Why does everyone who seems to make an impact wear these hats?" Jones inquired. Anto looked at Jones for a moment putting his hat onto the empty wall hook next to the picture of the Jaguar. The Spirit of Music laughed at Jones, "You see, life is interesting. Even though we watch over this world in silence and help others. Hats are kind of like an empty canvas.

CHAPTER TWELVE – SCATTERED INFILTRATION

The hat can be formed to be anything you want it to be." After a moment the man pulled out another hat of the same caliber off of his hat that he had hung up on the wall, "This hat is yours." Anto gave a brand-new brown hat of the same type he had to Jones. "Where did it come from?" Jones asked. He hadn't noticed it before hanging on the hook in the house next to the picture. Anto took his hat back off of the wall and put it on top of his head. He then adjusted the brim in various ways. After a few moments, he urged Jones to look at the ever-forming brown fedora hat that gave him various looks. "See? If we form it this way, the hat will do what we want it to. Things are created much the same way. This is why we wear the hat." Anto said. Jones smiled, "You know I've always wanted to see an orchestra playing within the stars."

The Spirit of Music's eyes lit up, "You really are a peculiar one." He got out a blank canvas, "I will paint. I will paint a piano in the sky in reality on this canvas. Maybe in our dreams, we will get to experience what you have again." Jones took the brown hat and put it on his head. "What do you look like?" Jones asked a serious question to the man. "Close your eyes and picture a blue octopus with nine tentacles and a saw for a mouth," he replied. Jones saw it in his mind as the Spirit of Music spoke away about the wonders of the world. "I'm glad you're peaceful creatures," Jones said as the Spirit of Music laughed at his joke. "Remember Jones, you must blend in with society or you will not be accepted," Anto warned. Jones walked back out of the small apartment. He waved goodbye to the man knowing he would see him again from time to time. Jones bent his hat up walking out in his coat as one of the kids walked up to him. "Hey mister, will you kick the ball for us?" the kid asked.

The woman who gardened with sheers smiled at him, as her face now looking almost dissolved, slowly clipped the grass. "A troll of some sort," Jones quietly said to himself. The Spirit of Music said into Jones's mind, "And our caretaker." With the kid still waiting, Jones replied, "I'm sorry I can't play ball, I have to go." Jones eyed the old steel toy with a magnet that made it spin around both sides going back and forth in the boy's hand. "But… you're bored with this thing, right?" Jones gestured to the boy. The kid gave the toy over to Jones, "If you throw it up like this." Jones demonstrated, "You can catch it. Then you don't even need me here to have fun." The kid smiled, "Hey thanks Mr.!" Jones patted the kid on the head who headed back to his friends playing ball. Jones walked back to find Ottie. "Woah, Dude! What are you wearing?" exclaimed Ottie, starting to freak out. "Can you drop me off at the Aztec Cards gaming cafe? Dude, that guy was crazy huh? You literally almost fought him." Jones turned towards Ottie, "I'm your guardian here man, just trying to guide you." Ottie scratched his head. "What? Whatever Dude, are you okay?" The two of them started driving, "Feeling better than most." Jones smiled.

Ottie quieted down but looked at Jones, "Seriously Dude, you're freaking me out." The two of them started driving towards The Cards, "Woah! Slow down, man!" Ottie shouted as Jones drove too fast for his liking. Jones pulled over to the curb and parked not wanting to argue. "Bro, the fuck is wrong with you?" Ottie said, shaking. Jones drove towards the Aztec Cards parking lot and got out of the car running in his slippers back and forth. "See? I'm your guardian!" Jones shouted at Ottie as he ran faster than usual. "I'm going to go get some smokes, dude. Fuck this. I'm going to go play cards. Just stay away from me for a while." Ottie got out of the car. He didn't come back. Night had fallen as Jones drove around. Seeing a bar lit up with street lights that flickered in rainbow colors and hearing loud laughter coming from a bar across the street, Jones knew to follow the music. Jones had his brown hat on and was dressed in his cashmere wool coat. He wandered into the bar as a man with a hat smoked an E-cigarette puffing out purple smoke. Many of the people were speaking French as the fire came out of the rocks that sat on top of the cement fire pit. The whole thing was surrounded in flames as Jones picked up one of the rocks. "Be careful or you might burn yourself." A man with a brown hat laughed at him.

CHAPTER TWELVE – SCATTERED INFILTRATION

He spoke French as a beautiful woman stood by his side. Jones picked up the rock as the fire almost seemed fake to him. Yet the fire was very much real. One of the rocks slightly singed his hand. "I Told you so. Extra hot, right?" the man stated. He looked like an old pilot from the movies, but he was young with a great mustache. "Welcome to the party — a paradise away from paradise." Jones smiled back laughing at the joke, "Alright, so what is this place really?" Jones asked. The man laughed, "Well we're linguists for the military. We're all practicing our French." This time Jones laughed, "I see." he said knowing now where he was as he threw the rock back into the fire. Another man sat on the bench dressed in all black as live music played in the background. Jones had never seen three drums fully electrical with one guitar before. The men started playing as Jones got up to dance in the front. The rest of the people followed him as if to understand that he was heading the galactic missions, changing the world as he went along. Here Jones felt free, away from responsibilities as he didn't feel the need to hide from the public eye. Jones could be himself. Parties went all up and down the block as people stormed in different bars within the lit-up street. Technology that he hadn't seen before ran around the block as everyone stayed extremely clean. Drinking didn't seem to be a big deal around the town, and drugs were not apparent in the life around here.

"Shirts must say what people represent around here." Jones thought to himself as two heads turned to hear what he said. He forgot for a moment that the galaxy could hear his mind. A car drove by as he ran in his flip-flops as fast as he could almost keeping up with the car that passed by. He shouted 'wait' to try to get some answers, yet the car filled with people didn't stop. "I've never seen such a place," Jones said to himself, huffing after his run. He turned around. A woman with bright red hair and a man dressed as a Pope holding a staff stood outside, his clothing embroidered with gold on pure white cloth. Within the embroidery, a symbol swirled up and around as the circle in the middle met in symmetry. An ancient symbol was written completely connected through the clothing he wore.

"It's thanksgiving, not a costume party," Jones said quietly to himself. "Hi, who are you?" the lady asked Jones as she smiled. She had red hair and a voice that spoke softly, almost as if the words of kindness fell across Jones. The man had a stern look on his face.

"I'm Father Time. If you'll excuse me, we must get going. I'm sorry we cannot talk more. You will not see me again." he said gruffly to Jones. Jones wanted to ask more questions. As soon as he had turned, he turned around again and the two of them were completely gone. No car, no walking. Jones searched for them inside but found nothing. Jones realized it was getting late. He went back inside the bar that had now mostly cleared out sitting across the bench line where the rocks were once on fire. The cold slowly went through the open roof. "Hey kid, I saw what you were doing. If you need any help around here, feel free to ask." a man with a scar on his face said who sat next to him in a black shirt. Jones shook his hand. He felt no fear against people anymore. Jones felt disconnected from the 'old world' and felt comfortable exploring his newfound homes. After a quick conversation, he left to go back to his car. He drove down towards the gas station as many new items he had never seen before hid inside of it. He wanted to explore them. "Share the road, Jones. Whatever you take from here will be created and promoted tomorrow. Each idea is made by someone. It's up to you to create and lead us." the Spirit of Music's voice echoed in Jones' head.

"You know, how come there's never any chicken sausage combined?" Jones asked a man who was picking out his food at the gas station. The man mumbled back to Jones, "Hey that's a great idea." Staring over at Jones, the cashier behind the register smiled and waved. Jones picked out dome gum that he had never seen before. "Interesting, but good choice." the Spirit of Music echoed through his head. Jones smiled as he finished filling his tank of gas. While getting on the road back towards home, his phone on the Waze app said 'searching'. As he drove forward though, the GPS had already found his home. "I heard you were having CIA troubles so I

CHAPTER TWELVE – SCATTERED INFILTRATION

disconnected you. Now you won't have to worry about them for a while when going places using your powers." Nepharius' voice this time reached Jones. "As promised, the trail, right?" The voice flowed through his mind as Jones drove on his way home speedin back through the fog as not a single car passed by on the road. Almost as if the galaxy knew he had to get home at a semi-reasonable hour. Jones got home in half the time it usually took to get to the general area.

Jones walked in the front door as his mother sat in her office as if she was researching what could be his issue. Jones went into his room hiding the brown hat in the closet as he hung his coat up to dry. Now that he had his cane and hat, he was ready to start across the major journey. All Jones needed to do now was to create the universal car. He looked up at the poster where a Jeep was located at the top right of his room. "Yeah, it has to be yellow like before, run on music, and have a happy exterior. A Jeep carries four people with an open free roof." Jones thought about it to himself. "It also needs to have a bright leather interior with pilot dials in the front." he smiled as he pictured it in his mind. "I've got to find the people who can make this happen." Jones lies on his bed slowly drifting off to sleep. He knew where to go with a mission, but had no idea what would happen next. The next day as Jones woke up, his mother came into his room.

"Jones, you need help. I'm taking you to a therapist." his mother went towards the phone to make the call. Jones quickly put on his clothes and went towards the front door. "I'm going out. I don't need a therapist! Don't tell me I'm crazy because I have ideas I want to try! he shouted at her, slamming the door behind him. The door shut as the leaves from the wind landed on the ground. Each leaf pointed towards the next one in a shape as the wind blew the direction in which Jones should walk. Jones went out towards the hillside that he and Ottie had skateboarded. The car marks from Jones' previous drive to Monterey Bay still showed in the road. Gravel sat around the two tire slots. Jones realized that his actions of speeding in the world had to go somewhere. The slots were a representation of that. He started jogging as a neighborly woman jogged with him, however, he got tired after a short moment because of his lack of sleep. He ordered himself an Uber ride down to the old Veterans Center Hall out of curiosity, hoping for the continued solitude that it might provide him. Jones walked into the front entrance of the Veterans Center where a worker sat. The place was filled with old pictures of successful war veterans.

"What are you doing here?" the younger woman asked him. "Oh, I was curious about this place. What do you do here?" Jones asked curiously. She had a bright smile and friendly energy. Instead of kicking Jones out, she let him in. "We do catered events and sometimes Bingo Night for Old War Veterans." she proudly said. Jones smiled back as he looked across the room. A bar sat in the back as three Old War Veterans sat around the table telling their stories. The lady turned around, "Alright, you have to leave soon as there's work to be done." "How do you stay so fit and look so young?" Jones asked the lady. She laughed, "Lots of creams and not eating meat has helped me throughout the years. And I suppose good genetics too." Jones smiled as he explored the inside more — nice leather chairs along with a marble floor complemented the outside hallway with a large floor-to-ceiling glass window view. The long hallway leads into meeting rooms each with double wooden doors intricately designed. Two glass doors led outside back into the parking lot where Jones had walked from. As Jones exited the building three strange men sat out by a yellow car.

These strange men were all wearing felt brown hats as a yellow Jeep sat in the parking lot. Two of the men did not have a clipboard with pen and paper to write down what they were doing; nothing in fact except for their bodies moving around the car as if they were fixing and building it. The much older gentleman stood on the side smiling, with a cane, as blue veins popped out of his face. He was well beyond the normal age you would see. "What's going on out here?" Jones asked the group. The older gentleman

CHAPTER TWELVE – SCATTERED INFILTRATION

turned towards Jones, almost surprised that Jones could see them. The older gentleman stood there as his two men walked around the yellow Jeep going over every area and possibility, memorizing every detail. "Why am I helping build this car?" the older gentleman said. "Can I go for a ride in it when it's finished?" Jones asked curiously. He walked over to take a closer look. Inside the Jeep on the dashboard were pilot's dials outlined in beige from the first generation of airplanes.

"You know, one day if the spare tire just came off and could latch onto the wheels automatically instead of manually replacing it, that would be awesome," Jones said to the older gentleman. After chuckling, the older gentleman put his finger up to his mouth to shush Jones. "Watch them. You might learn something," he said to Jones with his eyes smiling. "After these two are done looking at the car maybe you may have a ride." Jones sat in the parking lot watching the strange men add their designs through some mysterious method. Eventually, Jones felt too startled, "I'm going to go now, there's more work to be done." Jones took a step back rejecting the offer to ride in the car. His dream felt too real, too soon. The older gentleman called out, "Be safe out there!" as Jones had already left the Veterans Center Hall rear parking lot. Jones had experienced something special but didn't know what. He felt he should have gone in that car, yet he didn't. Jones walked further into town where people started to notice him. He was thirsty after walking and his mind was working too fast. As he walked down the street, he started putting ideas into his phone. For each idea, he would think of every pro and con to every possibility: 'Farts that don't smell would be funny.'; 'Futuristic lamp posts that illuminate blue light instead of white lights.'; and 'Music in the concrete where you can step on every block, everywhere instead of just steps that light up in different colors as a person stepped on each square.' "Alright, that's enough for the moment," Jones said to himself.

Jones ran off further from his house towards BART as his mom texted him. "Jones, we have an appointment set for tomorrow. Where are you?"

Ms. P texted. Jones ignored the text message as he heard the BART train come closer to him. Feeling caged in by the small town, he went off to the station. Jones walked up from the backside stairs to the station entrance. As he barely had enough cash to get him on the train, the ticket machine gave him a one-way trip. The crowd sat silently on the BART train like a man with tattoos, wearing a giant felt hat, sitting in the very back of the car. His family sat in the back too watching Jones as he practiced gymnastics from bar to bar. People watched him silently as one woman stood up. "You know this is BART, right?" the woman said to Jones. Jones replied sarcastically, "Yeah, no one cares right?" Jones looked at the man in the back who laughed, "Do your thing. No one cares." he said. The woman got off at the next BART stop scowling at Jones.

Jones had a free day. There were no club events that he was aware of. It dawned on him that he hadn't checked his emails in a while so he pulled out his iPhone. "We're traveling next to the tropical islands! By now superstar, you should be able to come here." Nepharius sent in a text message. "Remember that movie? It's about time. I hope you've been practicing with the music, movie, and stuff I've been telling you about." Jones complained, texting back, "I need more time! I haven't even walked the trail yet." Nepharius replied, "You already know!" All of the interactions happened in a flash as Jones closed his eyes testing out the dance steps on BART — practicing and singing the song he had in his headphones. "Hey, I know that song. Keep practicing!" encouragement was shouted out from one of the Watchers on the BART train. Feeling tired, Jones finally sat down after spinning. Using his hands in an infinity sign as if to say he understood the Galactic language, he stopped. The BART also stopped, not moving along over the normal allotted time.

Jones got off the BART in San Francisco and strolled The Embarcadero on a sunny day looking for places to train himself further. Jones arrived at Pier 39 where he noticed cement blocks spaced evenly across the pedestrian entryway. He realized that this would be a perfect place to train where

CHAPTER TWELVE – SCATTERED INFILTRATION

he could jump across each cement block. Jones looked out across the San Francisco Bay, seeing the waves lightly wash up against the metal bar that separated the sea and the pathway. A newscaster sat out there as Jones went over to a man suntanning on his back dressed in many different colors. "What's going on here?" Jones asked the man suntanning as he eyeballed one of the sculptures that he had never noticed before showing how DNA connected. The Double Helix sculpture had a button that said 'press me', but it was seemingly unresponsive to the touch. "Well apparently someone got shot. A woman, I think. She was with her grandfather." the man said.

Jones stopped jumping over from cement block to cement block as the lights from the newscaster's set lit up. "Hey kid, you've gotta move soon." the newscaster said politely. Jones leaped over the metal railing bar that prevented people from falling into the Bay from the Pier but failed, falling backward on his butt in between the walkway and the cement block. The crowd that was watching him jump said "Ow!" in concern. Feeling his phone buzz in his pocket, Jones loaded up his iPhone and started watching BMX bikers ride their bikes on that very same slim bar, almost as if challenging him. "Can our hero do it?" the text read. But Jones needed more practice. Feeling that too many people were watching him, Jones stopped. The newscaster standing nearby said, "Wear a helmet! You should practice somewhere safer." Feeling concerned now, Jones looked up at the man as he reached down to help Jones. "Need a hand?" the newscaster asked. Jones took the newscaster's hand as he got helped to his feet. "Don't you want to comment on this important matter?" the newscaster asked Jones.

Jones shook his head no, afraid to be on T.V. "No, it's a tragedy and we really should be safer." was the only reply Jones said before the T.V. newscast started. Jones went towards the dock where he practiced the same moves again, this time stepping on a spinning chair and jumping to the next chair. He stopped to notice the clouds around him. San Francisco had become his playground. He would prove that there were secrets hidden away to the people in the city and that ideas could be formed off what existed. Jones thought to himself for a moment, "The Exploratorium. That is where I should go next." The place had changed a lot since he last went inside, with the building now glowing from LED lights from the outside, and as sculptures lay inside the building grounds within a plaza. Jones realized that the Exploratorium was a breeding ground for knowledge, each sign representing ways in which humanity used to matter to develop the technology. Outside of the Exploratorium on the side of the building, Jones saw a steel plate painted green with scripture that could be read. Each symbol seems to mean something from ancient times with no description.

Behind the building, an SS Coast Guard ship appeared in view, docked up against the corner pier. Jones closed his eyes as a bird came into his mind, showing him the way to more knowledge. "I'll call him Bird, bird my guide," Jones said to himself. Back towards the pier, a photographer was taking pictures of the birds. A water bottle, half-drunk, lies over on a green table further away. "I'm telling you, sir, we're all technically gods. We're all creators." Jones said to the photographer. The old man shook his head. "Look, I'll get water in under five seconds." Jones boasted. The man smiled, "Prove it." he said. Jones ran to the table out of sight and came right back, "See? It's even still good to drink." Jones drank it right in front of the man. "I suppose so." the man said with a gruff voice as he went back to filming the birds. Jones decided that he would get more information at night, after all the ship was right there, right behind the Exploratorium. However, what most interested Jones was the steel plate painted green with the etched scripture that he saw earlier on the side of the Exploratorium building.

Jones started to walk towards the SS Coast Guard ship down the alleyway. A second green metal plate with an etched scripture came into view, also behind the Exploratorium. Jones studied the moons and the triangles on the two etched green steel plates. There was no explanatory sign. He

CHAPTER TWELVE – SCATTERED INFILTRATION

assumed that the scripture must say something important; and that it was built by someone who knew the ancient language. As the sun slowly went down, Jones went back to the main entrance of the Exploratorium next to the dock. The clock struck 7:00 PM as he walked over to the sculptures in the plaza outside.

The wind picked up, blowing a water bottle and a napkin next to the fence across the way. Jones saw the wind roll the water bottle as the trash pointed towards the green gate saying to go that way. The wind kept blowing the napkin in a pattern suggesting Jones look around him. Jones went over to the stone sculpture in the ground lit with LED lights and stood on top of it. A car drove past him as he concentrated on standing on one foot on the top point of the stone sculpture. "Kamehameha!" someone in the car shouted laughing as it passed by. Jones lost his concentration for a moment and fell on the sculpture face first. Without a scratch, he got up and balanced again gathering his focus. The bird appeared in his mind flying across the ocean again. Jones opened his eyes. He walked over towards the green steel plate with etched symbols as a man dressed in all black made a call on the phone nearby. The man had black shoes on and did not want to be seen. Jones followed the man towards the SS Coast Guard ship which was moored at the dock. A chain blocked the entryway of the walkway to the ship at the pier. There was another chain at the ship with a simple sign saying 'Do Not Board' blocking off civilians from coming aboard.

Jones went under the chain, up the walkway, and onto the SS Coast Guard ship. Jones went towards the first door. As he was opening it up to enter, a scientist he hadn't seen before stood on deck outside the door. Jones went inside and down the hatch ladder to were a cook in the Coast Guard was making food on the ship. "Hey, you the new recruit?" the cook asked Jones, smiling, offering warmth. Jones hadn't said anything yet as he climbed down the ladder from the hatch. "You don't talk much, huh?" the cook continued. Jones replied nicely, "Well, why a cook?" asking out of curiosity. The cook laughed, "Food for the crew. Of course!" The cook grew curious, "So what placement are you from?" Jones knew he was in trouble, "I'm lost actually." The cook, now alerted, walked up to him, "You need to get off this ship now!" noticing that Jones didn't have any Coast Guard uniform clothing on. Nepharius's voice rang through his mind, "Tell him Retragrammatron and special agent." The Coast Guard cook took a step back as Jones repeated these words aloud. "Alright, I'll walk you off the ship politely. Don't come back here without clearance!" The Coast Guard cook escorted Jones to the deck. The scientist he had never met before held his thumb up to Jones. "He's part of the crew!" the scientist said, trying to save Jones to keep him aboard. The Coast Guard cook replied in return, "He already told the truth that he's not." Jones walked off the ship towards the dock where an Exploratorium security guard met with him. "What are you doing here?" asked the security guard, hinting at a possible arrest. Jones simply replied, "Looking for the world's experts." As Jones walked politely with the security guard Jones asked him, "Do you believe in the vibration of sound?"

The security guard laughed, "That's how I know you're telling the truth. We're walking at the same speed. Don't let us catch you back here. Get authorized." Jones slowly walked away looking back towards the place. "I suppose that's a mystery for another time." he thought to himself. He walked towards the BART as his phone showed a low battery. Feeling hungry he saw a grocery truck unloading strawberries and an assortment of other fruit. "Hey, may I have one? I'm really hungry!" Jones shouted. The delivery man looked up for a moment, "Yeah, here." The man handed Jones three bananas out of a crate that had been opened. Jones walked along looking for people who were heading to the BART too as he had lost his way. Two men started talking nearby so Jones stopped to ask for directions, "Hey, guys want a banana?" Jones offered as he ate another one himself. One of the men took the last banana and thanked him, "Yeah! We'll see you around!" Into the distance, the men faded as Jones continued towards BART. After a few minutes of wandering around Jones heard all

CHAPTER TWELVE – SCATTERED INFILTRATION

of the lights going off, sounding like machine guns firing from far away. Jones couldn't take the sound around him anymore. He finally reached the BART entry and went down the escalator. "Hey! You're the guy who gave us the banana." the two men laughed, already on the BART platform. "Simply trying to get home for today," Jones said, laughing back.

Jones sat down on the BART train and slowly relaxed his mind. The events that took place in succession had worn him out completely. He realized he didn't have enough money on his ticket to get off BART at his stop. As the train arrived, Jones got off and exited going down towards the fence. Four boys stood outside of the BART station dressed as if they were from the past in 1980's jackets. They were giving money to one of their friends. "Hey, you don't have enough to get off BART, huh?" one of the boys said looking at Jones. Jones shook his head 'No'. "Here you go." said the boy handing Jones some coins. The change still had not been enough, but Jones thanked the four boys anyway. The female station agent at the BART Exit looked at the situation when Jones tried to exit with the insufficient fare on his ticket.

"Just go through the door," she said pointing towards it. "It's fine." Jones hesitated, "I guess it's those galaxy discounts and karma." he said to himself. As the BART gate shut behind him, there were taxis waiting curbside ready to take paying customers. An old man with glasses sat in the first car, filled with snacks among other things.

"Hop on in," he said to Jones. Jones explained the situation as the man started up the taxi. "It's alright. Just put it on the IOU. $10." he said smiling. "What's your story, sir?" Jones asked curiously. Jones could feel the energy. The man had some true history. "Well, I'm an old War Veteran." he smiled at Jones in the rearview mirror as he cleaned his glasses. "Just biding my time doing this job." Jones pictured a ship painted on the water as the man described his journeys. When they arrived at this house, the driver also showed him various pictures on his phone. "Alright, we're here. Good night." said the driver. Jones thanked the man and walked slowly towards the door. The City and his adventures were more than what he was ready for. As Jones waddled into the house feeling completely drained, his mother took one look at Jones and continued to stare at him. "Where have you been?" she queried with alarm.

Jones looked around for a moment before answering, "For a walk in the City." Jones was really testing out theories he saw on YouTube and trying to locate experts in the world of his own reality. Ms. P., Jones' mom, backed off a little, "Tomorrow, don't go anywhere far, please. We have an appointment at 3:00 PM." Jones replied, "Okay, mom." then turned to enter his bedroom and collapsed on his bed. Shortly after this, Mira came into Jones' mind, "Told you. If you meddle too much here, the CIA will come after you." Mira said in a sad tone. "Now they've been notified. You'll be going to therapy. Jones, if this continues any further you may be locked away for a very long time." Jones shook his head 'No'. There was still so much more to do and explore. He floated, contemplating the next move as Mira sat there from across the table. "What's your plan, Jones?" Mira asked. Jones contemplated the question for a moment, "The world just has to see Mira, see that this world exists."

Jones floated calmly as the table disappeared. "Good luck," Mira said, "I've got a Nepharius to catch." Jones' dream disappeared into the night as worries filled his head. The feeling of being lost in between life on Earth and his universal world that connected the two planes of space hit him as hard as the realities of tomorrow would.

Chapter Thirteen – Therapeutic Judgment

The next day Jones woke up. The sun was shining brightly on his window. There didn't seem to be a rain cloud in sight. Jones's mother looked at him from the kitchen. "Today you will be seeing a therapist named Ms. Orin." she reminded him. Jones didn't object as he got out of bed. "Okay," he replied. "I'll beat them at their own game." Jones thought to himself. Therapy for people like Jones sounded more like a prison to lock away those who had imagination and ideas. "We're going at 3:00 PM today so this time don't go anywhere." Ms. P. said, a bit more sternly. Jones nodded in agreement as he picked up the cane and went out to the backyard. Jones angled himself at the very back of the pool in direct line of sight to the sun. As all of the triangles connected towards the wooden post in the backyard, he followed the triangle that his hands made as if he were looking through binoculars. Jones looked down at the pool as little droplets sat at the bottom. Among those little droplets, the sun's shadow also hit the other side of the pool. He stared at the sun holding up his cane almost as if he was moving the actual sun as the shadows followed Jones's movements. The entire world went red in his vision. After trying a few times, he gave up on the idea for the moment that his ability to move things through the connection of shadows might be plausible. He followed the same patterns among the wind towards the back of the yard by the family boat.

A wooden post stood alone as Jones climbed it to try to look out while balancing atop the post. The post broke and Jones fell taking no damage.Realizing that the physical capabilities of his travels were limited, Jones retired back indoors. The clock almost struck 3:00 PM. "It's time to go." his mother said, calling him into her car. "Okay, but can you at least roll down the windows? I don't feel so good." Jones asked. His mom did so as they started their drive. Jones stuck his hand out the window making a wave almost as if to follow the wind through the windows. His mom closed the sunroof and windows as the car neared the freeway. "Open the window," Jones asked politely. His mother retorted, "No, we are on the freeway." Ms. P. then locked the doors afraid that Jones might try to open them. "Can we at least listen to music?" Jones asked as his senses went wild. She didn't comment, feeling annoyed at Jones's antics, "No, not right now." she said. Once in the parking garage, Jones blurted out, "Turn here." As he had felt the wind previously, Jones sensed a parking space open in the garage.

"See I told you," Jones said as his mother looked at him in awe for a moment. Every other parking space was taken beside one open spot, so Jones informed her accordingly. "Okay, we need to cross here." Ms. P. said, pointing towards the road as two red cars on either side of them stood stationary. "Here?" Jones asked as he darted straight across the road without looking. "Watch where you're crossing!" Ms. P. shouted as she chased behind him across the street. Jones could feel the energy of the world around him. He didn't feel the need to look 'both ways' as on pure belief alone, he felt separated from the Earth plane. In Jones's mind, nothing could touch him besides his own allowance of damage to his world. "Damnit, Jones!! I told you to wait!" Ms. P. stated angrily when she caught up to Jones. She was getting frustrated and scared of his antics. Jones waited near the elevator that led up the building. "In here?" Jones questioned. She answered, "Yes, let's get you checked in for your appointment. If you keep acting like this, they will put you away. And for good! I'm trying to keep you out." his mom warned. Jones coughed,

CHAPTER THIRTEEN – THERAPEUTIC JUDGMENT

"Well…"

Jones didn't have much to say as they rode up the elevator to the third floor of the building. He walked out of the elevator past a water fountain where people waited in line to check in. "Next please." the woman said from behind the desk, almost as if every person in line was a customer rather than a patient in need. Jones went up to the counter as the lady eyeballed him. "Fill this sheet out." she sighed as Jones took it and went to go sit down. Basic questions like, 'Do you feel like harming yourself or anyone else?' Appeared on the sheet with scaled numbers below each question. A man sat next to Jones ranting about a magazine and how the person on the cover had become fat. He angrily sat by like a tinder box ready to explode. Jones wanted nothing more than to get out of the place, even though it was supposed to be comforting. He felt trapped as if the world had been closing in on him. "I need some water and to go to the restroom," complained as he finished the sheet, handing it to his mom. Ms. P. looked over at him reaching for the clipboard with the completed questionnaire, "Alright, be quick. Don't forget your meeting."

Jones walked towards the restroom reading the exit signs of the building. From not being able to focus, layouts of buildings were becoming crystal clear lately. He bent over to taste some water as one of the doctors walked by smiling. Jones didn't make eye contact. "Alright, Ms. Orin is ready for you." the Check-In lady said as Jones walked back into the waiting area, calming his nerves. Jones had put on his iPod headphones to block out the sound, helping him focus as the rest of the building echoed with noise. The violin music kept him sane as he could hear the emotion serenely playing through the headphones. Jones walked down the hallway to where the cherry wood door opened. A little dolphin sat on the right side where Ms. Orin's office was located. "Good to meet you. How are you doing?" Ms. Orin said with a slight smile. Jones, not knowing what to say, looked straight back at her, studying her every move. "You'll be seeing a doctor in a bit, but I'm here to get to know you." Ms. Orin continued trying to make conversation. Jones thought for a moment about his past, "I feel like I don't fit in lately." he said. Orin replied, "Why not?"

Jones said in reply, "The world seems so bland lately. I want to do something new. I want to work. I feel far behind." Jones began talking. He figured that at least this way maybe he could stay out of trouble with them. He knew this was his prison, yet the other world was calling. After a few minutes of conversation, she typed some words into her computer. "Okay, it's time for you to see Doctor K.," Ms. Orin said, directing him down the hallway. Jones walked with his hat pulled further down, seeing a room setup with chairs in a circle where people were already gathered. He had yet to be indoctrinated into these "appointments." Doctor K. looked at Jones and the notes in his system. "Based on the notes, take this and this." Doctor K. handed Jones two bottles of pills and a starter dose of one pill each. Jones didn't want to. He took the bag but would refuse to take the yellow pill he held in his hand. "So, what do people believe when they come in here anyway?" Jones asked Doctor K., trying not to cause trouble while trying to satisfy his curiosity. Doctor K. looked at Jones, "Some people believe they are being chased by the CIA, some people believe they are angels, vampires, or take on different personas. Most of them get influenced by the books they read." Jones thought about it for a moment, "Why?" he asked.

The doctor looked at him for a moment. He grew curious of Jones, noting that none of his patients asked him these questions before. "You're a peculiar guy, aren't you? Asking why leads you down the pathways you want to go." Doctor K. said kindly. Jones replied, "Do you like music?" Doctor K. looked back at Jones, "My grandfather used to work with Elvis back in the day." Jones lit up. At least this deciding factor in his life had a joy for music. "I see. Wow! Really cool!" Jones replied. "Alright, come back in a few days." Doctor K. said, watching over him from afar. Jones took the bag of medication but wasn't going to take the pills prescribed. His mother escorted him back to the car where Jones explained the wind to

CHAPTER THIRTEEN – THERAPEUTIC JUDGMENT

her. He didn't say a word to Ms. P. about his visits with Ms. Orin, the therapist, or Doctor K., the psychiatrist. "I used to sail too, Jones." Ms. P. chatted brightly. "Sometimes you have to walk against the headwinds and stay out of the shadows too. Just because you walk in the shadows doesn't mean you're hidden from plain sight. There are two sides to everything."

She scolded Jones as people walked off to the edge of the sidewalk into the shadows as they neared them. Jones instinctively knew where to go based on the 'perfect balance' that had been running through his mind. "The police called by the way. Your court date for paying off that ticket you and Ottie got is coming up. We have to attend Superior Court in a couple of weeks." Ms. P. stated in a matter-of-fact tone. Jones had forgotten about that incident in all the craziness of his journeys. He nodded his head 'yes' slightly as red cars suddenly filled the space stopping Jones from walking across certain lines. Jones got in the car as his mother drove him towards home. However, he didn't want to stay indoors. As soon as he was back inside the house, he walked outside the back door. The geometrical theory he saw on YouTube was at play. Each leaf pointed towards a hand-crafted bird 'mailbox' with an owl emblem on it. "I guess 'pros' get their mail this way," Jones said to himself. Jones walked towards the Iron Trail which took him back behind the trees. An old man walked on the trail alone with yellow teeth and a hat. Sir, I'm sort of documenting my journeys. Can I film you?" Jones inquired.

The man said, 'No." politely, but cackled, "Yeah, I know who you are talking about. That man's ideas were stolen. He's building a machine for the other guy." The old man stood under an oak tree and continued, "You though, kid, you're like a black hole. You absorb information and spit it back out." The old man laughed as he walked away. The oak tree that he had been standing near lay dying from poison. A golf ball from the golf course rested right by the base of the oak tree. Jones looked behind him as the old man was completely gone from sight a few minutes after he had passed by him. No one else stood on the sidewalk; no one was around. Following the direction of the leaves and wind, they pointed Jones towards town. Jones, walking in his slippers, began following more of the Iron Trail that Nepharius had pointed out to him. Jones spotted a Valkyrie symbol holding a place of honor down the street next to a large hospital. Jones was to talk about Retragrammatron to the experts, soliciting sales in a way, regarding the movies and concerts that would be in great need of the experts' skill sets. Jones had started his walk with his sweater on. After feeling tired he stopped to rest along a wall near a warning sign that read 'Do not stand here. You may get shocked.' Jones stood on top of the wall feeling the energy going through his body. His slippers had not melted by the electricity. Jones was ready to move again, charged by the generator below him. When Jones was rested and ready to move again, he dashed off down the street, veering off left to explore houses that seemed to have antiques and artifacts inside of them. Stress seemed not to be welcomed in the neighborhood.

Jones peered inside the window of one home of interest where he saw a woman quietly reading a book in detail, almost as if to do research. She seemed to not notice him as he slowly crept around the corner of the house and through the side gate where the screen door was open. But Jones stepped on a twig and it cracked loudly. The lady looked up from her reading, "Hey!" she shouted as her pupils dilated. Jones ran out of the gate and through the street looking for an escape before she could alert her neighbors. Jones walked further into the neighborhood where another trailhead began. An Army Base was off to the left as trash from the reservoir dam pointed him forward through two cones. The wind blew again telling him to look up. The address Nepharius sent to Jones appeared on his phone as he neared the school. A text message also appeared, "Remember to go to the cross street, the house by the lemon trees". Looking up Jones continued walking through the school campus with the wind directing him where to go. Children sat on the outdoor benches, tables, and sidelines as teachers were instructing an outdoor class. "That's a beautiful turtle." the teacher said to one kid as another kid walked

CHAPTER THIRTEEN – THERAPEUTIC JUDGMENT

by them. The second kid started punching the turtle. "Yeah! You get that turtle." the teacher egged them on.

"What is this school?" Jones asked out of curiosity, as it was hidden behind the Army Base. "This is a place where we teach kids who are a bit special." the teacher smiled. Jones walked on the property going over to where two older teachers sat, "Mind if I watch?" he asked politely. The teacher working with the boys and the turtle walked over to Jones and asked him politely, "Why are you here?" Jones replied, "I am interested in the mysteries behind places like this." The man laughed as another woman came over. "This woman is a mystery. She swam across the ocean as far as the eye can see." the teacher said, smiling. Jones could see their eye pupils pulsating on their stress levels. He had uncovered a welcoming place, but a place where he shouldn't return. "I heard you walked pretty far. That's impressive. Come on back soon and we'll have a chat." the teacher continued with a welcoming tone. "If you'll excuse me now, I have to teach dance to some of these youngsters." The teachers went back to doing their routine class sessions as Jones left the campus. He thought about the address Nepharius had given him and his encounter with the old man on the Iron Trail. "A black hole, huh? Thought I was an Arbiter." Jones said to himself curiously.

Jones retraced his steps back through the neighborhood towards the address and cross street given, looking for the house with the lemon trees. A lady was standing out front. "Why are you here?" she asked. Jones said, "Retragrammatron. It comes from Tetra-." The lady cut him off, "Never return here again!" she warned Jones. Jones realized he had failed his first mission. As he wandered down the road seven policemen showed up. Jones sat on a log. "Sir, we heard you were soliciting here, knocking on doors. Do you have a permit?" the policeman asked. Jones shook his head 'No'. The policeman looked him in the eye after hearing a call over his radio,

"Do you have any weapons on you? Any of the sort?" he asked. Jones shook his head 'No' again. "I was simply trying to get the word out there, is all," he replied. The policeman looked towards his comrades, baffled at the simplistic replies. "I'm a trusted policeman. Leave here and don't come back. No soliciting without a permit. Consider this a warning." he warned Jones. Jones walked off out of the neighborhood as the policemen got in their cars and left.

He wandered back towards the Iron Trail walking to his house. By now his feet were dirty and covered with blisters. However, as he got in the shower, he noticed that his feet would heal at a pace more quickly than natural. He took out his phone to film himself but to no avail. He didn't catch anything. After he got out of the shower, he put on some music trying to relax. Nepharius called him, "Are you training Jones? I've just interviewed the man who climbed Mount Everest in his shorts. You should learn these types of things." Jones replied, "How's the movie coming along?" Nepharius laughed, "Good. I'm teaching them all sorts of things. It's going to be great. You already know what to do." Exhausted, Jones passed out on his bed. What did time truly mean in his world at this point? He felt lost. Drifting through his dream state, the three men he saw building the yellow car appeared. "Hop in." one of the men smiled as Jones got in the yellow jeep. Music played in the background as he flew through the galaxy almost as if the flying car was prepared for space travel.

"You have to learn to blend in better with society." one of the men suggested laughing. "We're watching over you." the other one said. "You have a lot to accomplish yet." Jones woke up and saw it was already morning. He felt as if time skipped through to the next day. He went over to start brushing his teeth and get ready for the day. This time Jones took a normal hot shower trying to recuperate his mind as yesterday's actions had taken him on a long journey. Jones put on his brown felt hat and a T-shirt that said 'dangerous'. "This will get the message across today," Jones said to himself. "I'll go out again!" he said aloud, checking outside. His mother interjected, "Try not to stay out too late. Where are you going?" Ms. P. questioned

CHAPTER THIRTEEN – THERAPEUTIC JUDGMENT

him. "To San Francisco," Jones said in return, being direct with her. He went out the door as she sighed. Jones started walking down the street as a bright red tree stood out vibrantly against the green lawn. Nature felt like a whole new world as he walked past the animals that stopped to stare at him. "Okay," he said to himself as he started jogging to town where the Veterans Center is located. A woman jogged up beside him from behind. "Let's jog together!" Jones offered not realizing how out of shape he had become. The lady slowed to jog along with him, "Really? You want to jog with me?" She talked for a bit, but Jones's lungs gave out and he stopped after a short while.

"I'm sorry. I can't. I'm a bit too out of shape." Jones lied as he huffed.

She laughed, "No problem. Where are you headed? Want me to call an Uber for you?" Jones shook his head 'No' and started walking forward. After a few minutes of solitude, the yellow car drove past him with the same three men again. "Wait!" Jones shouted, "I'd like to go for a ride!" The men turned around and smiled, "Not yet Jones!" As they drove off into the distance waving their brown hats. Jones kept walking towards the BART listening to music to keep himself focused on the task. He needed to Add Fare at the station, paying money before getting on the train. This time Jones did not make any special training movements and sat quietly on the train contemplating the possibilities of what he could find hidden away in the city. San Francisco was a plethora of historic information written on the walls within each sculpture or building. Even the chairs were given donation names to be explored.

After a while, Jones got off of BART as the red sensors lit up for him again if he had gone too far. The people of the galaxy were guiding him again. He got off to walk towards the first sculpture that intrigued him. A giant bow shooting towards the sky, placed in the middle of the parking area on the Embarcadero. Clouds seemed to follow the same pattern as Jones walked through the city following the slight wind that went by. A French man with his class was practicing interpretive dance similar to the way

Jones had. "Would you like to give it a try?" the teacher offered. Jones shook his head, "Thanks, I'm better off watching." The people followed each of the instructor's steps on the grass as Jones waited. He had grown more interested in the city's history. Jones walked through the giant clock tower where information was written on the floor about the building. "I bet there's some deep-rooted secret here," Jones mumbled to himself. After getting a coffee, Jones sang some old-time songs to himself, practicing his skill sets. He walked further towards a closed-down mall.

Scriptures were written on the mid level as a sign read, 'Closed Due to Drought'. Jones thought, "The rain masters aren't here right now." Jones walked on. He saw a pyramid sculpture, brightly painted with bluefish swimming up towards the top point of the pyramid crowned with a gold star. The ceramic sculpture sat nicely in the middle of the square near the San Francisco CIA building. As Jones walked up to the sculpture, he saw a kid with his father playing catch. Jones stopped to read the sculpture sign scripture. It was suggesting that if he could run up the sculpture to the uppermost point, Jones would be able to make it rain. He would be able to move the clouds in front of the sun. The air temperature would drop allowing the rain to be released from the clouds. "Well California does need rain," he said to himself, smiling at the thought. Jones ran around the oblong statue gathering speed intending to run up the side to the top as the kid followed suit. After feeling at a loss Jones stopped.

"Even if I did make it rain, no one would believe it," Jones said to himself.
    The father called his kid over as he sensed something was wrong with Jones and was fearful about the situation. Jones understood and took a breather, looking towards the government building. His phone showed a low percentage battery. So, Jones walked across the square and into the CIA building. He sat on the chair where the front desk man could see him. "I need a charger for my phone," Jones said. The man looked at him in wonderment. "Alright." the front desk man said as Jones sat down ready to charge his phone. "That scripture outside has something to do with

CHAPTER THIRTEEN – THERAPEUTIC JUDGMENT

rain you know," Jones said aloud while recalling the four people playing music on the square. The painting inside the lobby of the CIA building had been plastered on each wall representing different emotions to call upon the rain. And he thought about the mall stating that it was closed until further notice due to drought. "What does it mean? Do you know?" the front desk man asked curiously. "Not yet," Jones replied.

After a few minutes, Jones's phone was charged. The man asked him to politely leave the premises. "It's getting late, please leave if your phone is charged sir." the front desk man said. Jones smiled in return, "Hey thanks." As Jones walked back outside of the building, the man with his child was now gone. He trudged further on to other parts of the city viewing problems in areas where he thought things could be improved. "If BART was more like a maglev train maybe we wouldn't have so many issues." Jones thought to himself. Grandiose ideas kept coming to Jones's mind, "And that giant mall that's still open. Some LED lights on the elevator would be nice. It would be awesome if some of these squares made music as you walked through them." He kept thinking to himself as the notes on his phone converged. It was as if Jones was writing on it directly. He could now upload his thoughts and other stuff to the internet, connected through the big technological companies. Someone wanted Jones to succeed. Something or someone was consistently watching over him beyond the galaxy eye that had been put on his back. Feeling tired from walking through the city for a few hours, Jones headed back towards BART. A Watcher walked past him dragging a mattress and a sleeping bag as he waved. "How are you doing brother?" the Watcher questioned Jones as if he knew him. Jones looked up and simply replied, "Good." The man nodded and continued walking.

Now the entire city started to gain traction knowing who Jones might be. He walked faster towards the BART when two men came out of the back of a meat shop walking on either side of him. The two men were singing songs commonly used in the Mafia. They dressed in all white.

Jones showed no fear while quickly walking ahead of them not wanting to be involved with them at the moment. Rather than entering the BART Embarcadero Station entrance, Jones walked towards the Ferry Building and the Embarcadero Plaza. There he saw a large patterned circle in the very center of the square with two large obelisk sculptures aligned to each side. He encountered a bicycle gang dressed in matching leather jackets. Glass bottles were littered in the middle of the patterned circle. Jones gained an interest in trying to balance himself on a bottle as he took one and stood on it. He was afraid at first but the bottle supported his weight. Eventually, the bottle broke under his foot giving him a minor cut on his toes. Jones looked down expecting blood, but the cut healed up quickly almost as if nothing had happened. He went over to the steps and stood on the bottles as each one knocked over breaking. "Hey, come on man! Don't be doing that here! People skateboard and stuff you know?" one biker said with a little bit of anger.

Jones picked up the pieces of his bottles as the gang surrounded him. "Alright, I'll pick it up," Jones said as he put each bottle in its place. Then he took out a Sharpie and wrote 'Vextrous' on one of the bottles exclaiming he was here as the leader of Nebulous. The bike gang backed away. Jones took out his phone to make a quick phone call to Ottie. He decided it wasn't safe anymore and started to head back to the BART. He wanted to get home out of the craziness which was the city. He ran towards the train after taking the stairs down just as it arrived. Not wanting to stick around, he jumped into the car.

His stream of conciseness ideas began to flow into his mind again. "You know BART should really have gates on the edges and light up at night for people down here.", Jones said to himself, noticing that people never lined up towards the black spots where the doorways opened. Another man boarded the same BART car with a black hat and a feather on it. "Ah, another demi-human!" he said politely, smiling as his teeth were stained yellow. The man smelled like he hadn't taken a bath in a while. "What?"

CHAPTER THIRTEEN – THERAPEUTIC JUDGMENT

Jones said, turning around towards the sound.

"I see you. The unnatural right?" the man said again, catching Jones's attention this time. "You mean you know of it?" Jones asked curiously as to the man's stature. "I've been studying scriptures and experiences on the unnatural for the last twenty years of my life." he cackled. "Welcome to the world of enlightenment." the man said as he got off BART. His black feather hat pointed away this time as the man strongly represented the feeling of death. Jones figured he'd better be careful around the gentleman so as to not upset him. The man walked off the BART train towards home laughing and singing. Jones got off at his stop. This time he had enough fare on his BART pass to get out of the gate. The same Station Agent lady eyed him as he passed through. Jones wandered home in the dark wearing his hat and blue-tinted glasses. The one bar in town seemed to be open as Jones wandered in. "What can I get you?" the bartender asked as a man with tattoos sat on the side. "Just a glass of water," Jones replied as the bartender handed him a glass. Jones chugged it and then threw the glass up catching it as he put it back down on the bar. "Don't do that please." the bartender laughed. The guy next to him with tattoos smiled.

Jones asked the guy next to him, "What do you think of the new technological world?" The man turned towards Jones, "I don't want to live in your world, man. I'm a dinosaur." Jones laughed as he walked out towards the local CVS across the street. He wandered in, needing to go to the restroom. The paper towels and a container of blue soap were mounted on the wall by the toilet. "I bet this tastes like blueberries." Jones thought to himself. He reached down and tried a small bit of it on his tongue. "Guess not. It'd be awesome if this soap was edible and it cleaned your hands and mouth too." Jones thought to himself. After using the restroom and flushing the toilet, the police showed up in front of the CVS door just as Jones walked out of the restroom. "What were you doing in there?" a policeman asked Jones. "I'm trusted."

Jones replied swiftly, "What? Just using the restroom." The policeman looked baffled, "This guy is completely normal. Let's move on guys". The policeman walked out the door as the woman at the cash register apologized profusely to Jones.

Jones began walking towards home. He saw a small stone near the door of a fitness center and picked it up. He threw it up as high as he could and watched it fall back to earth, spacing out thinking about the possibilities of his newfound abilities. "Gravity really is quite unsolved. It will be nice when I can travel up, like that car." Jones stated to himself. Jones saw a man walking by. He followed him briefly as the man turned to go inside of his house. Jones walked up to his house and knocked right after the man closed the door. "Hey, got any water?" Jones asked. The man invited Jones in after giving him a once over, deciphering if Jones was dangerous or not. "Yeah, I got some water." the man said. Without hesitation, the man seemed to understand Jones in his state of mind. SouthPark played in the background on the T.V. "I was there once. I understand how you feel." the man said, "Got out of the Army not too long ago." "That's a nice wardrobe." Jones complimented the Veteran as he looked at the suits hanging in the Veteran's open closet "Yeah, not bad, huh?" the man smiled.

"If you could do anything right now, what would you do?" Jones asked, trying to make conversation. "Don't worry man, relax a little. I was where you are myself just a bit ago. My wish? That I could be a good Veteran and help animals all day. That's my long-term goal, you know?" he said smiling. Jones smiled as he put down the water glass, "Thanks for the drink. I should get going. Work hard towards it and you will probably have that you know." Jones walked out of the man's front door in a feeling he needed to hide from the world. He ran back towards home in his slippers and jeans as the night fell. After a long journey back, he finally arrived. Jones opened the door exhausted. "We've been watching you." the voice echoed. The sound filled Jones's head as the people sat on the roof scurrying back and forth. The bushes moved throughout the night as Jones tried to sleep. "Go away! You're keeping me up." Jones waved at the

CHAPTER THIRTEEN – THERAPEUTIC JUDGMENT

people and the bushes. The sound of scurrying faded away as the bushes shook. After a long night's sleep, Jones woke up the next day getting ready as fast as he could. He headed outside before his mother could call out to him. He found a bamboo stick in the street. When Jones moved it, the hole in the stick would make a sound almost as if it was whistling like an instrument. "This is totally a mini flute," Jones said as he walked through the street carrying the bamboo stick.

Unable to drive, Jones called upon an Uber which took him to the center of Walnut Creek Mall. He sat looking for other people like him. A peculiar old man sat in the Starbucks as he was doing statistical research. Jones walked over to him and started up a conversation. "What are the world's biggest problems?" Jones asked the man. "Hey there, youngster. A name could be a start." the old man said. Jones reached out his hand, "Jones. And you are?" Jones replied cordially. The man laughed, "Bons the name. What can I do for you, Jones?" Jones smiled, "Hi, Bons. I'm looking for a job, but please answer the question first." The man smiled, "Well overpopulation is a big one along with the way electronics are affecting our youth. How do we expect to finish anything when people can't even finish a comic book?" the man responded.

"Yeah, I think distractions will be a huge issue, I mean most of us can't even use a road map thanks to the consistent use of GPS," Jones replied. Bons laughed again, "You're pretty sharp. I do need a pilot to fly for me if you're interested in the job." Jones smiled. Bons meant serious business. "I walk from my house to Starbucks at 6:00 AM every day. Come by sometime." Bons offered. Jones looked around feeling shy. "My guy out there is with his family right now. He's my private security. I have to talk to him. Sorry, but I must cut our conversation short." Bons said to Jones.

Jones politely thanked the man for the opportunity and walked away. He sipped his coffee as he passed by another window that had the same yellow Jeep displayed on it. The cafe was filled with people. It reminded him of his earlier encounter with the three men who had driven away. Jones stared up at the sky for a moment as he wandered further down the Iron Trail back over to the golf course. Three protesters sat outside the golf course. As Jones felt tired, he asked if he could sit by them. The big building of the main hospital showed on the horizon behind him. "What are you protesting?" Jones asked as the sun beat down on the bench. The man drank from a gallon bottle of water. "Fair wages!" he said. "This place has been robbing us for ages." Jones wandered towards the hospital building through the parking lot as a security guard in a red uniform stood outside. Inside the building, it said, 'Restricted. Special Treatment. Discovery Only.' Jones walked up towards the security guard as the man waved him away, "Do you have a patient in here to see?" he asked.

Jones shook his head 'No'. The man waved him away again as Jones walked out for a moment. When he came back down the pathway, the man left the post while the door was opened by a lady who opened it from the inside. Jones walked inside. Three doors sat in the entryway with code locks on them – 'Venus', 'Mars', 'Stardust' written on the doors. "Huh?" Jones said to himself as he walked further in past the soda machine. The doctor's door was open. Jones snuck in to look at the papers in detail. A small key lay on the table. The energy around him made him feel off-balance here. Jones headed back out through the main door sneaking around the building on the premise towards the utilities that controlled the whole hospital. Jones went slowly under the shadowed trees avoiding people as he hid under the pine. He looked at the instructions, interested in how the place worked. He could view every screw to its last detail. After checking to see how the technology was built, Jones went out from around the back of the hospital. "This could be heavily improved. I'm not sure how yet, but I'll find an idea." Jones said to himself, walking on the premises. "Stop right there! Head of Security!" the man shouted at Jones. Jones stopped in his tracks on the cement path as twelve big security guards surrounded him. "What were you doing near the utilities?" the Head of Security asked.

Jones replied, "Just checking it out." The man looked at him making a

CHAPTER THIRTEEN – THERAPEUTIC JUDGMENT

judgment call, "Do you need treatment?" the Head of Security asked him, being concerned. Jones could feel the energy coming towards him. He had to somehow escape. "No sir. Thanks for the offer". Jones replied. The Head of Security turned around, "Don't let us catch you again! Geo, escort him off the premises!" he said with authority. Jones warned, "Alright, but don't touch me or you might get shocked!" Filled with energy, he walked up next to the Head of Security. "I won't touch you. As soon as we get to the end of the property. Just get out of here." he sneered. They walked towards the end of the premise as Jones went up the hillside around the corner slowly. He heard cops showing up at the hospital from far away. Jones had to think fast. He ran around the corner down the hillside hopping a fence into a neighbor's yard. A dog barked at him as he knocked over a trash can.

"Sorry just passing through!" Jones yelled as the old lady watched him in awe. He ran further into the neighborhood away from the noise as the cops slowly went the other way. Feeling exhausted, Jones eyed a peach on the ground that had fallen from a tree. Jones ate it. "At least this is still good," Jones said to himself. He had to find a charger as his phone had died. He had to call his mom to get him out of this location. Jones sat down to think for a moment. As he looked down — a cup with ketchup had stained the cement. "Patterns, right?" Jones thought to himself. He remembered the mailman who was driving the cars. The ketchup was in the middle of the road with tire marks on it. The mailman directly ran over the ketchup, the same way he had assumed. A man approached from behind Jones. "Hiya. You lost?" he said to Jones as Jones sat on the edge of his property. "Yeah, I need to make a phone call. I walked all the way from the school." Jones replied. "That's a far walk," the man said. "What did you do?" Jones asked with curiosity. The man sat around on his chair, "Well you see, I used to race cars for a living. Now I'm simply living here. Got my dogs and I'm pretty happy."

Jones smiled back. "Alright." Jones charged his phone and he was able to call his mom. Ms. P. arrived later to pick him up. Jones's feet were stained with bruises from running away, partly filled with cuts. "Where have you been?" she asked, trying to be understanding. "Just exploring," Jones replied quietly. His mother was now extremely worried. She hid her emotions. Police sirens faded in the background as they had given up on finding Jones. His mother drove him home. "Jones you can't keep going out like this without proper treatment. Have you taken your pills?" his mother asked him with concern? Jones lied and said "Yes" as he started flushing them down the toilet each time. His mother had been keeping track and told him the importance of continuing to take them. But Jones didn't want to lose the power which he had obtained. He didn't want to lose his other world. Jones's mom thought he was taking his pills as she slowly backed off wondering why he was still acting the way he was. Jones didn't want to be inside the house. He started to dislike being at home. He wanted the feeling of freedom. Jones got cleaned up and went back outside in his slippers in the dead of the night running around the neighborhood trying to keep up with his abilities. Trying to train his body like Nepharius ordered to withstand the cold. To become something more using the 'human mind'. Jones now ran to get home fearing that the people of the night would prey on his own sanctuary. After a while, Jones went back home and lay in his bed thinking of more ideas. He was starting to break down as his mind was becoming more and more scattered with all of the unfinished ideas. Jones was now out of control as not only sleep but also his ability to properly function started to fade.

Chapter Fourteen – Drowning Trap

The next day Jones woke up late. The clock hit 2:00 PM as the sun had been up for hours. He strayed off to the side of his bed not wanting to get up to see the world outside. He knew that he was caught with no way out this time. "It's time for your new Group Therapy Program." his mom said gently. Ms. P. went over to him to look him in the eyes as he got up slowly to get dressed for the day. "Alright," Jones said complying as he put on his hat. He left the cane behind by the doorway. Details flashed through his mind as the wind pointed south this time, always blowing away from the direction Jones had been heading. He got into his mom's car waiting in the driveway. "Drop me off and I'll go by myself this time." Jones offered. His mother looked over at Jones checking on him, "Okay, but don't miss your appointment." Ms. P started up her car as classical music began playing. As they neared the building where the appointment was, she stopped the car in the parking lot and let him out. "Call me when you're done," she said brightly. Jones nodded as he walked into the building. A man with long hair, all dressed in purple sat in a wheelchair. As Jones walked into the building lobby, he crossed his hands.

"A Watcher? Here?" Jones said quietly to himself as they went up the elevator together. Using the same techniques to shut out the world through his headphones he walked up to the desk where the lady checked him in. This time the building was completely silent. "Welcome!" said the

Psychologist leading the group. She sat in the room as men and women sat in a circle. "Today we'll be doing a drawing exercise." the Psychologist said, "You'll introduce yourselves and speak your name. Then we will be drawing our worst fears. Who would like to go first?" Jones watched the Psychologist cross her legs and copy her. "Hi, I'm Yessi. I like to cook and bake pancakes. I'm really happy about cooking." Yessi wore a bow in her hair and was wearing a black dress. The smile on her face faded as she looked around. "Very good, Yessi. And how about you?" the Psychologist asked as she pointed to a man wearing a gray hat. "Hi, I'm Jay. I make music and I'm glad to almost be done here," he said as the Psychologist looked over at him. "Sounds good, Jay. See, that wasn't so hard, right?" the Psychologist said encouragingly.

The Psychologist moved on to the next woman who was older than the others in the circle. She was dressed in all red with a clear glass cane that went from her hand down to the floor. It was almost as if she was from the 101 Dalmatians story. The older lady simply replied, "Oh, you poor soul; having this job as a Psychologist." The Psychologist scrunched up her face in confusion. Her eyes had bags underneath them as if she hadn't slept in days. The next person in the circle was the man dressed in purple. He sat in his wheelchair right across from Jones. He began talking slowly. "My name is Jon. I'm an older musician by trade and here to say hello." "Very good, Jon. And next." said the Psychologist. As everyone else in the circle said their names, the Psychologist finally finished. "Okay, it's break time. Feel free to roam for fifteen minutes and be back here." said the Psychologist. Jones walked over to Jon as he wheeled out of the room going towards one of the comfortable chairs that were set up outside. "So, you made music?" Jones asked Jon politely. "Yeah, I used to do bass a lot," Jon replied. Jones looked him in the eye, "I noticed you were making triangles with your hands in a pattern. Show me the signs." Jones said being direct.

The man's eyes perked up as he slowly put his hands in three different

CHAPTER FOURTEEN – DROWNING TRAP

patterns. "If you successfully get three people sitting in a triangle to do this with all signs matching, things will happen as you want them to," Jon said briefly. Jones sat there for a moment memorizing the hand signs as the rest of the group participants began coming back to the Group Therapy room to sit down. Jones and Jon got up to join them. "Okay everyone, it's drawing time. Please take the clipboard and a piece of paper." the Psychologist instructed the group. Jones volunteered to grab all of the clipboards available in different colors and hand them around the circle. He sat directly across from Jon. The two of them and the Psychologist formed a giant triangle within the circle. Pointing his legs in a cross towards the Psychologist and Jon, Jones attempted to make a successful triangle with the Psychologist as she talked. Without her noticing, Jones did the hand signs. "Everyone, begin to draw. What do you see in your drawing?" the Psychologist asked.

As everyone started to draw, the Psychologist crossed over her legs as Jones kept trying to make everyone match her actions. Yessi finished drawing first holding up a piece of paper that showed scissors on it. Jay drew a jazz saxophone and Jon drew a house. Right then as the Psychologist was about to make everyone talk about how their drawings made them feel, Jones successfully matched up everything with the Psychologist. Suddenly, the two doors of the Group Therapy room opened at the same time as two new people flooded through into the room. Three people got out of their chairs at the same time, walked in a small circle, and went over to get water. The Psychologist's face grew confused for a moment as natural chaos came about the room. By matching up the energy within the room it shifted towards Jones's train of thought giving him control over the situation. "Let's take another quick break." the Psychologist said, scratching her leg feeling uncomfortable for the first time.

Normalcy didn't match up so well. Jones, this time left his clipboard on his chair, having drawn nothing on the sheet of paper. He walked down the stairs of the building. This time, looking up at the sky running over to a wall where the clouds told him to run, run as fast as he could, Jones got on the wall and started dancing joyously as another Watcher walked by. "I see you!" she said laughing as Jones smiled. The wall was paper-thin, but it didn't bother him. He jumped down the other side towards the Iron Trail that ran behind the Center, running all the way into a gated neighborhood off to the left where a man with a leaf blower blew the leaves. The leaves kept going in a circle as Jones danced in them as if they were the wind gearing up to run fast again, trying to gain energy to see a different world — his world. However, to no avail, it did not work. Jones felt drained as he tried again. "Hey, what are you doing?" A neighbor in the gated community said as Jones hid in the shadows under the tree. "Hanging around," Jones said. The man pointed, "Get out of here."

Jones walked away slowly back towards the Therapy Center. An old veteran stood outside with her dog smoking a cigarette. Jones sat down for a minute feeling broken as he started to return to reality. "Hey." she said as she walked over to him, "Got any spare change?" He looked over at her for a moment, "I don't, but what brought you out here?" Jones asked. Her dog walked over to him and licked his foot. "Well, I used to work for the NYPD, but after a while, the place I was living in said I had to get rid of my dog if I wanted to stay there. So, I chose my dog," she said smiling as she stood outside with the lighter. Jones thought for a moment, he didn't know what to say. Here he was messing around in parallelism. People were struggling all over, stuck in this actual state of physicality. Jones had decided at that moment that the stress he was causing because of Nepharius was more than he bargained for. Spontaneously, Jones hugged the woman, "I don't have spare change, but I hope you will feel better." Jones said sincerely.

The old veteran thanked Jones as he walked back to the Therapy Center. This was the first time Jones had felt sentimental in a long time, reconnecting with the world around him. Walking back up the stairs of the building, Jones went into the Group Therapy room again and sat down

CHAPTER FOURTEEN – DROWNING TRAP

in the circle. "Why the scissors, Yessi?" the Psychologist asked. She had already started as Jones was late getting back into the room. "Well, the scissors are here because they represent how I feel. I feel as if the world is cutting me consistently." Yessi said. Jones looked back to his right at Jon who was falling asleep in his chair. "Jay?" the Psychologist asked as she moved around the circle. "The saxophone represents what I want in life," he said smiling as if he was graduating from a therapy session. Jon mumbled half asleep in his wheelchair. Jones's ability to understand the Watchers was fading. He could so easily understand them before so he knew that his power was coming to a close. It was only a matter of time before it struck. The Psychologist finished the session, "Alright everybody, now get up. It's over for today." she said, exhausted. Jones walked out of the building to go sit on the bench as he watched people walk by aimlessly. His true depression hit now realizing that the world around him was the world that he created to escape. None of the world around him existed. Jones sat waiting for his mother to pick him up. She called his phone, "Tomorrow is your court date. Don't go out anywhere. I'll be there in five minutes." Ms. P. showed up as promised to drive him home and Jones got into the car feeling defeated. Jones didn't feel like going out this time. The sun shined lightly down as it slowly went over the horizon. His email, filled with spam, made him turn it off as the titles asked where he was going and where he had gone. As the night fell, Jones got in his car and floored it, driving down uninvited to Monterey Bay. After a few hours, he arrived as he drove through the fog which seemed to save him time. Seeing that his car was low on gas, he pulled into the same gas station as the time before, next to where a stylized star sign could be seen from the highway near the mall.

The old man working the cash register looked at him with pity as he pointed to the hot dog. The whole galaxy seemed to know the trouble that Jones was having. Jones pointed to the hot dog, 'Free?' Jones asked himself. The man slowly shook his head in a yes motion. Jones took it and ate it as he smiled bleakly to himself, "Hmm, chicken mixed with sausage."

Jones said aloud. Jones went back out to his car as he slowly drove back home that night. He was barely able to function as he collapsed on his bed. The next day was Jones's fateful day, the day he had made his one and only mistake. He remembered that day to its fullest extent because that was the day his freedom got taken from him. "Jones, it's time to go. You're going to be late." Ms. P. urged him to get moving faster as he got dressed in his fancy shoes and long shorts.

Jones got in the car as his mom drove him to the Solano County Superior Court in Vallejo. Jones and Ottie had gotten the actual moving violation ticket before the whole journey to LA began. By making a wrong left turn, Jones had gone into an alleyway where he hadn't seen the policeman. The ticket went unpaid and the situation built up over time. Today was his day to contest this ticket and tell his side of the story. Jones jumped out of the car as his mother tried to figure out where to park her car. Several gangsters eyeballed the 'fancy' car out by the brown house on the curbside; as Jones's mom's car drove by. She crossed into the courthouse entryway. His mother parked outside on the street as the chief of police road up on his motorcycle to the front of the courthouse.

Jones slid his shoes across the smooth concrete as he went towards the front door of the Solano County Superior Court House. "Behave Jones!!" Ms. P scolded Jones as she caught up to him and they went through the door to the front of the Court House together. The security guard looked at him with a glare almost as if to pity and scold him at the same time. "Please remove all of your stuff." the Security Guard requested. Jones had two pennies in his pocket along with a belt on his Dockers. As he placed the items on the conveyor belt, the man told him to move forward. Each of the hallways was empty; the courtroom had no more than ten people there. Jones and his mother sat in the middle row, waiting for the case to be called. Another man sat behind them with dreads. Viewing the courtroom from the back, the police force showed up in full, sitting in their chairs in uniform all erect. After a few moments, it was Jones's turn. "Fake being sick." Nepharius's voice rang in his head. "I don't want to,"

CHAPTER FOURTEEN – DROWNING TRAP

Jones said in return. "I said fake it!" ordered Nepharius.

Jones started coughing unwillingly as his name was called, first in small amounts. The whole world went still as the voice got louder and louder. "Jones T. Harver. Stand up please." the Judge said. "Yes, I'm right here, Sir," Jones said weakly. He mumbled as he heard, "Mr. Harver." Jones coughed loudly as his finger went up to the call acknowledging his name. The entire crowd looked at him riveted. Then, Jones sunk slowly down onto the Court Room floor passing out. The entire courtroom was tricked. They thought it was real. "Good job Jones. You're free for a while." Nepharius said. Two Court policemen picked Jones up and put him onto a bench at the side of the CourtRoom where Jones lay in a stupor. "We need a paramedic here, NOW!" the two policemen called out. The wood grain of the bench in front of Jones's eyes stood out at him. Jones had coughed due to either a lack of sleep or the forces that be, either way, he was in trouble. "Get this man out of here!" the policeman pointed as Jones's mother gasped. The paramedics wheeled him out on a gurney putting restraints around him as the ambulance showed up out front. Ms. P. followed the ambulance in her car. Off to the Emergency Room in Vallejo for evaluation.

"Did you smoke anything?" the paramedics asked inside the Ambulance ride. Jones acted and lied, "A blue rock of some sort, some called it moonstone." he said. The paramedics reported that possibly methamphetamines or ecstasy mixed with heroin had entered his body upon admission to the Emergency Room in Vallejo. Little did they know that Jones was referring to the galaxy, actual moonstones passed around to expand their horizons of communication with other galactic planets. People using moonstones to understand one another's languages. The yellow straps went off the back of the bed as Jones faded to unconsciousness. A few moments later he opened his eyes. He was on the bed with his mother sitting nearby. A red laser was taped to his finger. A nurse came by with some water. "Drink this." the nurse said.

Jones looked at the water and smiled, "I guess this could be used in a bouncy ball." Jones moved his finger around while looking at the ceiling, tracking the red laser light, and surveying the room. The nurse laughed out loud. And for the first time, his mother's stress broke. "Where are we?" Jones asked his mom. "Jones, you're in the hospital. You fell in the CourtRoom, remember?" she said gently, reminding him of what he already knew. "Oh yeah," Jones replied quietly. Jones's mind started to wander thinking of multiple thoughts simultaneously. As the nurse wiped down the green side chair seat, a city-scape briefly appeared on the chair seat through the water that was wiped. Jones had now fully hallucinated the galaxy, visualizing it in reality fully for the first time. Then the cityscape disappeared. "You should restrain me," Jones said to the nurse as they escorted him over to the bed and put the straps on him.

His mother waited in the Cafeteria as instructed. Jones looked over at his wrist and that's when it happened, that fateful moment where he broke from reality. "I need water." Jones pleaded to the nurse as his lips dried up, almost as if his brain was overheating. "Patient in waiting number 1,937,928,882" read on his patient wristband that the doctor had clipped onto his arm. His mind started racing faster. Jones's lips turned a pale white. He was feeling dehydrated. The rule where Jones had told himself he must wait before others overextended rattled through his mind. "Wait Jones." the nurse said aloud. Then Jones lost his mind, yelling as he tried to break out of the straps that held him to the bed. "Hold him down!" said all in the room. Seven pairs of hands all held onto Jones as he was breaking free in a frenzy. And then silence. Jones fainted right then and there on the bed.

Chapter Fifteen – Grand Escapist

"Hey, roommate! How is the reading going?" Jones asked his roommate as Jones came back around the corner from his meal. "Kind of hungry." the roommate replied. "Can I keep reading? I don't feel like mingling with the rest of the chumps here. He paused for a moment, "I didn't know you were in a psychiatric ward once before." Jones sighed as he walked back into the room. He sat on the bed next to the desk. "Yes, that fateful day is when I ended up caught by them, I'm sure you know from reading my Journal. I woke up and I couldn't convince anyone to believe my story. I was in a double room, next to a gentleman who was so depressed he wouldn't even get out of bed. We were in a Locked Ward behind four sets of locked doors. In this place, they call it a 5250 hold, but in galactic space, it is called a prison of the mind. A prison in space is meant to stop baddies like me I suppose." Jones said in a matter-of-fact tone. So how did you get out?" the roommate asked.

"Keep reading and you'll find out," Jones replied as he sat on the bed picking up the nearest book looking for clues. The roommate turned towards Jones and began reading the Journal out loud: Jones walked by as a man saluted him. "Welcome back Boss." Instantly recognizing him as a high-ranking member of the crew. Jones got up, getting out of bed for the first time, dressed in all brown. A kid with a hat sat on a couch as if they were surveying the area, reading people's minds as the people in the Locked Ward walked by one another. Two nurses sat up front at the desk feeding pills of lithium to patients. Jones had to take the blue pill and yellow pill as the nurse watched. Jones wandered over to a private door where he would meet the doctor for the first time. "I'm Doctor W. You are to take this pill and this pill once a day. You have bipolar and psychotic tendencies at this current moment in time. Let me ask you, Jones, do you know how fast your mind was going?" Dr. W. inquired. Jones shook his head, "You tell me. How fast?" The doctor smiled viciously, "Mach 3. We just need to slow it down and have you fixed up a bit." Jones smiled back, "What fixing? All I've been doing is developing the world around me. Doctor W. cut him off, "Jones, do not confuse bipolar tendencies with intelligence! We are done here! You are not intelligent!" he said empathetically and angrily. Jones got up walking out of the office.

"Not intelligent, huh? I'll make it out of here." Jones said quietly to himself. Surely this Locked Ward had to have some sort of way out. Jones would have to poke around for information to find his way forward. He sat down on the bed in his room where one other roommate lay. No shavers were allowed. Only a single book and a toothbrush were all a person could carry here. Jones realized his phone was gone. In complete lockdown, a man lay on the other bed in the room. "What landed you here?" Jones asked his roommate curiously. The man said, "I'm Gary and… 'Meh'." he sighed, not bothered to reply fully. "What's up with that guy?" Jones asked one of the people in the hallway as they headed to lunch. The person started speaking really fast, almost so fast that Jones had trouble picking up his words. "Oh, Gary? He hasn't been out of bed in a week already," he said. Jones leaned in, "A week?" he said concerned. Jones didn't want to question how long these two had been in here. He knew that it would be one for the books. A nurse called a lady over that Jones saw on his first day as a patient. She screamed at the nurse.

"No, I won't take your stupid pills!" she screeched as she started to run down the hallway tearing away at what little window coverings existed. Jones noticed the red runway pathway with umbrellas for eating outside

CHAPTER FIFTEEN – GRAND ESCAPIST

as the rest of the place was well barred behind four locked metal doors. A security guard chased this lady down and held her as she screamed in rebuttal. The security guard poked her with a syringe injecting her with lithium as she squirmed on the ground. "Are you going to be good and listen or do we have to keep giving you injections? We can do this the hard way or the easy way!" The Security Guard said loudly for all nearby to hear. The Security Guard seemed frustrated with his daily work as Jones watched from the sidelines. "Jones! It's your turn to take your two pills." said the Nurse.

After seeing what had just happened to the lady on the floor, Jones realized his worst nightmare had become a reality. He took the blue and the yellow pills. Instantly the two hit his brain making him hungry and slow. He couldn't think at the fast pace as he was functioning at before. "It's now time for lunch." announced the staff. "Macaroni and cheese available on a table outside. Soon we will do exercises. Zaya will play guitar for us." More announcements by staff were made. Jones tried to make sense of what was going on as he was handed a packet detailing 'Today's Daily Routines'. "This is supposed to be healing?" Jones said to himself quietly. "I feel more like I'm in an Orwellian 1984 Animal Farm." As Jones sat down quietly eating by himself, Zaya the guitarist walked up to Jones and sat down next to him. A giant man with a white beard made bird noises in the background. "Hi, I'm Zaya," she said. She was short in height and was wearing tattered clothing. One of her eyes was slightly different in color than the other. To Jones, she needed company and was ousted from the rest of the people around them.

Jones introduced himself and then picked up his fork and finished eating. "How long have these people been locked up?" Jones asked Zara, starting to question the sanity of the place where he had no more than a couple of hours to himself since arrival. He continued, "Has anyone ever gotten out of here?" Jones asked Zaya. Meanwhile, Jones began to plan his escape route with the possibility of climbing one of the white umbrellas over the wall to freedom. "One man escaped a long time ago. He climbed the roof and ran away." Zaya said without emotion. Jones commented sarcastically, "Oh great." Looking around, Jones felt that escaping wouldn't work. Jones would have to play by their rules. He was, after all, in their territory. As Jones finished up his meal, two nurses went around to gather up the emptied plates taking no chances. Everyone was pampered like a baby. Jones already hated the place. He could feel that he had been misplaced; forced into a ward to 're-correct his brain'. As nurses attempted to study the disconnects behind each individual persona that had developed, Jones sat there studying the nurses.

"Okay, now everyone, we will have a 30-minute workout session." the head nurse said. Zaya went up to the front of the class where an instructor, who was half asleep, started to direct them. "Today you will be doing jumping jacks. I will count to thirty. If you feel tired, please do not participate further." the instructor stated. The instructor nodded at Zaya as she played the guitar. Everyone did as they were told - half drained and half brain dead. Jones joined in the crowd as the drugs hit further into his system. He struggled to keep up with the jumping jacks and the workout session, eventually sitting down in the white chair directly behind him. After a few minutes, it was over. The giant man with a white beard, standing in the background, sat down next to Jones. "When do we go home, usually?" Jones asked the giant man, trying to figure it out. "We're never getting out." the man cackled as he made more bird noises.

Most of the people left the man alone in his corner. He had been too far gone to be recovered. Now, it was due to being in there too long. Jones got up and backed away from the man, looking towards the door that led back inside. He sat on the wooden table where the man who spoke too fast came to join in. "Antsy," he said as he shook Jones's hand. Zaya followed behind coming up to Jones. She had taken a liking to him because Jones was nice to her. If anything, Jones knew that Zaya may be his key to getting out of the Locked Ward, back to civilization, before he would

CHAPTER FIFTEEN – GRAND ESCAPIST

be fed so many pills. Jones didn't even know who he was anymore. This was Mira's warning; this was the CIA's holding house. Jones sighed to himself. Seeing the box of crayons lying on the table, and getting out a piece of paper, Jones started to draw. "What else is around here?" Jones asked aloud as he drew. Antsy spoke up, "A 30-minute routine, a piano. Sometimes we get to go workout and sometimes we hang around after eating." "Slow down there, Antsy," a nurse's voice came from the glass wall watching them. "I can't," Jones said repeating himself three times as he walked back towards his room, but first he grabbed the box of crayons. Jones kept on drawing, trying to keep his mind focused on the blank sheet of paper that lay ahead of him. Nothing was coming to mind as Zaya looked at his doodles. "Jones, what are you drawing?" she questioned him as he wasn't thinking of anything. Another older woman sat over to his right. She started drawing too. She tapped Jones on the shoulder.

"Look," she said, only able to speak a word or two. It was a picture of the earth with the emotion 'enraptured' enveloping earth that went up towards the sun. Jones nodded his head smiling; admiring the work, but not understanding for a moment. "Who am I? Where am I?" a third woman queried as she walked up to Jones after spinning around like a butterfly. "You're in a ward," Jones said bluntly. "A ward?" she said looking around confused. "Yeah! Your name is…?" Jones asked, questioning her. At that moment she seemed to snap out of her daze. "Elly? Oh my god, how long have I been here?" Elly said, snapping out of her spinning around looking straight at Jones. Her legs looked like they hadn't been shaved in a while as she had hair growth everywhere.

"I'm not sure, but at least three weeks," Jones replied. "That's how long I have been here." Many others stopped their activities and watched them speaking to each other. "Thank you. You've saved me," she said, shaking Jones's hand. "I've got to make a call." Elly went over to the phone that stood in the hallway of the Ward across from the Nurses Station. There was no privacy. Jones watched her dial out. Elly spoke to her parents, who were surprised that she was even capable of contacting them. For the first time in a while, Jones felt like he had been free, that there was probably a way out of this place if he followed their rules. He looked over to Antsy who walked away towards his room as Zaya walked over to Jones. "So, you like music too, huh?" Zaya asked Jones. Jones didn't remember mentioning that he had done so. "Yeah, I love it. I heard there's a piano in here?" Jones walked over to the door that was at half-mast. "Hey shut that door!" one of the nurses shouted from the Nursing Station window as Jones went into the room with the piano.

Jones pushed the door closed, shutting his eyes in relief. He then stopped the door from closing with his hands as another man came into the room. "Don't do that." the man said. Jones stood by the doorway, "Do what?" he asked. The man stood there waving his hand towards the door, "I saw you starting to put a lock on the door. Don't do that!" he said agitatedly. The man went over to the green couch and sat down as Jones walked to the piano bench. "I just want to play." Jones said, trying to reason with him, "What's your name?" The man looked up after scratching his leg, "Tober." he said distractedly, as the old man looked out the window at the sun. "I lost my wife recently." He leaned back as Jones played the first few notes on the piano. Zaya laughed, "You two are funny." The man looked back as he scratched his skin off more. It slowly fell to the ground. "God has been telling me to find the well. If I could get back to that damned well, I'd be young again. The people here won't let me out of here so I'm starting to rot." Tober said in the background as Jones kept on playing without speaking. The only place where the sun shined in all day consistently was in that room next to the green couch. Yet everyone else was too euthanized by pills to realize this room even existed. This room kept Jones sane and focused.

Zaya reached over the bench at the end of the piano and started playing at a rapid speed. She was musically inclined in both the guitar and piano as Jones sat aside watching her play. "What do you consider yourself?"

CHAPTER FIFTEEN – GRAND ESCAPIST

Jones asked her jokingly. "I don't know. Perhaps I'm a little demon sent here to protect you." Zaya said in reply. "You're nice to me where my family isn't. I guess I'm here to watch over you." She looked down to the ground. "You know, or something." Jones sat and listened to Tober and Zaya express their thoughts as he took back over the piano. He was very impressed by Zaya's playing skills and wanted to learn from her. "How do you play separately like that?" Jones asked. "I can't seem to play one hand at a different tempo from the other." She reached over to the base of the piano. "Well, you just start with the bass notes down here because each song has to have bass. Then you just alternate like this." She alternated her fingers hitting the bass lines on the piano. "Now try to add in your second hand." She started playing while alternating as the professionals did. Her hands moved at a speed faster than Jones was naturally used to seeing. Tober sat in the back of the couch slowly falling asleep. "You know, I see in four dimensions," Tober said aloud.

Jones turned around, "Do you make stuff then?" Jones asked, curious as to learn Tober's reply. Cautiously Jones listened in. "Well, I used to be a carpenter," Tober said as Zaya continued playing the piano. Jones's interest grew for a moment as he kept this statement in mind. "It's time for dinner!" the Head Nurse shouted. As the crowd hustled back towards the eating area tables, Tober found a clear table and sat down. Oranges were delivered in front of them as people bickered and laughed about their journeys and ideas. Tober tried to draw what seemed to be a cabinet drawer on a sheet of paper in front of him. "You know Tober, that's not four dimensions," Jones said to him, trying to reassure him that his skillset in drawing wasn't showing through. Tober looked back at Jones for a moment. "I can't see in three dimensions anymore. I can only see in four dimensions." Jones thought for a moment about this statement. He thought about how he was convinced and out of focus on his own head. "I may have a solution for you." Tober kept on rambling about Church and randomized idealisms as Jones took an unpeeled orange from the dish. "Tober! Watch very closely. Look at this orange." Jones picked up the orange and started throwing it back and forth between his hands as Tober tried to make sense of it.

"Okay, but I'm following the orange and… oh my!" exclaimed Tober. After a few minutes of Tober's head going back and forth, he looked at his paper again. "Now draw something." encouraged Jones. Tober gasped as if he had found a newfound vision. He put down the crayon and started to draw. Tober's drawings got better and better. "You're helping me. What do you want from me?" Tober asked. Jones replied, "You're a carpenter, right?" questioning Tober as he sat there listening. "Yeah, I am," replied Tober. Replying directly, "Well alright then, I'd like a gold piano, custom-built, when we get out of here." smiled Jones. Tober looked at him, "Alright, anything to get me out of this place." The man went back to eating and drawing as he smiled at his newfound ability. Elly came around the corner, staring at her dish for a moment. Her mother had just come to visit her. She was now talking about leaving the building. She went to her room to get one of her books, clearly no longer enjoying the fact that she was in there. She preferred reading her books as she hung out, trying not to converse with too many people.

Jones surveyed the room looking straight ahead as one of the nurses came up to the crowd. "Now we're going to exercise. Line up single file line one after another." said the nurse. Jones and most of the crowd lined up as all of them followed the head nurse down the hallway where one of the lock-down doors was opened for them to pass through. Another person from a different sector stared at them all as they looked towards the crowd as they passed by. Jones remembered a Theory he had watched on YouTube as he walked down the carpeted hallways towards the exercise room. 'Connections - they can be made through the mind. Made by understanding one's energy and matching that with another.' Jones let these thoughts go as quickly as he remembered them. He couldn't speak about this Theory here. Jones knew he was being monitored. "You all have 30 minutes." said the instructor. Two treadmills sat next to a T.V.

CHAPTER FIFTEEN – GRAND ESCAPIST

In the opposite room there was table hockey and various exercise balls in the corner. "Zaya, I challenge you to a game of table hockey!" Jones said as Zaya looked over at him laughing. Jones wanted to test out the equipment and get a feeling for the surroundings. Zaya went around to the other side of the table and got into her zone hitting the hockey puck first. Jones guarded his end, hitting the hockey puck back across the table as the puck picked up speed. The two of them started hitting the puck faster and faster, not slowing down as it went across the table. The energy picked up around Jones as the room lights flickered each time the hockey puck was hit. As the puck slid across the table back and forth the lights now sparked until Jones hit the puck right into the corner pocket. The hockey puck flew off the table, its green circle flying through the air as it almost hit Zaya.

She laughed as the nurse scolded them for playing too hard. Everyone else watched for a moment, noticing that Jones wasn't normal. The Watchers in the room smiled as if he was in control of the place now. Jones knew that he would be able to get what he needed. He would be able to break free of the lockdown. "Okay that's enough." the nurse said, "Everyone head back, as it's time to rest. Tomorrow we will wake up and do the same routine. There will be a dance instructor coming in as part of music therapy." Everyone stood in line and followed the nurse back to their locked area. Jones didn't want to attempt to escape as he knew the lockdown would be too much for him to get through. He weighed climbing the umbrellas by the track option, or simply running out the door when brought through to the other side of the locked doors for exercise. But he had found a better way — Jones would beat the facility at its own game. Pioneering the plan in his head, Jones got ready for bed. As he went over to the other side of the room, Gary still lay there looking at the wall and sighed. Jones brushed his teeth and then got into his bed. As he lay there looking at the ceiling dreaming about nothing, the pills were taking effect on his mind. His imagination was fading.

The next day, Jones woke up bright and early. Apples had already been placed on the desk next to him as he went to use the shower. "Mind if I?" Jones asked Gary who sat there depressed in bed. Gary sighed and mumbled, "Yeah, go ahead." Jones went over and prepared for the day. He wasn't allowed to shave as nurses sat in fear of their 'test subjects' using shavers as a weapon. Jones took a bite of one of the apples after brushing his teeth. He heard the morning call from down the hallway. "Everyone, it's time for your dance lessons and then therapy sessions." the nurse said. It seemed the routine had continued through the Ward as the same song played. "Now everyone, get into a circle and dance. Follow me, just like last time." said the instructor. Jones sat there for a moment as he had already gained the trust of others. "Can we listen to different music?" Jones asked, looking at the dance instructor. She looked back at Jones eyeing him as he snapped his fingers to a different beat. Other people in the room started to vocalize their feelings as well. "Yeah, the same songs over and over are boring." someone said. The dance instructor gave in, "Okay, what would you like to hear?" she asked the crowd of people. "A different song is fine. It doesn't matter." Jones said, trying to direct a minuscule change in the ward's environment.

The dance instructor said, "Okay, next time when we come back, I will do that." Then she picked up the CD player that was on the table and started walking out the door. Jones turned to Zaya, "Do you go through this every single day?" he asked. She laughed again, "Yeah, we do." Zaya replied. Jones sighed, "Anybody would go crazy in here. By doing the same routine over and over with no change." Jones noticed a feedback sheet that was left on the table. None of the feedback sheets had been filled out in years. "Jones you have a visitor." said the Head Nurse. His mother was standing at the Nurses Station. She came to see him and asked to speak privately. As they have no meeting rooms and counselors watch everyone at all times, he led his mother out to the red track in the sun in the middle of the locked ward. She sat down at one of the picnic tables with a fixed smile and a very worried look on her face. "Jones, I'm trying to get you out

CHAPTER FIFTEEN – GRAND ESCAPIST

of here. You have to pay attention to your surroundings." Ms. P. started. Jones looked back at his mother, "My surroundings? I have already told you how I can go into the future by running fast. Watch my hands. See how they disappear?" Jones moved his hands at fast speed in front of his mother's face, not remembering that the pills had already taken effect. Jones had lost his communication with the outside world.

His mother looked at him with love, but in a confused way, trying to understand the world that Jones's mind had become stuck in. "I'll come back in a week when I know more. You are supposed to have a hearing about your release." Ms. P. said. Jones sighed as he watched her walk through the locked doors after giving him a hug and turning, able to leave the place. Jones stared aimlessly at the sky as he tried to run around the track gaining speed to garner the same effects as when he was free. However, Jones had zero success. He walked back inside over to the room with the piano, playing notes to keep himself sane and connected to the world around him. With each note that Jones hit he was able to focus, but the pills dulled his thoughts. "Remember you have to play along to beat them at their own game," Jones repeated to himself, over and over to try to stay conscious. Jones walked back to his room, trying to avoid the routine that the place set him through. Gary sat up in the bed for the first time, "Piano. Dance." he said. These two words described how he felt. Jones understood the old man as Gary stared into Jones' eyes, half-smiling for the first time in two weeks. "Oh, you want to? Play the piano and dance?" asked Jones. The man slowly got out of bed and looked at himself in the mirror. He began brushing his teeth.

Jones watched silently. "Meh… maybe tomorrow," Gary said as he went back towards the bed to go lay down. Jones felt obligated to help this man heal. It seemed that the man responded to music. "What's your favorite song?" Jones asked him out of curiosity. "I don't know, something nice," Gary said to the wall, turning around and laying back in bed to sleep. Jones figured he would request a new song tomorrow. After all, Watchers tended to love new songs. It was their way of communicating with one another, especially through titles of songs. A title that held the emotion with it afterward was the easiest way in which one could understand another in the galactic world. Jones knew that by including this he would be able to stir up communication again. Jones walked out of the bedroom, back over to the table where two people sat on the couch nearby. A new person had entered the building. "Hey look at this new guy," Jones commented from the side of the couch to the two people on the couch. One man wore a hat, sitting towards the end of the couch that pointed towards the T.V. The red track sat behind them both. "Why are you here?" Jones asked the man with a blue baseball cap out of curiosity. "Magic." the man replied jokingly. Jones decided he would sit down next to him and play along. "Name's Jones," Jones said. "Name's Pan. No wait, call me Jack. You'll be Pan, let's make this interesting" said the man with the blue baseball cap.

"Okay, call me Peter Pan. This matches your magic comment doesn't it?" Jones said laughing. "If anyone gives you trouble here, I'll help you. I kinda like you already." Jack said willingly. "These pills make us go crazy, but they put us in here when we're depressed. How does that even help us?" He wasn't happy that he had to be there, even for a short amount of time. Jones sat there and listened to him rant, nodding his head slowly, "Well I suppose." he said in return. "Let's sit outside." The large man with the white beard sat in the back making bird noises again. He was there because he had punched his best friend in the face. Jones had overheard the conversation from Antsy prior. Antsy seemed to know about everyone's business who in turn told everyone else due to his incapability of shutting up. Jones sat there in the sun, attempting to gain some peace of mind to think. But he couldn't gather his thoughts. As another plate was put in front of him, this time meatloaf, Jones ate. For some reason the nurses wanted the patients to eat a lot more than normal. The pills were making Jones even more hungry each day. "Peter Pan, stop eating so much!" Jack offered, trying to help Jones moderate his weight.

CHAPTER FIFTEEN – GRAND ESCAPIST

"Alright," Jones said, as he sat there, eyeing him down. "I'll try not to." All of the white walls and windows gave Jones the same sense that he was getting nowhere. The place felt designed to break spirits rather than heal them. "Hey, Peter Pan, where are you going?" Jack shouted as Jones went over to the piano room where Tober sat. "That man went pee in the sink last night you know!" Jack continued as his voice faded out. Soon after, a distant voice came from the hallway as Jones shut the door and started playing. Slowly, his fingers could only play by muscle memory running over the same three keys in an arpeggiated manner. Tober sat there scratching his foot. "Stop doing that." a nurse said, looking into the door, scolding Tober as he sat there. "Let me out of here and I'll stop." Tober retaliated. Jones kept on playing, trying to stay sane regardless of what had been going on around him. Zaya opened the door, "Can I play?" she asked Jones. Jones nodded, unable to fully converse. Zaya didn't seem to be taking any pills at all. She was filled with energy as she played the same song over and over again. Jones's mind slowly woke up as he listened, sitting on the piano bench. Growing frustrated with the setting, Jones took over slamming the notes down on the piano.

"What happened to the beautiful playing?" the nurse asked. "You sound frustrated." A pen and paper sat there as the nurse documented Jones's actions down on a sheet of paper. Jones was being studied by his every move and knew it. He had gained some freedom for not acting up and playing along with their games. Jones got back up saying nothing. He went back towards where more commotion had gone on. A security guard stood at the front of the lockdown doors surveying the area. He could see white daisies sticking out of the ground towards the sky as the nurse rotated everyone again. A half-finished puzzle lay on the table as someone had tried to finish a game. Scattered with ideas and odd people, Jones couldn't make sense of the place anymore. Another man walked by him. The guy who had saluted Jones on his first day had been transferred to a different section of the building. Jones sat there feeling alone. All he had left was the piano and Zaya. Elly had been cured and was released.

It looked as if Tober was on his way to being released too. Jones's mind wandered and headed back to his room. He thought many of the nurses and doctors resembled people he had met outside of the ward, almost as if the people inside had direct resemblances to those outside. Jones laid back down in his room with nothing further to do. He stared at the ceiling waiting for tomorrow to come.

Chapter Sixteen – Musical Heart

The next day Jones got out of bed trying to coax Gary into standing up again. Gary sat there for a moment. "Join us. It will be fun." Jones said as he tried to make direct conversation. This time the music therapist played a different song from the distant hallway. Gary got out of bed and started to move towards the noise. Gasps came from everyone as Gary appeared. The therapist was surprised. "Oh my god, he's up and dancing?" the music therapist said to herself, surveying the area. Gary replied, "Yeah." he said, smiling a little bit. "So, you're healing then?" the therapist asked. As Jones went down the hallway to join in, he was pleased that his coaxing worked. The night before he had told Gary that the only way he would get released would be if he danced. The two had struck a deal previously, that Jones would get him a new song played. That gained his trust. That small step allowed Jones to blend in further. With the Locked Ward's staff expectations of patients, the set routines and mundane scheduling to keep patients grounded, and the use of mind-numbing medications — all were designed to allow patients to be studied.

Jones felt like a rat trapped inside a cage. As part of the galactic people and all that Jones stood for in his world, he was afraid that his thinking was being repressed. Watchers who had been helping him were also being held captive. The Ward was preventing Jones and the Watchers from escaping towards home or back into their galaxies. Jones felt the burden he shouldered as thoughts continuously poured through his mind: "Yes, that's right - holding people in locked wards without proper treatment is being overlooked. As if a person is sweeping dust under the rug. The staff captures patients' imaginations. These people are subduing us to a point where there is a lack of even the simplest thought. These damn wards are making us into walking zombies that don't know who we are or why we are here by the end of this so-called treatment." Jones finished his thoughts becoming distracted as he saw Gary dancing. He smiled again as he realized Gary was being freed from his repressed mind, being freed from this place. "Yeah! Go Gary Go!" Jones shouted, laughing as he danced alongside Gary. "Jones looks like he's healing too." one of the nurses observed. After spending two weeks inside of the Ward, Jones had set himself up to know every name, acting within the routines, while placing his imagination on hold and making connections with patients and doctors alike. Jones would be able to go back and collect all of his data after it was all over.

A nurse walked up to Jones, "Today you graduate from the routine." Jones could only think enough to put his thumb up. He was going to have to figure out a way to get off the sedating pills to get out of the Ward. At Jones' hearing for release, he learned that Doctor K., his psychiatrist from the Outpatient Therapy office, had written a letter demanding the release of Jones. This was coupled with his mother's basic coaching skills and knowledge of the California Mental Health State Law, Section 5250. This Section details the grounds for holding a patient against their will and patient advocacy policies. These two factors require that the facility relinquish the outcomes of all studies about their patients; in other words, did the facility programs make their patients better? As the facility was slowly losing their test subjects due to Jones' antics, they decided they could no longer keep him there. The facility tried to transfer him to an affiliate, but this move was intercepted by legalities. Doctor W., head Psychiatrist of the Locked Ward, waved his arms in anger at Jones during the 5250 hearing. Trying to keep his composure as he knew Jones had

CHAPTER SIXTEEN – MUSICAL HEART

won, he nodded at Jones and acknowledged that he had successfully beat the galactic prison system. On a parallel path, Mira, the CIA informant who had predicted Jones' demise by getting too close to understanding energy, had now realized through Jones' harmless interactions with her, that they were following a dead trace to try to capture Nepharius. At least, that's the impression that Jones had given her.

As Jones walked towards the front of the locked doors Zaya waited for him, "Goodbye Jones." she said. Zaya's parents came into the Locked Ward to talk to her as she was also being released soon. By Zaya's good deeds Jones was protected while in the Locked Ward. She did her duty. The universe seemed to be rooting for Jones at this point as everywhere he went, he was surrounded by people who supported him. As the four locked-down doors unlocked, a taxi cab prepared to take Jones back to where he thought would be his home. He treaded forward to the cab, after signing the release forms in his name. "Ah, freedom!" Jones said to himself. "Finally! I get to feel the sun on my own skin on my own terms." The sun shined down as a sense of warmth hit Jones' body. He saw the taxi cab, except it was no normal taxi cab. It had a symbol on the back — a triangle as if it was transportation for people that needed to hide from the world. A man walked up to Jones and smiled, "We have specific instructions to take you to another place where you'll have more freedom." He was dressed in a white shirt and wore a white hat. He wasn't forceful, but clearly, he was prepared to chase Jones in the event of Jones running the other way.

Jones had not seen this type of vehicle before. The transportation, all painted in silver and black, shined brightly. The rims smaller than the entire van were noticeable. Jones spotted the triangular caution symbol on the back as his bag was placed in the cargo area. He hopped into the taxi where six empty gray seats were. The taxi cab driver sat alone upfront. As the man pressed the 'Push to Start' button he started to talk, "How are you feeling?" he asked Jones. He stared briefly back at him in the rearview mirror, as if he was driving Jones to the airport. Jones was impressed by how smoothly the large van drove as he expected the ride to be bumpy. "I'm feeling well, thanks. You?" Jones asked in return, not sure why the taxi driver was making small talk. "Are you able to think well lately?" the driver started to pry, almost as if he was one of the doctors watching after Jones. "Well, I suppose so. But these pills are blocking off my imagination."

Jones replied directly to the Taxi driver turned psychiatrist. "That's alright. That will fade in a few weeks." The taxi driver-psychiatrist reassured Jones, who had already put on ten pounds, after being fed the most fattening foods possible during his stay in the Ward. "You're in what's called sleep debt. Have you ever thought about what that means?" the psychiatrist asked. The Taxi driver was trying to make sure that Jones understood where his questioning was headed. "No! Sleep debt?" Jones asked. "Sleep debt is when someone hasn't slept for a long time. The body falls behind and, in the mind, you might start to hallucinate. Ever hear of that?" The taxi driver was friendly, almost too friendly. "Where are we going?" Jones asked, trying to make sense of his situation as he was driven away from the front doors of the Locked Ward. "I thought I was going home." For a moment Jones didn't care as he was already being watched by the galaxy, though they wanted little to do with him now that he was currently captured. In reality, the galactic people hid in disguise trying to break him out slowly from the clutches of the studies. "We're headed to Angel Housing. Much less commotion there." the Taxi driver said in reply. As Jones sat in the Taxi buckled into the back seat, he silently looked towards the side doors of the car. He was unable to see out the window at the sun that had just shined down at him outside of the Locked Ward.

After what seemed to Jones to be a long drive towards Sonoma, the car stopped. "Alright, you'll be staying here at this location for a couple of weeks. Check yourself in." said the Taxi Driver-Psychiatrist. "You will be protected here, you know…from them." The Taxi Driver got out of the car to greet a slender woman. She had long brown hair and blue eyes. "Come on Jones. Get out of the car. Put your clothes and personal things

CHAPTER SIXTEEN – MUSICAL HEART

upstairs. We already cleaned the room out for you. Each one of you has your separate rooms here." said the slender woman with a welcoming voice. She waved Jones forward as Jones shook her hand. At least staying at this residential care center, he wasn't in lockdown. He could feel that there was a lower level of security. He would only be watched briefly here rather than every waking moment. "What's your name?" Jones asked politely, trying to make peace with the situation he had been placed in. "Gilly," she said in return. "Head upstairs and unpack your things." Jones realized he still had a bag of items from when he fainted in the Courtroom. The memory passed through Jones' mind as he slowly went upstairs. As he looked through the bag, his brown hat was not there. However, a sweater and change of clothes were there. One pair of broken glasses that he had put on earlier and one shaver were left untouched. His phone and pair of headphones were also stuck within the bag. The feeling of what had recently happened felt long ago as he shuffled through his items. "Where's my hat?" he said quietly to himself attempting to get settled.

Aloe sunscreen lies in the desk drawer along with a small selection of shampoos when Jones would be able to take a shower. His beard had grown too long to be able to be clean-shaven. Now spiky, the beard would have to be buzzed off first, so Jones left the razor on the counter not bothering. Seeing the Aloe sunscreen brought back another memory. During his time in the Ward, Zaya told him a bit of information, "You know, if you want your hair back, all you need to do is use Aloe from the natural plant. I've seen that stuff be used on the scalp and people had silky hair afterward." Jones smiled at the thought. He missed his hair and Zaya too. Jones quickly unpacked and got into a pair of shorts that were left for him on the bed. He assumed the shorts had a monitor in them and that was how the place would be able to keep track of him every step of the way. As he went back downstairs, he saw three chairs that sat outside the glass door to the backyard. The place was as if he was living in a small college house again. The only difference was that most sharp objects were locked away as if the people living there were little kids, not college students.

A lady was sitting out by the chairs smoking a cigarette as Jones made his way outside. She was pacing back and forth while talking to her mother over the phone. This woman was much older than Jones. "Hey! Newcomer!" she said to Jones, noticing him right as she hung up. "Hey," Jones said, feeling shy about the situation, not knowing what to expect. "I've been watching you. You're a pretty interesting guy," she said. "Name's Bey." as she reached out to shake his hand. "Bey?" Jones said in return, "Do you rap or something?" She laughed as she delivered a short rap, "I used to!" She smiled nicely, seemingly hyped up on cigarettes and coffee. "So, what got you in here?" Jones asked. She replied quickly with no hesitation while laughing, "Ran from the cops. I was hiding from them for three weeks. I forgot what for though. It was weird, I felt like I was going through time and space itself for a while."

Bey wasn't a galactic watcher. Although the way Bey spoke hinted at a connection. Jones could tell that she had similar connections to galactic space without realizing it. Another person who could see the parallelisms as he might be able to. He figured that she was harmless as he looked at the wooden gate covered by trees that blocked off anyone from seeing inside. Jones went over and started looking at the rocks that stuck slightly out of the ground. Feeling bored, he hopped from rock to rock as Bey sat down smoking her cigarette observing. "How about you?" She asked Jones trying to understand the situation. "Well, kinda similar. At this point, I want to get back home." Jones said. "It's not so free here." Bey laughed, "True, but much better than elsewhere!" Jones shook off the thought. This time there were no security guards, only two staff that walked around the house. The other two roommates staying at the house had yet to wake up. Jones wandered back towards the house as he looked back out the door from the inside trying to understand where he was.

"We're going to serve lunch soon." one of the staff said, looking directly at Jones as she guided him regarding the routine. "So, do we clean our own dishes here or do you have to take care of us as if we were three years old

CHAPTER SIXTEEN – MUSICAL HEART

again?" asked Jones sarcastically. She laughed at Jones' remark. "No, more like five years old. You can call me Stacy." Stacy held a buttered knife in her hand as she reached over to a piece of toast that sat on a plate. "Jones, why don't you take a bit of toast and eat? It seems you've been overeating. We'll go outside and get some exercise in a moment." Stacy said kindly. Jones looked out the window again towards where a larger apartment complex was. A park must be nearby in the distance as he could hear teens shooting basketball hoops and children swinging on swings. Stacy looked at Jones as he had sat down by the kitchen table to eat. The peacefulness that pursued in the eerie quietness gave Jones a melancholy feel about the residential care place as he bit into his toast. He savored the feeling of being able to finally walk around on his own accord with the little space that residents were allowed to go. A man came through the front door of the house carrying pesticides on the back of him. To Jones, chemicals usually would give off an obvious smell of danger but as the man sprayed the rose bushes on the outside of the house, the smell of root beer rose into the air. Jones tried to make sense of it as he had expected a terrible smell. "Yeah. Next, candy canes are going to start coming out of the bushes too." Jones joked to himself as the voices from the galactic intercom were no longer communicating directly into Jones' head.

Bey stared at Jones as she went back inside to sit on the couch. She began writing down rap bars while talking about her lack of being able to go home. Jones sat there contemplating his next move in silence as the man with the weed killer quickly finished his job wandering back through and out the front door of the house. Another man trudged down the stairs towards the couch. This time the steps came from the room above near his. Jones expected the footsteps to be from someone who was also high energy but this man was old. He looked to be about eighty as he stumbled towards the couch. "Ah, a newcomer I see. Stacy, did you get my toast?" the man asked, acknowledging Jones at the same time as he sat on the couch. Jones looked towards the man feeling peculiar about the whole situation. "Yeah, I'm a bit new. Do you like music?" Jones asked. Jones' mindset was always on following the music as the sound had always taken him somewhere new, somewhere towards the life of the party. The man sat down and started his story, "Well when I was a young boy, I used to sing a lot." Jones quickly interrupted him, "Your toast?" Jones pointed to the man's lunch plate on the kitchen table. "Oh, right, my toast." the old man looked over at the table briefly and back at the couch.

"I almost forgot to ask, what's your name?" Jones wondered as he surveyed the man making sure that he would be friendly towards Jones rather than a nuisance. "Well, it's George." the man said looking back over at the toast as he got up to go eat. Stacy called out Gilly's name to help the old man as she put out his pills in front of him with some water. "Take this," Stacy said firmly. The man took the pill with little hesitation as he quickly ate the toast. Crumbs with bits of jam fell onto the decorative plate. Gilly came over and cleaned the plate, placing it softly into the sink. "Now, where was I?" George said aloud. "Ah, yes I was always a decent singer you see. I have my guitar here." He pointed to a carrying case that was off to the side near the T.V. and the glass door that led to the backyard. Jones looked at George, interested in his story, "Well I never really learned how to sing..." Jones hesitated, trailing off. George replied, "You know how you sing, right? Just take your finger and stick it inside of your ear so you can hear yourself. Make a little AH sound of the note you're trying to hit. When you feel you've matched up! Voila!" he laughed a hearty laugh. Jones hadn't heard of this technique before. As he tried to use it landing a similar note of the scaling system. Now singing, "Do-re-mi-fa-so-la. Hey, you're right!" Jones exclaimed.

It wasn't long before they connected through music. Jones didn't realize, however, that by him being there, a commotion was soon to follow. One more resident had been sleeping upstairs close by and could hear the new voice singing. Jones headed back upstairs to his room. He took the bottle of sunscreen with aloe in it towards his head. He spiked up the remaining hair that he had. After coming back down, he received several

CHAPTER SIXTEEN – MUSICAL HEART

looks. "What are you doing?" Stacy asked. Jones explained what he had heard about using aloe to restore hair growth from Zaya's explanation in the Locked Ward. Elly had also told him about natural healing as that was how she operated within the world. Jones recalled his conversation with Elly, "Argon oil will specifically help and naturally heal you as well. I can feel your energy. Write me some time." Elly's voice rang through Jones's head. He looked back towards his now spiky hair in the mirror, wearing sunscreen almost as hair gel. It hardened as if there was no difference between the shampoo he was using and this sunscreen. Stacy looked over at Jones, surveying him for a moment. She sighed, "You're weird but suit yourself." She went back over to the table to clean up. Bey called Jones over, "Hey! When we go outside for our walk, we can hang out on the swings! That will be fun."

Jones was still trying to understand where he was and what to expect as the day went, further along, waiting for the midafternoon to come up. In the Angel Housing, it was almost as if time itself had stopped. The outside world meant nothing more than the sun rising and falling as sound and noise almost felt nonexistent to him. Was this a healing house? Was he studying? Jones couldn't make heads or tails of the place as he went over to where the door and gate locks were. He supposed that the place was meant to treat them as if they were regressed children. "I suppose that's how I will treat this place. Gilly must be a galactic angel. After all, we are in a place named Angel Housing." Jones thought to himself as the T.V. sat quiet, untouched. "Jones, we have to be sure you get more rest," Stacy yelled out from the kitchen, her voice brisk, making sure that the routines were properly followed. "Remember, you're in sleep debt. You have a lot to pay back towards all of that sleep you've been lacking."

Jones sat there smiling and then headed back to the chairs that sat outside in the sun trying to gain enough energy to move around. He hadn't felt the weight of the sleep debt on his shoulders until Stacy mentioned the possibility of it. The roses now looked more beautiful to him as he noticed their yellow and red sprouts. He began questioning if his ideas would ever come to life under the supervision of an enclosed world, the world hidden away in its own reality. The final roommate awoke as he walked down the stairs wearing a green cap with blonde hair showing underneath. The man headed directly outside and started doing several pushups as he pulled out a cigarette. The people surrounding Jones were stressed by the life they had surrounding them. "Hi, Jones," he said, introducing himself to the man with the blonde hair starting to smoke. "Hey." the man said, not wanting to respond further. "Do you like anime?" Jones asked, trying to start a conversation as the man wore a shirt with various video-game characters on it. "Oh, bro! Of course, I do! The name is Axel." his face lit up from a cautious, sour look to a full-on smile. "So, what brought you here?" Jones asked out of curiosity trying to figure out who was a watcher and who was simply in here from their connections. Jones started to realize he wasn't alone in the galactic world. "Axel is a cool name by the way!" Jones said, trying to encourage him to talk.

"Yeah, man. I'm here because I had no place to go. I was living under a bridge and I don't get along with my Pops, you know?" Axel continued, "Just wanted to play some video games and keep away from Pops. Didn't feel like home was home anymore." Jones couldn't relate as he listened to Axel's story about how he landed himself inside of the Angel Housing placement. Jones stared for a moment, trying to change the subject when he noticed Axel had a tattoo drawing on his arm. "Whoa! Is that?" Jones asked, looking amusedly at the videogame character. "Yeah, it is!" he said smiling. "Sick!" said Jones as he admired the blonde-haired video character wearing a green sock hat carrying a steel sword sitting on Axel's arm. Jones also noticed a triangle drawn on Axel's other arm. This was the first time Jones saw a tattoo so formant. A message suggesting that he might know about galactic space. "Hey, we are getting ready to go exercise and draw for a bit," Axel stated as he seemed to know the routine of the place. Jones responded with a nod. "Okay, everyone. Time to go for a walk." Gilly said as Stacy started cooking again.

CHAPTER SIXTEEN – MUSICAL HEART

The four residents lined up at the front door as Gilly escorted them out unlocking the door. They headed towards the park where big trees stuck out above the rooflines. George walked ahead singing to himself while Bey looked at the sky blissfully. Axel walked behind with Jones, conversing a little bit about their favorite T.V. shows.

Bey called out, "Hey look at that!" The branches of the trees in the park hung lower than usual as the gloominess teemed over the sidewalk. Almost as if the group from Angel Housing had a disease, people waved from a distance. Jones simply smiled back, walking and feeling the sun as he made his way through the park around the corner towards a neighborhood. Gilly stopped for a moment, "Now we don't usually do this walk, but our instructor will be showing up in a moment to take us through the neighborhood." she smiled. "So, for now here's some chalk to draw on the sidewalk along with the swings if you get bored." The entire park was empty as Gilly handed each of them some chalk. "Now if this was candy, I'd eat it," Bey remarked jokingly as she started to draw. Axel followed shortly behind as George decided to rest over by a tree. Axel drew the same character that was on his arm as Jones grabbed a piece of chalk. He started to draw an eyeball much like the one in the masthead of Nebulous Magazine. He wrote under it 'Musical Warrior', smiling to himself at the thought of helping develop the Universe around him. Bey looked up for a moment as she finished her drawing of a few scribbles. Axel finished his drawing, demonstrating his artistry skill. "Wow!" Jones said surprised by Axel's vigor and abilities to draw. Bey tapped on Jones' shoulder, "Hey, let's go to the swings." Jones shrugged as he figured there would be no harm in it. After all, he was still in captivity under watch. "Alright." Jones agreed as he went towards the swing and sat on it. Bey sat on the other swing next to him. Each swing had old steel chains with a black swing below them. The two of them started to rock back and forth. "Hey Bey, you know when I was a kid, I used to swing trying to see how far I could jump after I was at the peak." Jones laughed. Bey looked back over at him and laughed, filled with energy as she tried to see how high she could swing. Bey went faster and faster, getting higher and higher as she made goofy noises each time trying to add comedy to the situation that they were stuck in. Jones stopped trying as he was getting too high while Bey continued on. The metal chains started to smack up against one another. "Hey Bey, you should slow down," Jones warned as she kept going, testing the boundaries of the swing. As Bey was coming down her foot hit the wood chips spiraling the swing out of control. She fell off. The swing continued as it wrapped around the bar up top, now fully out of commission. Jones went over to Bey and helped her up. "Are you okay?" Jones asked, concerned about her wellbeing. After all, Jones had coaxed her on to test her capabilities and how far she would go. He didn't expect her not to listen.

"That was really fun," she said jokingly as Jones went back over and started walking towards the group. An older lady with gray hair arrived waving at Gilly. "Thanks for watching over these four while I was gone," she said mysteriously. The instructor surveyed the situation. She had kind eyes. George got up from his rest and gathered around her. Jones and Bey treaded slowly towards the group, with Jones trying to gain an idea of what was going on. "Right the neighborhood," Jones said to himself remembering Gilly's words as he gathered up behind the instructor. Jones, Axel, and Bey all started walking behind the instructor as George followed behind feeling tired. "I'm going back to the house," George said, hoping to catch a break from the exercise. The instructor looked at him for a moment thinking about the situation. "George, try to walk a little first. If you feel tired then we will take you back" the instructor said. George waved back to her, "Bah, I'm not in the mood for a walk." Jones looked up towards the sky wondering how his day would be moving along. The instructor and the rest of them started walking through the neighborhood as Jones looked at the green bush standing right in front of him. He blinked twice. The green bush turned pink, as purple flowers sprouted out of the bush. Purple needlegrass surrounded the bush keeping Jones from approaching the plant to pick the leaves.

"Do you walk this path often?" Jones asked the instructor curious about

CHAPTER SIXTEEN – MUSICAL HEART

why the four of them were walking this pathway. "No, not usually," she said nonchalantly. "This is the first time we've been this way." Jones quieted down wondering if that was the case. After every unusual situation he had been in, the people always seemed to be disappearing or retiring on him. Jones and the others quietly walked further down the road as houses were painted in various colors. The instructor stopped for a moment as she eyeballed the tree. "Huh, I wonder what kind of tree that is?" the instructor asked. The tree stood out aflame as if it was growing copper inside of it. As the group walked further into the neighborhood, a star sat in the middle of the road showcasing flowers as if it were a giant cookie box. Jones didn't understand. He walked around the star getting a full angle of it. "What? Planter boxes don't usually look like this. Next, we'll have statues with flowers on them and names written out in cement letters." Jones said half-jokingly and half out loud. The instructor laughed overhearing Jones as the group walked further. Jones had stared at the sun directly turning the whole world red and the sun green due to the colors, but nothing like this had ever happened before. Reality had already mixed with his galactic world, these plants becoming all too real in a mixture he thought he had put behind him. As the group continued to walk and eye the scenery, new species of plants that he didn't recognize kept appearing in various lawns throughout the neighborhood.

Jones turned to Bey, "Ever seen something like this before?" he asked her, remembering the pink bush and copper tree they had passed earlier. She quietly shook her head no. "So, it's not only me seeing these things," Jones said in awe. "Okay, we have to get you back now." the instructor interrupted. She turned around towards the end of the neighborhood cul-de-sac. She noticed that Jones had been returning to galactic space. She smiled feeling accomplished that the walk had met its goal. "I've been around here many times, but never in this part," Axel said as he felt attached to the area. "Time to go Axel and don't think about going back here because construction is happening tomorrow. The whole area is going to be renovated." The instructor called out to him as everyone walked side by side turning around. Jones couldn't comprehend what had happened. He was looking for the pink bushes he passed by earlier but to no avail. The bushes showed as plain green. The woman with gray hair walked them back towards Gilly who was standing outside the house. Jones felt a sense of healing and distraught mixed between worlds.

"Hey, Gilly," Jones asked her with curiosity, wondering if she was part of the world too. "Yes Jones?" she replied calmly. "Gilly, what are you going to do after this job?" Jones asked, testing out her knowledge of the world. "I'm going back to school in Oregon. I have studies to finish," she replied. Jones was right. Retirement followed him into the shadows between light, dark, and the balance of chi that he had been saying to everyone. These people were still there for him and solely because Jones needed to be watched over. Jones walked back into the house as the instructor was greeted by Stacy. "Good to see you, it's been a long time!" Stacy exclaimed, letting it slip out. Jones went over to the couch to sit down as Axel turned on the T.V. popping in the anime series. "You've never seen this have you?" Axel asked Jones. As Jones sat there in his thoughts trying to make sense of the situation, he finally responded, "No, I haven't." Jones's hair was no longer spiky as he stopped using the aloe sunscreen and started to use shampoo properly. Jones continued to want to read everything in detail, but his need for taking it literally slowly vanished. Red no longer meant always dangerous. Yellow didn't always mean happy anymore and shirts didn't represent who people were. Jones sat there for a moment relaxing as George went back upstairs to sleep. Bey went back outside to catch the sun that was waiting for her.

Jones's roommate turned to him, eyeing him for a moment. "I don't quite understand. Is this where you first started to document your journey? Why did you wait so long?" he asked. Jones sat in the psych ward pondering the question for a moment. "Well, it didn't occur to me as with most people, to write down their journeys as they happened. Since we can't document everything that happens, I figured I would try. At that moment I decided to

CHAPTER SIXTEEN – MUSICAL HEART

write. For you, for me, for those who must know. Many secrets are hidden in books, right?" Jones replied. Jones got up out of the bed and picked up a pen twirling it around. "Are you going to keep reading?" he asked the roommate. His roommate sat there, "Can I have that pudding, Jones? I'm a bit hungrier now." A staff member overheard the two, "Next time eat your lunch on time Le- ", the staff member warned. The roommate quickly cut her off, "No problem, alright." he replied. The roommate turned back to Jones," I'd like to hear about your first-time writing. You know, revelations and all of that." he said. Jones looked directly at the roommate, "Let's keep reading then. Sounds like you're up for it." The roommate picked up Jones' journal again, turning the next page. He started narrating over the words that Jones started to write while inside the residential care facility. Jones started to write while anime played in the background. He was reminiscing about his journey to himself. He sat down taking a pen and paper to write in his journal for the first time.

The Watchers Way – My Journal Page 1

Back when I was in Monterey Bay, I had climbed the hillside when the clouds and sun mixed. Two kids sat on the hillside. Out of their curiosity, they were trying to break into the same world as mine. "That popstar is a werewolf," one kid yelled, calling out to me. "We're actually 30 and 40 years old and we've been reborn", the other kid followed up yelling as they approached me. When I told them to go back into their house, the two children refused. Since they were a part of the Spirit of Music's neighborhood, it only made sense that the two would say ridiculous statements. Later one of them texted me, somehow obtaining my number from a person around that area. He asked me for help, texting that he was stuck, saying he had tried lack of sleep and that he was now stuck in the forest. "There's a bear here and an evil man. Help me please!" The texts appeared on my phone. So, I texted him back that he was in his own mind and to follow his footsteps home. I advised the kid to stay away from the bear and to not keep track of the bear following him. If he ignored the bear, it would eventually disappear, leaving him alone.

Later on, the child texted that he had made his way home successfully. He said that I was right and he thanked me. Axel looked over Jones' shoulder as he wrote, "What the fuck are you writing about?" he laughed as he read what Jones had written. Jones recalled his journey, "Just a tidbit that happened while I was visiting an old friend in Monterey Bay." Axel smiled, "Watch the Anime, will you? This part is really cool. You're going to miss them warring over different universes and being the destroyer of worlds." Jones looked back at the T.V. He put his pen down and sat back, watching as he relaxed back into the couch. He crumpled up the paper and threw it away. "Yeah, sounds good to me!" Jones said aloud. After a while of watching the two of them went to the kitchen where dinner was now being served. Stacy yelled out calling everyone to the table. She sighed as she got out various foods in containers from the fridge. "This time everyone will get their food from the containers and clean up after themselves. If you cannot do that then I will have to send you to your room." Stacy said nicely, but firmly. Everyone nodded following instructions as the dinner was laid out on the plates. Jones was no longer taking the strong pills as the dosages had been lowered. "After dinner, we have to give you these Jones. I know you're not a fan, but give us an easy time and take them." Stacy announced, being direct and to the point. Jones didn't want to argue as he could taste freedom by doing as he was told. Soon he would be out and not have to follow anybody's direction. "What's this?" Jones asked making small talk with Stacy as she looked back over at him. "Nevermind looks good," Jones said, taking the plate to sit down. "Gravy and mashed potatoes are over there." Stacy pointed to the containers as he got back up grabbing a glass of milk. Chicken also sat on the counter.

"Finally, a real meal. Not this packaged stuff." Jones said happily, eating as he felt like he hadn't been feeding his body ever since he was captured. Bey played a song with the title "Food is good." Trying to communicate her feelings without saying a word at all. Watchers often communicated

CHAPTER SIXTEEN – MUSICAL HEART

this way Jones had learned after each quiet encounter "Jones!" Mira went through his mind as he took a bite. "Jones, this place is meant to normalize you, to get rid of your imagination and blend you back into society." Jones replied in his thoughts, "Why are you helping me still? I thought you had lost interest." Mira replied with no hesitation whispering in his mind, "I'm doing this because Nepharius is still out there, stealing from our sacred places. Atlantis is burning." "You know that place is underwater, right?" Jones said in return. "Underwater because they disobeyed their vows and went to war." Mira replied, "Yes, Atlantis is literally burning. Nepharius has stolen the relics making himself more powerful, untouchable almost." Jones replied, "I have no intentions of stopping that space pirate. It's you who got me in here!" Jones raised his voice in his mind. "Shh, or they will hear you," Mira said. "Jones?" Stacy said, tapping him. "Are you going to eat your food?" She leaned in to see if he was paying attention. "Yeah of course! I was already scarfing it down, see?" Jones showed the plate mostly eaten. "Looked like you were daydreaming," Stacy replied curiously.

"I've got the dishes!" Bey offered taking up all the plates as Jones got back to eating, finishing down his last few bites. "I need to rest!" Jones exclaimed as he went up towards his room. "Take this before you go." Stacy took the yellow and blue pills mixing them together as she put water next to him in a paper cup. "Right." Jones took the pills as instructed, his mind going back as if a limiter had been put on his imagination. Although the alarm clock sat on his table slightly off from time where time was irrelevant. In the house, Jones still paid attention to the sun going down. "It'll be night soon," Jones said to himself laying on the bed. "I suppose I'll have to explore more tomorrow about these people." Jones slowly closed his eyes, falling asleep into nothingness. His thoughts were being blocked as his body drifted off into a deep sleep. "Time to catch up on that sleep debt," he said to himself, chuckling at the thought of the coined term. "I owe it to myself".

Chapter Seventeen – Imagination Reincarnation

The next day, Jones woke up bright and early as he looked outside at the sun that shined down into his room across the bed. He was prepared for another warm day as he slid out of his pajamas and put on a T-shirt and shorts. Warm water came out of the sink as Jones splashed a little on his face. He stumbled down the stairway towards the front of the house to where George sat on the couch already playing a musical tune. "Heya, George!" Jones said, waving to him. "What?" George asked in reply. "I said good morning!" Jones replied with the same cheerful tone of voice, trying not to startle George who was strumming the guitar. "Oh, hey Jones, I'm having a guest of mine visit from Church today," George said, turning towards him, now paying attention. Jones sat on the couch as he reached for peanuts set out in the glass bowl. "From Church?" Jones sat, questioning George. "Yeah, he's almost here," said George. Jones looked around in question as everyone else seemed to be asleep or in the kitchen.

"Well, alright," Jones said, abruptly closing the conversation. Right as the words left Jones' lips a man knocked on the door. "That must be him," George said as Stacy went over to the front to greet the visitor. He came in wearing a bright red shirt and a black felt hat. The man also had a guitar on his back as he came into pat George on the back. "Tim, how are you?" George said as he smiled towards Tim's company. Gilly shut

CHAPTER SEVENTEEN – IMAGINATION REINCARNATION

the front door as Stacy went back to the kitchen. Tim had to sign a guest sheet of paper showing he had come. "Well, you sell yourself to the Devil and the Devil's going to come and get you. Ain't that right George?" Tim said jokingly as he strung a note on the guitar. "I hear your name is Jones. Can you sing too?" Tim looked over at Jones. Jones replied to the man, noticing the energy around Tim. Risks were a big part of this man's life. "Yeah, George taught me a little about how to sing on key." Jones stuck one finger in his ear and sang out a note. "Not bad. Let's sing for a while together." Tim requested. Jones got off the couch and went over to the sun. Tim sat down on the couch next to George with his guitar. The two of them started singing as Jones sat in a nearby chair writing down lyrics from thoughts in his head.

George strummed the guitar slowly at first as Tim encouraged the playing to go faster. Jones started singing along trying to keep up. He hit each note as he sat idly by singing songs he didn't know well. He knew that if he wanted to get better, he would have to practice. This was one of the best ways to do so for Jones. Tim started strumming the guitar faster and faster as George sang along. "Keep up ya' old bean," Tim said laughing. He gave off the feeling of a man who stole others' time and soul through music. Jones had enough as he stood up to go upstairs. An hour had passed and there was still more to explore within the house. "Hey, Jones!" Bey waved him over, "I'm headed home tomorrow so it looks like I'll be seeing you later!" she said smiling hyped up on coffee. Jones looked back at her, "Alright, stay off those swings." he said, unable to imagine or conjure up much as the pills were still in effect in his system. Bey laughed, "I'm not leaving yet dummy. We still have time to hang out." As Jones had been stuck in a place, her leaving meant a new roommate would be coming in tomorrow. Jones looked towards the pieces of papers and drawings within the house as Stacy came over to where the scissors were locked away. "What do you need out of here?" Stacy asked him. Jones sat for a moment, "Nothing actually, I was wondering what all of these drawings represented."

Stacy turned towards Jones as if she had not been asked this question before. "They're drawn by previous adults who have been here. Drawing therapy is a thing you know," she replied. Axel, waking up, came down the stairs to join in with the commotion, "This lithium is too strong Stacy." he said the first thing. "We'll see if we can lower your dosage in a day or two," replied Stacy. Axel complained that he couldn't think, the same as Jones had been saying. Bey paced quickly back and forth. "I can't wait to see my daughter!" she said excitedly. Jones didn't know what to say. All of the drawings spoke to him from the walls as this Residential Care house had been around for a long, long time. "Jones, it seems you're almost caught up on your sleep debt and functioning in society. I'll have a call in to have you picked up and taken back home in a couple of days." Stacy said. This brought Jones out of his reverie. Jones had just begun to grow used to the place and it started to feel like home. Jones went over to Axel and smiled at him as Axel smiled back. The two of them bonded over small talk and sharing of their stories. "This sucks! Man, as soon as I leave this place, I'll have nowhere to go." Axel sighed looking back at Jones. "Well, how about your dad's?" Jones asked. Axel stood there for a moment dreading the words that he had just heard.

"My dad's not chill, man. I'm telling you. It will be hard." Axel continued. Jones thought for a moment as the artist struggled with the thought of going home. "Isn't going home better than trying to live under a bridge? Right?" Jones threw this out there, questioning Axel's position. "Yeah, well, maybe," Axel replied, thinking about getting back in touch with his father. Jones felt bad as he continued to stare at the paintings on the wall. "That's the way life goes, I suppose. What are you going to do when you get out of here?" Jones questioned Axel again, hoping for a more optimistic response. "Like I said man, go back under the bridge. It's my only home. I'll give my Pops a call, but I doubt—," said Axel, who stopped for a moment. It was clear he didn't want to continue the conversation. "Let's just sit down and finish watching some Anime." His brain churned about the thought of having to rekindle back with society. Over the next few hours, the four of

CHAPTER SEVENTEEN – IMAGINATION REINCARNATION

them talked, playing board games and sitting down discussing the dosages of their medications. The four residents had brought together a symbiosis and in a short bonding time, they also healed together as the day went by. Since Bey was leaving tomorrow, Jones figured he wouldn't be seeing her again. Jones was dead wrong on that premise. As night fell, he went up the stairs to his room. The pictures on the wall downstairs became clear in his mind as the pills let up a bit. Although he had gained a lot of weight and his beard started growing in, Jones refused to let his imagination falter. Merging the drawings in his mind and giving them actions in his head, pieces faded in and out as his thoughts wandered. Jones was falling asleep.

"With all this power and knowledge, there is no way I can let up here," Jones said to himself quietly as he turned over trying to get comfortable. Down the hallway, a resident started to yell in their sleep. Jones put on his headphones to drown out the noise closing his eyes. "Are they really healing us here?" Jones asked himself, questioning his sanity. "Am I really the insane one, or are all these people around me the insane ones? Keeping the world plain as it is? Or not developing each small piece of it by every action we do?" Which is worse?" Jones wasn't sure if he should let the galactic space world go at this point. There was so much to accomplish from all walks of life. He knew he could lead from the front if given the right tools and chance from the watchers. As he laid there within his head thinking of what little he could, he was continuing to question himself and imagine the paintings on the wall downstairs. Suddenly a man from the sandwich shop in Monterey Bay popped into his head. Clear as a day as Jones was in his dream state. Jones also remembered walking into a small shop that had a black and grey sweater for sale, and a hoodie that could come off at will when worn. The shop sold clothing from the future as if unreleased works in progress were being displayed to the world. This shop was hidden away in a small sector of the mall. "There must be some way people energize themselves and get around quickly over here," Jones said to himself in his dreams, reminiscing further about what happened in Monterey.

The shop owner walked over to Jones as he sat there looking back at him. "Can I help you sir?" the man asked Jones. "Yeah, I'm Vextrous Fortunata, Fortunata for short. I'm looking at those sweaters over there. Got a heater in them?" he asked the shop owner. The man laughed, "No. But for you, only fifteen bucks instead of thirty." Jones remembered the shop owner as he lay in his bed at Angel Housing in a semi- dream state. "Only fifteen? Alright!" Jones said excitedly grabbing the sweater, paying for it, and running towards the door. Jones walked from there over to the sandwich shop. "Make me something new," Jones said to the man across the other side of the counter as the guy looked back at him. "Well, here's my favorite. It's not on the menu." The man got to work making the sandwich faster than normal. Jones knew he had hit the jackpot of watchers and galactic beings at this Mall. "I need to use the restroom," Jones said to the man making his food. "Yeah, right around the corner," said the sandwich shop man.

Jones wandered looking for the teleportation device. He figured it was somewhere hidden away as an average everyday item. He wandered in and out around the store trying to take a quick peek before the man finished making his sandwich. Jones didn't want to get caught. He paid normally as he had attracted too much attention already. "Alright. Thanks!" Jones said to the man walking out of the store. Jones had failed to find the teleportation device as he sat on a star in the patio area outside of the shops staring up at the sky. The star embedded in the ground in giant red and black had the same location as the stars up in the sky. Jones wondered if this was how the watchers communicated in their free time as they worked their way around the town. Jones woke up from his thoughts, looked at the clock, and saw it was already morning at Angel Housing. By the time he wandered downstairs, Bey was at the front door talking to her mother who had arrived to pick her up. She was all packed and ready to drive home. "See you soon Jones!" Bey said as she waved goodbye.

Jones waved back at Bey not expecting much as another lady came through

CHAPTER SEVENTEEN – IMAGINATION REINCARNATION

the door. This time the lady had curly white hair and was much older. Her eyes drooped down as if she hadn't slept decently in years. The dark tones under her eyes stared back at Jones as he sat on the couch. "Hi, I'm Jones. What type of music do you like?" Jones asked, trying to be friendly. "Motown. I just want my peace and quiet. Everyone around me is dead. Nothing matters. Motown keeps me sane." the lady replied. Jones had nothing further to say. He had listened to her rant and he didn't want to upset the lady more. Jones for the first time didn't want to get to know the lady either. "Oh, sorry about that," Jones said, trying to offer comfort as he backed away towards the other side of the room. George was already in the common room and had permission to bring a couple more friends over this time. George was a much louder guy as he and his friends began playing music. The old lady told George to keep the music down as the new resident was unable to stabilize. "Keep it down or I'll scream" she yelled. Stacy intervened trying to keep the two residents calm at that moment. This was the first time that Jones visualized anger at Angel Housing as he could feel the negative energy pass over to him. Stacy moved swiftly, breaking the two apart.

"George, go outside, please!" Stacy said in a tone that was understood by everyone. Without questioning or even fighting back, George led his friends outside to chat up and play music. At this point, Jones wanted to leave. He felt there was no more reason for him to be a resident there as he was now functioning fully. "Hey Stacy, my time is up, tomorrow right? Jones asked her, hoping for a good response. "Yeah actually, you've got today being one of your final days," Stacy replied. "I'm not going anywhere else after this, right?" Jones questioned making sure this time he would be fully free of the studies done by the nurses in the building. "We have everything we need to know about you. When you are released you will be going back into therapy sessions. You will need to attend them like classes, but you are free to roam as you wish." Stacy continued. Jones got a clear answer as if he was being treated as a probationary criminal. He had nothing to reply to her as he shivered at the idea of having to be in that situation again. Jones sat there for a moment accepting that the world was moving forward regardless of his participation. By now the galactic watchers must have lost interest in him, going back to their realm. However, each of them still seemed to support him periodically from behind the scenes.

Although he had currently failed at his promise, he wasn't ready to give up on the dreams of imagination that had been taken from him. Jones was determined to reignite the comfortability of ideas into the next realm. Was it the informational age that kept everyone in a cluttered society from organizing and comparing the best? Was it the failure of capital hoarded by those at the top? Was it that those at the bottom didn't know how to play the game of life to get their ideas out there? The more Jones thought, the deeper his ideas spread, destroying his confidence in restoring the progression of humanity forward. "I'm just one man." Jones thought to himself. "What can one person do?" Axel overheard Jones mumbling to himself. "Sometimes one person has to inspire others. That's it. One person doesn't have to do anything but inspire others." Axel offered in return. Axel was trying to council Jones through as he saw him deteriorating. Jones looked over at Axel. "This place needs us more than it realizes. Why are we stuck here?" asked Jones rhetorically.

Axel turned towards Jones. "You can say the weirdest pain in the ass things sometimes dude," Axel said smiling. Jones felt a sense of gratitude and melancholy. Axel got up and went over to start drawing again. Then he headed outside to smoke another cigarette. Jones, feeling defeated, went back upstairs as he could hear George playing a song outside. "Ignore it. Ignore this way." George sang, almost as if he was trying to tell Jones his direct feelings. "Remember the end goal. Show people. Show them Jones." a familiar voice went through his head as he faded out from where he was a resident at Angel Housing. "Tomorrow. Tomorrow I will be out of here." Jones vowed. He walked over to the glass windows that looked outside as the quietness shadowed the house. The nurses were winning.

Chapter Eighteen – Chase

The next day Jones woke up to a knock on his door. Stacy called Jones' name with annoyance in her tone. "You're late Jones! Someone is here and is picking you up." Stacy said through the door. Jones called out, "Alright, let me just pack!" He needed to buy himself time to get ready. Over the two weeks of living at Angel Housing, Stacy had grown close to Jones. She tried to keep him orderly. But he needed time to organize his thoughts as well as his possessions. "Okay!!" Stacy replied storming downstairs into the front rooms. Jones, being able to connect with everybody and anybody around, had ended up turning the place towards his favor. He was happy about that. Jones quickly tossed all of his stuff in a tan carrying bag and went rushing downstairs. "Dad?" Jones exclaimed. He was surprised to see his father standing there at the front door. "Ms. P is on vacation so I'm here to pick you up and stay at the house for the week. We'll talk when you get into the car." his father said.

Jones shrugged as he wasn't sure what to expect. They walked over to the rental car as he opened up the passenger side door. "So, you're officially out." his dad looked at him, noticing that his hair had grown longer with a beard that hadn't really grown since he had seen him last. Jones wasn't sure what to say as he hid his face in shame. "A haircut is in order, I suppose." is the only reply Jones had as his father drove them back to the house. "Doctor K. tells me your therapy isn't done yet. You still have to attend the Therapist Office weekly for sessions." his dad said. "Yeah, Stacy told me," Jones replied in short. "Let's get you some lunch." his dad said after they arrived home. He got out roast beef and coleslaw and toasted it with cheese atop some making open-face sandwiches. The tension between the two of them was clear as Jones began to realize what steps his parents had taken to get him out of the mess (5250 Locked Ward of the State) and back into their custody. "Can you drive yourself to therapy?" his father asked. Jones nodded yes, as he was less zombified after two weeks at Residential Care. As he picked up the sandwich, Jones responded, "Yeah I'll go tomorrow." he said.

"Glad you're out Jones. Good to have you back." said his dad. The microwave dinged announcing his father's melted sandwich. Jones had nothing to say further so he gave a slight smile. Although he was no longer cornered by his thoughts, the galactic space kept calling him back to them, even if he was free. Jones found his iPhone in his bedroom. It had been taken from him when he entered the Locked Ward and Ms. P had kept it plugged into the wall to charge at home these past weeks. Jones grabbed the phone and announced that he was going for a walk. He headed outside as his dad flipped on the T.V. in the family room. The weather had turned colder as the months went by. Jones was so caught up in thought he hadn't noticed the changes around him. As he walked down the road filled with wind and leaves, he no longer felt the world changing around him. Jones walked forward looking for the watchers or experiences he could interact with from his world. He tried to call out to Mira but his attempt did not affect her. "Take a break, Jones. You've been working too hard trying to change the world around you." a familiar voice sounded in his head.

A spam email came up on his phone right when he thought he was out of luck: "Nepharius show canceled. Ends in disaster." Jones eyed the email as it described the musician falling on stage. Jones closed his eyes as he sat on the corner bench in town watching people walk by. The whole town seemed quiet and uninterested in Jones where watchers had turned to him before. A man walked up to Jones asking for spare change but Jones

CHAPTER EIGHTEEN – CHASE

couldn't understand him as he had before. "I'm sorry, I can't understand you," Jones said as the man pulled back his outstretched hands. The man sighed and tapped Jones' shoulder. Smiling, the man spoke inaudibly. "I don't have any spare change," Jones said as he got up. The man sighed, walking away and mumbling to himself. Seemingly unhappy that he wasn't understood.

Jones walked further down the road to sit on the bench in the park. The old sign marked with an arch-looking symbol doused in red and the red star graffitied on the wall that glistened brightly and in plain sight of the old movie theater were now gone. In their place was a simple broken-down building. Jones checked his spam email again: "If you have a sex offender in your area, get notified today!" his spam email had turned back into normality too, with no secret messages. Jones sighed as he slowly looked across the park where two fathers and their kids played together with each other. He watched for a moment thinking to himself, "I wonder if their imaginations will flourish in society today. We need new ideas." Jones got up after a moment and walked back down the road towards his own house. He stopped as a text message popped up: "The Spirit of Music would like to meet with you." Jones received a second text with a photo of a painting of the orchestra in the galaxy. "Your idea was beautiful." the text said as piano music played in the background. Jones felt a little better. "I can't come down now. Not for a while. But someday." Jones texted back.

"We'll always be watching you." was the response. Jones laughed. He wondered what else had changed during his time 'away' as he realized a haircut and a shave was much needed. When Jones reached his home, he went into the bathroom picking up a razor. But he wasn't able to shave off his beard as it had grown long and thick. "Spiky," Jones said to himself uncomfortably. "Jones, be sure to rest soon." his dad called out from the other room as Jones reached over for the yellow pill. Jones took one small dose as he sat in his room drifting off looking at the setting sun. He started reading all of the text messages that had accumulated on his phone from people he had met. He was trying to figure out if the world he had discovered was real or all in his mind. Was his mind projecting what he wished the world might be? "Bah, does it matter if it's not here?" Jones rolled over thinking to himself a moment. Text messages between Jones and Nepharius began to appear. "The magazine is complete!" an exclamation said from the last time the two of them had spoken via text. A picture of the Jeep next to Einstein sat near the ceiling of Jones' bedroom. He looked around his room and the contents. "This hat! I don't deserve this brown felt hat!" Jones said to himself. He retired the hat to the poster board pole that he decided to use as his hat hanger.

Jones rolled over and tried to sleep, dreaming of nothing. In his mind, he asked himself, "Had anything really ever been completed? What was all this for?" These were his final thoughts for the day. The next day Jones went over to the bathroom sink and scratched his beard. He went into the shower and started washing with the soap thinking about the time he felt like tasting it. "Wonder if it's possible to eat what we use? A society like that would be so useful." Jones said to himself as he finished showering. "Hey, dad. Can you take me to the barber?" Jones shouted out loud as his dad woke up from the couch. "Alright. What time?" his dad asked. Jones looked at his phone which now had many of his ideas in his Notepad area. The iCloud was now connected with his iPhone so he could upload whatever he wrote. "Huh? That's weird." Jones said to himself. He called back out loud to his dad, "In about twenty minutes." Jones smiled realizing that his family was still by his side. Jones got ready and headed out to the car where his dad waited. "Your mother is on vacation in Europe, so that's why I am here." his father explained. Jones no longer felt the claustrophobic feeling by having the windows closed while in the car. "Oh, so that's why. You mentioned it when you picked me up. Remember?" Jones replied. "Yeah, you're lucky she was able to get to you. We didn't have custody of you anymore. You became a ward of the State of California. We had no rights, even though we are your parents, your legal guardians, and are paying for your health insurance." his father said, trying not to

CHAPTER EIGHTEEN – CHASE

sound harsh.

Jones quietly sat there thinking and recalculating all of the trouble he had gone through getting in there in the first place. After a few minutes, they arrived at the barbershop. "We will be right with you." a lady at the front desk said as another man sat down next to Jones. He wore the same running shoes as could be seen in the advertisement on the wall of the barbershop. "Jump higher?" Jones thought to himself as he recalled seeing this advertisement another time on a large billboard while driving his car. The lady called Jones up to the front desk. She sat him down in the chair shortly after. "We'll need to use a buzzer for that beard first," she said. Then you can switch to a razor afterward. "That's okay." Jones quickly replied. Jones laid back as the barber started cutting his hair. He was remembering himself driving the silver car down to a car factory where he was trying to meet Gautty, the billionaire who had recently been developing new car types. Jones stood there in the parking lot looking up at the sky as a security guard in a red jacket approached him. "Can I help you?" the security guard asked. Jones stood there, "I'm going to stay here until I can meet Gautty." The security guard laughed as another man walked up to him, "What are you? Some kind of alien?"

At that moment Jones' phone went blank, completely disconnected. The security guard looked at the other man as Jones gave a distrusting face."Come on, let's grab a burrito. Kid, stay as long as you like," they said to Jones. Jones sat in his silver car parked in the factory parking lot as the spam email showed up on his phone: "I'm sorry, I can't make it." Eventually, Jones left the parking lot driving back towards his home thinking of other ways to find the men building that universal car. "Alright," Jones said to himself. "Sir, your haircut's almost done." the female barber said.

Jones came out of his thoughts. "One or two?" the barber asked him again, pointing the mirror at his neck. "Two is less short." "Let's get shorter," Jones replied as she continued to clip his hair. It was almost time for Jones to go to therapy. His dad sat there and read the magazine as the lady finished the haircut. "Have a wonderful day!" she said smiling to son in the chair and father who paid. Jones replied as people usually do when coming in and out of the haircut shop. The normalcy was hard to get used to. "Jones, feel better?" his dad asked. He was curious as to how Jones took his first outing in a month. "Yeah, I feel as if I've been reborn again." Jones perked up.

They drove back home as the clock reached 2:00 PM. His dad parked the rental car as Jones went over to the silver car in the driveway. Jones drove himself to his therapy session, thinking inside of his head about Ms. Orin and Doctor K. "Remember our offer." Ms. Orin had said to Jones almost two months ago now. After a short drive into the parking lot, Jones sat outside for a moment eyeing the traffic going by. The shadows followed the cars in perfect succession. He got out of the car after parking in the open spot right in the middle of the lot. He walked up the long flight of stairs straight into the receptionist area. Jones didn't see the receptionist that he saw before as someone new sat there smiling. "Four minutes." the receptionist said as Jones sat down. "And Ms. Orin will be ready for you soon." Jones stared around the room at the people waiting for their appointments. They looked beat up, whereas one woman sat there with her comfortable shoes on. "How are ya' kid?" the woman said, looking over at him. She had a crutch in one hand and a broken foot cast over her left shoe.

"I'm alright. Trying to get through the day." Jones said in reply. "How are you?" She looked at him with a warm smile, "Well I've seen you around. I'm here for me, working through my depression. Kids got me in a tassel." she said. "Name's Lin." holding out her hand towards Jones as he sat there. Jones shook her hand as he got called. "That's me." He got up and went through the door, past the hallway where group therapy was going on. As Jones passed by the open group therapy door, Bey sat in the chair hyped up on coffee. "Bey?" Jones exclaimed as peaked his head in the door. "Jones?" Bey shrieked, "Glad to see you!" Bey said from the room as the

CHAPTER EIGHTEEN – CHASE

rest of the crowd looked at the two of them. "I'll catch up with you in a moment," Jones said as the therapist told Bey to pay attention. "Third Floor's way more fun. Free coffee." Bey said, smiling as Jones laughed. Jones continued walking further down the hallway towards Ms. Orin's door, opening it and sitting down in the black chair. The window framed a mountain behind her desk chair in the corner of the building. Beautiful view. "Hey, Jones! How are you feeling?" Ms. Orin asked him curiously.

Jones was able to think clearly as he was now only taking a single small dosage of medication. "Well, I'm feeling alright," Jones said, not sure what to say or how much to say. "Anything you want to talk about?" Ms. Orin asked. "What about your goals?" Jones sat there for a moment contemplating why he was there. "Guess I can tell you more of my story," Jones said to Ms. Orin as they sat there facing each other. "At the peak of my…" Jones cleared his throat and started his story as Ms. Orin listened intently. "At the peak of my adventure down to Monterey Bay, I had driven there to meet the Spirit of Music. He had asked me to schedule a meeting with him sometime. As I drove hours down the road, the fog carried itself inland, coming in unannounced. The Road Warrior tab popped up on my WAZE as bikers and policemen all seemed to be lined up with one another pulled over on the side of the road while my car sped down through that fog in the middle of the night. The Spirit of Music wasn't too happy that I knocked on his door so late as he told me to go home, to get some rest and schedule rather than coming down again unannounced. Later that night I went into the gas station where I had gotten gas before and the man who had offered me a free hot dog looked at me in dismay, almost as if he knew I was going to be in here again. He handed me a hotdog that tasted more like a mixture of chicken sausage. I bit into it walking out without paying and without saying a word. After listening intently to Jones' story, Ms. Orin scribbled down some notes in her notepad.

"So, you're always a deep thinker? Thinking of ideas?" Ms. Orin asked curiously, looking at Jones as he looked out the window. "I feel as if I was taking the ideas someone else was making into a reality, into the world," Jones replied. Ms. Orin scratched her head, "You should apply for volunteer work Jones. Get productive to take your mind off things. I think it would help." Jones stared back for a moment. "Doctor K will see you now. We will talk again next week." Ms. Orin said. Jones walked further down the hallway towards where Doctor K was sitting in his office. "Hey! Good to see you, Jones. How have you been?" asked Doctor K. Jones sat there for a moment, "I've been well, Doctor K. Can I tell you more of my story?" Jones asked. Doctor K sat there for a moment contemplating, "The stories you have told me thus far are all fictional. But it's my job to listen to those in need." he said sitting back calmly, nodding to Jones to share his thoughts. "So, after I got back into town from my trip to Monterey Bay, you know, before I got locked up; I went into Walnut Creek where two men were handing out papers scrutinizing the president. One of the men sat there as he talked with me about saving the world. He gave me a CD and told me to upload it onto my computer. The Spirit of Music from Monterey Bay had told me his friends had something for me. I thought it was this CD."

Jones stated to Doctor K. Doctor K raised his eyebrows, "You were running into people during your episode?" Doctor K continued, "Sometimes people believe the CIA is chasing them or that demons and angels exist in the world. Some people believe they are one with the book they've read." Jones sat back and asked Doctor K. a question, "What about the pineal gland?" Doctor K shook his head, "It's simply a gland that produces melatonin that helps regulate sleep, nothing more." Jones wondered how many people believed in the pineal gland holding special powers, sometimes known as 'The Third Eye'. And how many were developing their spiritual aspect of life through their experiences and honing their Third Eye. "Jones, it seems you've calmed down from your episode. I'm going to take you off these pills fully and administer daily Intensive Outpatient Therapy (IOP) as the treatment plan. Why don't you head over to the door down the hallway – the IOP program will start shortly." Doctor K advised. Jones shook Doctor

CHAPTER EIGHTEEN – CHASE

K.'s hand, "Thank you. What's your last name anyway, Doctor K.?" Jones inquired. "It's K. Road, M.D." Doctor K. smiled as he walked out of his office down the hallway the other way, extending his belly. Jones went over to the door down the hallway as instructed. Bey sat in the corner still listening to the same lady as before. "Jones, why don't you take a seat?" the IOP Therapist suggested. Jones took a seat next to another woman. "Hi, I'm Pearl." she whispered, "I've got six different personalities and I swear my life is like a princess," she said happily rocking back and forth in her seat.

Jones replied swiftly, "Sounds intense, what's going on here?" Jones said to Pearl as he looked around the room. Another man sat next to Jones named Abe who looked like he hadn't showered in a while. In a high-pitched voice and smelling like coal, he said, "I'm Abe! I've got lots of friends in the computer industry and I'm here because I need this." He laughed to himself as he looked over to the right at one of the other men, "Oh, he's cute!" The therapist looked over at Jones, "Jones would you like to share?" Jones sat for a moment thinking of the world around him, "No, nothing at the moment." he said, trying to catch up to the exercises that were happening in the room. "You need some new slippers," Pearl said as she noticed Jones' slippers were worn so much that his toes stuck into the carpet around the edges. "I don't go shopping much. I don't really know how to—." Jones responded. Pearl cut him off, "After this let's go shopping! I'll show you how to get the best deal." Pearl responded warmly. Jones looked at her for a moment. He figured at least this would make therapy interesting. Bey waved at him from the other side of the room, "Hey Jones!" she said. The IOP Therapist put her finger up to her face frustrated with the group participants' actions with Jones's entrance into the group. "Shh!" she said, trying to get the group back under control.

The IOP Group participants sat down as the Therapist continued to ask her questions, writing down multiple exercises that the participants would be doing. Suddenly Abe stood up, "I need water." he said trying to get himself out of the session. Jones also called out the same need for some water. "Let's all take a break." The IOP Therapist noticed what had been going on around the room. Jones walked over towards the water cooler as Abe hit the button three times. "What are you doing?" Jones asked as Abe tried to get an angle on drinking the water. "I'm trying to call out as an emergency to my computer friends. I don't want to be here." Jones stared at Abe for a moment. "I simply want some water. Do you mind?" Jones said. Abe nodded as Jones took a sip of his water, thinking of the people in the room. Jones wasn't sure who to trust. He surveyed each area, studying their patterns of how each person interacted trying to make a proper decision. "Thanks!" Jones said as Abe went back to pressing the water cooler button like a telegraph keypad. Abe's hands were almost black and his weight bulged so big you could see the man was struggling to get a handle on himself. However, Abe seemed happy in his moments. Even in his 'state of emergency, he was consistently smiling. Jones walked into the break room where some people were conversing, some were drawing and others were sleeping. Another man sat in the back corner, eating peanuts and wearing a gray sweater on his head. He was the only awake person in there who didn't make running comments.

"How are you?" Jones asked the man in the back corner, sensing the relaxation in the back of the room. "Overly tired and depressed." the man said, "It's why I'm here. Want some?" The man offered Jones what little he had left in his bag of peanuts. Jones reached out and took the peanuts, "You know it's quite something, when people have so little to give, they still give. Sometimes I feel as if these people in their shitty situations have the most empathy out of anyone because they know how it feels to have nothing. They know how it feels when life is over for them, to simply survive in a communal setting." The man sat there listening intently to Jones as he half fell back asleep, "I'm out of peanuts. There's a store right down the street," he said. Jones got up and headed down the street with the man. As the two of them walked into the grocery store, the world around Jones didn't look the same as it had previously. The clouds no longer held

CHAPTER EIGHTEEN – CHASE

patterns connected to where he was supposed to go, trash meant trash and watchers had seamlessly gone back into hiding mumbling to one another or themselves on the street. As Jones grabbed a small bag of chips, the cashier looked directly at Jones, "That will be a full price of $1.17." she said. Jones asked the question to test out if he still known, "No discount today?" Jones inquired. The lady looked back at him as if he was crazy, "No sir, we have our grocery discounts and that's all." she smiled afterward reiterating the $1.17 price.

Jones walked out as the man caught up with him, "Peanuts?" the man offered again as Jones took a handful of peanuts that had lime seasoning. "Alright, yeah I'm pretty hungry anyway. Come on, we have to go back," said Jones. Jones followed the man back up the stairs towards the IOP Therapy room where everyone sat again. "There's a whiteboard in the room and some questions listed on the board." the IOP Therapist said as each person entered the room. "I want each of you to answer them." Jones went over to where pizza had been put in the room. On the board were written two problems: "What's the best way for space travel?" and "How do we take care of the world's overpopulation in fifty years?" Jones couldn't comprehend why these questions were on the board as he grabbed a slice of pizza. He sat there quietly listening to music as he drowned out the sound of others giving their defined answers. Jones was able to relax his mind while the others answered the questions as if nothing was wrong. "How is this therapeutic?" Jones asked himself as the IOP Therapist sat there with paintings on the wall of Mozart and Einstein. "Hmm, I guess this is therapeutic because it gets you to think." Jones knew at that moment he was still going to be studied. "I have nothing to contribute at this time," Jones said in retaliation.

After ten minutes the IOP Group participants walked back outside. Pearl sat there waving over Jones as Bey had already gone back upstairs for more coffee. "Hey, Jones! Let's go shopping for a new pair of slippers for you." Pearl said. Jones went downstairs with Pearl and headed towards her car.

The car had been beaten up and was old, but the interior was surprisingly clean to Jones. So, was Pearl another watcher disguising herself from the world? Jones didn't want to think about it. Pearl opened up immediately talking, "I can't wait to see him. You know I'm kind of a princess in a sense." she said dreamily. "He's in a wheelchair. He can't get out much, but the man owns a mansion. He's so caring. The last time I was with him in this bar, they were rude to him. So, he bought the entire bar and fired the owner and the bartender." she babbled on. Jones sat there in her car listening to the story. "Where should we go?" Jones asked as a clothing store passed by the window. "Let's go to the drugstore," Pearl said. "Pearl, why there?" Jones asked out of curiosity.

"Because the drugstore has the best deals on slippers, silly! Anyone knows that" replied Pearl smiling. They parked and walked towards the drugstore past a fountain that sat in the middle of the mall. Pearl had previously parked her car in what was seen as an empty parking lot. Jones stopped for a moment. "What is it?" Pearl asked, wondering why Jones suddenly seemed disturbed. Pearl could tell when Jones was feeling off, even in the short amount of time the two had talked. "A while ago, before I got picked up…" Pearl and Jones walked over to the bench and sat down. "There was this little girl and her mother. I was hopping on the cement blocks, practicing jumping from place to place, right over here for a while. This little girl had a bunch of superhero toys. She asked me, 'Which one is your favorite?' as she showed me each toy. I stood there balancing in my slippers on the edge of the wall, practicing to show the world." said Jones reminiscing. Jones continued, "I told the little girl, 'Why not like ourselves as our best superhero? But out of them, the middle ones are pretty cool.' The mother filmed the interaction." Pearl laughed, "So you were teaching her inspiration?"

Jones smiled, "I just wanted her to grow up believing in herself and her imagination." He sat there looking at the sky. Pearl asked, "Why are you bothered then?" Jones sat there, "I guess I'm bothered because maybe I

CHAPTER EIGHTEEN – CHASE

was telling her the wrong way to think. Or maybe I'm bothered because the mother looked at me as if I was insane. I was jumping from the cement blocks to the pots, from the pots over to the water fountain." Jones continued. Pearl laughed again as she patted Jones on the back, "I don't think you were wrong. Even if she does remember that for the rest of her life that's strength and belief. That Jones will go further than anything. Let's keep going and get you those slippers." They got up and started walking again. Pearl continued her story of how the man was a fashion designer from Italy. Regardless of her situation, Pearl seemed to have the same freedom. Jones and Pearl walked into the drugstore to where the slippers were. "See!" she said pointing towards the $10 slippers. "Woah, great quality for the price," Jones exclaimed as he saw them in blue and white.

They walked towards the check-out line and stood there for a moment as Jones took off his torn-up slippers. As soon as he purchased the new ones, he threw the old slippers away in the garbage can. "See? Isn't that much better Jones?" said Pearl warmly. Jones smiled, "Yup! As good as it's going to get." "See you in two days?" Pearl asked as Jones got back into her car. "Yeah, I'll be there!" Jones replied. Pearl drove them to where Jones' car was parked near the Therapist's Office. His car sat alone in the parking lot as the sun slowly went down behind the mountain. Jones thought back in time about a show he had gone to, Rusty's Tech Show. It seemed like a lifetime ago. "Hey Jones, spit a rap!" his friend Massie had said to him at Rusty's Tech Show. "I don't want to," Jones said out loud as he sat down on the curb in the Therapist Office parking lot. Back in his reverie, Jones was at the club at Rusty's Tech Show. A man sat down next to him outside smoking a menthol cigarette as he puffed mint into the air. He wore a ring with a golden piano on it. "Did you know gold piano strings have a better holding than copper or bronze?" the man said.

Jones sat there on the curb in the Therapist Office parking lot wearing his brown felt hat staring back at the man in his reverie listening intently.

"No. Had no idea." Jones said out loud as he noticed the man's earrings. Continuing his reverie, Jones walked back inside the dance area at the club at Rusty's Tech Show. The crowd gathered around, dancing in a big circle. The lights were blaring. Jones held up his finger with a number one sign as the rest of the people gathered around him. The men and women held up their fingers as the crowd got rowdier. The bass rumbled through the club as Jones could see the music waves pass by him in color as if he was seeing a light show indicating each frequency that passed by his face. "Jones?" A strange man said as Jones turned around towards the voice. The man had been playing the main bass on the stage prior as Jones sat there watching the show. Every time Jones went somewhere within the club, people who dressed in even crazier costumes seemed to hold more knowledge. It was there that Jones went upstairs to feel the real power of the place as the slow, sweet music had lulled Jones to sleep. This was while sitting next to his friend, Massi, who also started to pass out. A man in a fur coat sat next to the two of them, to watch over Jones as the security guard walked by. "You cool?" the man with the piano ring tapped Jones on the shoulder.

"You can't be falling asleep here you know." Jones nodded as the sleep deprivation had finally bested him. Even in his altered state of mind when he was sitting outside at the club talking to the other man with golden earrings and piano string information, he was still able to rap. Snapping out of his reverie, Jones noticed that Pearl had already driven out of the Therapist Office parking lot. Jones hadn't heard from Mira, nor received a single text from Nepharius as he sat there on the curb. Jones got into his car, stepped on the gas pedal, and headed for his house. Ms. P would be flying home soon from Europe. After arriving home, Jones walked in quietly towards the shower as his neurons fired off in his brain. The water dripped down slowly. Jones heard music in his brain from each water drop playing single notes. Jones skipped dinner and went right to bed as he prepared for another session. Jones woke up the next day as he headed to the Therapist Office. He was starting to enjoy attending the place as it seemed he was learning most from the people there themselves.

CHAPTER EIGHTEEN – CHASE

As Jones walked into the Therapist Office a man dressed in a full-body suit skeleton sat upstairs in the reception area. He took off his outer helmet as he waited in line.

"Woah, that's cool. Why are you wearing that?" Jones asked out of curiosity. "Name's Stint," the man said, "I sell weed and it's a motorcycle outfit." Jones shook his hand. "Add me some time on Messenger and we'll talk a while," Jones said briefly. The man was gone after he picked up his family member. "Jones, Ms. Orin is ready to see you." the receptionist announced. Jones got used to the routine of waiting and getting water by now. He had been there so many times. He understood the map and layout of the entire building. Jones sat down in front of his therapist Ms. Orin. "Doctor K. tells me you had a very interesting experience recently. Would you like to talk further about it?" coaxed Ms. Orin. She sat down at her desk facing Jones as Jones sat in a chair facing her. Jones sat thinking about it for a second before responding. "Well, Ms. Orin you see... I went down to this place in Monterey Bay, trying to understand the way our society worked. I had this friend, Jason..." Jones began. Jones started to reminisce his experience in Monterey Bay from a few months ago as Ms. Orin sat back and listened to him continuing the story: "Hi Jones, it's Jason. Are we meeting today?" Jason texted. Jones replied swiftly, "Yeah! Of course!" as he put on his brown felt hat and grabbed his cane trying to figure out what had happened that previous night in Monterey Bay. "I heard you were getting invited to join the Navy as a neurosurgeon." Jones texted Jason as he drove his car towards Monterey Bay. Jones felt confident being able to maneuver his car, texting at the same time while driving.

"Yeah, I'm always into interesting people. Let's grab a bite and talk for a while." Jason texted back. Jason sounded as if he had a lot to share. After a three-hour drive, Jones arrived across the way from the meeting place. The first thing he noticed was the generator connected to the mall with graffiti painted on it. However, instead of it being graffiti, the inner workings of the machine were painted on the outside in pure white graffiti paint over the green generator box. It was almost as if people wanted to inspire others to show them how things were built. Jones walked across the street past a yellow fire hydrant towards the mall where Jason waited by the main entry door. "Hey man! Right on time! Perfect with our walking vibration." Jason smiled. Jones started to talk, "So you're trained to see the patterns in people before they even happen. Does that make it boring for you?" Jones asked. Jason replied, "Well, our social security is documented by color, not just numbers. It's filed away in orange, green, blue, and patterns. I feel like the world doesn't really understand the way we work. It's all hidden from the public eye. For example, see that lady over there?" Jason pointed to her as she talked in an inaudible language. "She's about to put one foot right and move around that person over there who is walking too fast." Jones looked over to the left before it happened. Twenty seconds passed and the prediction happened exactly as he said. Jones became more intrigued.

"You know I was here a while back. Some people were talking in all French?" Jones observed. Jason seemed surprised, "Well the military linguistics section is based down here. That makes sense." Jason said. Jones right then realized he was being watched over by the space pirate Nepharius. The eye was following Jones around regardless of what he had done. That damned Nebulous eye! Ms. Orin held her hand up. "Wait, Jones. You believed an eye was following you and got involved with the military?" she asked him, questioning his sanity. "How did that affect you?" she asked. Jones looked back on it. "I was calm, I was excited to learn more. My world was becoming that reality." Jones replied. Ms. Orin nodded her head. "Continue with the story." Jones continued, "That was the first time I ended up posting on my social media Instagram account, # 'NoFilterShot', meaning nothing added to the pictures. The trend took off as I was being watched. Jason sat me down at the table as we talked about his experiences. We ended up going to the park afterward in town." Jones said. Jason walked into the ice cream shop, "Want one?" he said to Jones looking out towards the water. "Sure, why not," Jones said in return as a dog looked at the both of them. The dog started staring Jones down as if

CHAPTER EIGHTEEN – CHASE

to read his energy.

"Do you think our energy can be read?" Jones asked Jason as they sat in the ice cream shop enjoying their cones. "It's your sound and vibration. The waves that your brain is making continuously are literally communicating to the animals around you." Jason said, trying to put life into a simple perspective for Jones. The ice cream dripped over Jones' hand as he listened to the rest of what Jason was saying. "I should go," Jones said. Jason nodded, "It will be a while before you see me again, but if you have any trouble let me know." Jones didn't know how to fight, what was he fighting for? he asked himself. Ms. Orin stopped Jones, "Sounds like you had a real experience. Is this why you thought the CIA was chasing you? For the knowledge you carried?" she asked. Jones looked back at Ms. Orin for a moment and then rubbed his head as he stared at the floor. "Well…my phone lost communication but still worked everywhere I went." Jones continued. Ms. Orin laughed, "You mean your phone was pre-loading data?" she asked. Jones rubbed his head. "I'm not so sure. Every time I went past a policeman in places I wasn't supposed to be my phone went into incognito mode and my communications shut down. You know Bey had a similar…" Jones stopped. "Okay Jones, it's time for your next session. It looks like you have been resting well." Ms. Orin paused, "Head down and we'll talk later."

Jones walked back towards the IOP session where Pearl sat. Bey was not there as it seemed she had been released from the program. This time the IOP Therapist smiled as if she had gained control of the room. There were no more "weird" experiences happening in the room, no more coincidences. "I haven't slept well in days," Abe said as he sat there shaking. He had gone home and showered for the first time, no longer smelling like coal. The IOP Therapist pointed at him, "Then head to the break room, Abe!" she suggested. Abe got up as the rest of the room continued. The IOP Therapist went around the room asking about people's depression. "Would you like to share this time Jones?" she asked gently. This time

Jones sat up, "My name's Jones. I suffered from severe depression which led to something called psychosis. Some people come out of it; others never do." Jones stated matter-of-factly. The IOP Therapist exclaimed, "Aww." Jones continued, "When I was in that state of mind, it was as if I could distinguish between the quality of people and their craft or skills from those who were stuck within their minds. My empathy and energy levels fell off the charts." The IOP Therapist replied, "Um, okay…" The rest of the room participants understood what Jones was saying, nodding their heads and agreeing as if they were relating to his world.

Jones sat back down as Pearl stood up, "Name's Pearl, I'm in here because I've had a hard time lately at home and needed to get away from the stress for a while." The IOP Therapist nodded, "What stress were you feeling?" she asked. Pearl explained the stress of her daily life, with her family and her relationship with the man in the wheelchair. She stated that she felt she always would have to impress him to survive in their relationship. "You should think about yourself, Pearl and what your needs are." the IOP Therapist said, trying to relate. Pearl sat back down feeling upset as if the therapist didn't understand what she had to say. Pearl turned to Jones, "I think you do a better job at this than she does." she whispered as the IOP Therapist spoke about the next task. "Okay break time!" the IOP Therapist said as everyone got up out of their chairs. Jones walked outside, this time looking out towards the mountain as he went over to the bench where people generally sat. A man sat on the corner of the bench dressed in all black, wearing an old cap. He had a surprisingly clean demeanor as he smoked a cigarette. He was talking to himself. The man seemed distressed as if he had seen a murder. Jones walked over to the man and sat next to him. "Name's Jones," Jones said to the man while extending his hand. "Russel." the man said in return. "You seem worried," Jones said, trying to make conversation. "I'm not worried, I'm stressed. The world of research hasn't accepted my paper. The thieves, they stole it." he said as he chain-smoked more cigarettes. "20 years of research, you know?" Russel said angrily. He stumbled as he got up to walk, "Nice chatting with you. I

CHAPTER EIGHTEEN – CHASE

gotta go."

Russel walked off as Jones sat there wondering for a moment. All these lives that Jones has met - swirling, contemplating, and conversing with one another. Everyone has a story completely unknown without knowing the battle between the musical warriors and the corporate society that has been stealing their ideas. Mira appeared in Jones' mind, "Why are you giving up Jones? Nepharius hasn't given up yet." she warned. Jones sighed, "Whose side are you on Mira? Why haven't you contacted me until now?" Jones asked in his head. He looked at his watch and saw the therapy break time was almost up. "Side?" Mira laughed, "I don't pick sides, but for some reason, you Jones are different. You have the power to motivate this entire world. You've seen it haven't you?" Mira asked Jones as he sat there on the bench. "Seen what?" Jones asked in return. "The power to inspire others all at once. The idea of connection is so gigantic that it shifts the energy of people simultaneously. Here's a tip-off, Nepharius got out. The place couldn't hold him down at the Island of 300." Mira said. Jones looked at Mira for a moment. "The Island of 300?" he asked.

Mira explained, "Yes, it's an island where criminals are kept. A beautiful tropical place where a gigantic electric fence stops anyone from swimming away. I'm sure you've heard of Alcatraz Island, right?" Jones scratched his head. "Of course. Yeah, I have," he said. Mira's face went from a smile to a serious, scowling face, "Nepharius broke out. An island so far away. He went swimming towards Brazil. He has gained his full crew and is building that movie. Kid, it's dangerous for you. I've been trying to pull you out of this mess." she warned. Jones rubbed his eyes looking at the time, "I have to get back to therapy." Mira waved goodbye, "That eye is on your back. Remember that. Oh, and I've one more thing to say," she said as she faded into the galactic space within a glass-domed coffee shop, "Watchers are communicating with music and song titles. Keep an eye out for this, would you?" Jones walked back across the street. This time as the odd colored cars that had existed once had now disappeared. Nothing was coming in or out of the street. "It's starting up again," Jones said to himself. "What is all this therapy for?" He walked up the steps to get back to the room that hadn't seemed to skip a beat. "My name is Daryl." Jones heard from the room as he walked in to sit down.

"Hi, Daryl." The room echoed in succession as Daryl explained his troubles. "I work in construction and if you've ever heard the song called 'Not Going My Way' that's how I'm feeling at this moment in time." Daryl sat down in his chair twirling his hand with weird sunglasses on. Jones had remembered how out of designing the walking bridges along the Iron Trail had been. He had stared at the top of one bridge as the glass reflected nothing, Jones started thinking of ways to spruce it up. "Hey, Daryl." Jones leaned over to him to speak, "Don't you think the walking bridges near here are kind of bland? And the short walkways that lead up to them?" Daryl laughed, "Kind of." he replied. Jones asked him, "Why don't we have a community painting and art jobs project to spruce up the walking bridges. I mean even the glass could be a colorful see-through. It's all over churches and amusement parks. Why not take that boring, smooth, gray, bridge and coat it colorful?" Jones' mind started turning. Maybe, maybe on a smaller scale, he could inspire others to take on the challenges in their area of expertise. Daryl smiled, "That's one way to look at it. But I'm here to get away for a while, not to work." Jones leaned over, "Feeling like a 'Lack of Communication'?" he asked smiling. Daryl laughed louder, "Great song man. Yeah, I do." The IOP Therapist wrote down notes on her pad as Daryl went back into his depressed state of mind.

Jones was starting to better understand why Nepharius had called upon Jones to help him, it was to help Nepharius escape fully. Jones had the idea that the rest of the world had not been able to see as they had not been freed, not because they were unable to think of them by themselves. The slow development was not because of the lack of creativity. No wonder Watchers hid in broken-down cars with their tools hidden from society. The Watchers did not want to be known or noticed. Jones could feel the

CHAPTER EIGHTEEN – CHASE

sadness in Daryl's voice. "If only I was taken more seriously. I could bring my construction ideas up." Jones mumbled as he looked back over to where Pearl was sitting. "Heya Pearl!" she smiled as Jones called out her name. Crayons had been set on the table by the therapist. "Draw how you are feeling today." the IOP Therapist said to the crowd as the crayons were distributed evenly. Jones started drawing the car he saw on that day as he contemplated how flying cars would slowly work their way into society. Jet packs were already successfully underway. Jones knew that what he had witnessed that day was on a different level. He sat there smiling to himself as he imagined the encounter. Pearl looked at Jones, "You look like you've caught the biggest candy in the entire universe. What's that?" Pearl asked Jones as she pointed to the car drawn on a sheet of paper. "Can you ever imagine Pearl, that there are people out there who have created useful items far beyond most people's imagination?" Jones sat there as he wondered about it too. "Yeah, I have. My mind's kind of stuck on my prince though." Pearl laughed as Jones followed his gut feeling, he knew now that he could trust Pearl. "Ms. Orin would like to see you again Jones." the IOP Therapist said as she referred Jones back to her office. Jones slowly walked down the hallway remembering the exits of the building. After opening the door, he sat down in the chair facing out towards the mountain.

"Hey Jones, I have a little extra time. I wanted you to continue your story." Ms. Orin said warmly. As Jones sat down collecting his thoughts trying to reposition himself to not be thrown back in a locked ward, he looked down at his phone as an application popped up on his notes. The two big servers were now successfully connected. "That's right, the people watching me did tell me to think first before I click. Each click that I do puts my thoughts into reality. Otherwise, my thoughts go back to the beginning and do not get created and shared. Each click on my phone now explains what the server Application did." Jones explained. Ms. Orin looked at Jones as he was slightly mumbling to himself "What do you mean? Servers? App's?" she asked, trying to follow him. "Well, you see

Ms. Orin, during a point in time, I had reached out to one of my friends via Messenger. He worked very closely with people at the top of two separate software companies. When he sent out an email, they reached out to my iPhone for testing. Once when I went down to visit this friend, I was walking down the street. I got close to the building as a lady came down and shook my hand. She said she was selling the houses, but for me, it would be a very big discount. I claimed I was coming to work for the company. She said, "I know." It was as if she already knew my plans of why I was there with my friends. At the time none of it made sense. I felt welcomed and alienated at the same time." Jones explained. Jones continued to explain the situation about how he had been forwarding his ideas to various places that were watching over him as Ms. Orin sat there nodding. "So, in real-time, you were creating software with two separate software companies, simply by tapping on your phone? Do you mean you were testing to see how user-friendly it was becoming? Like for the user interface?" Ms. Orin interjected questioning Jones.

Jones nodded, "This relates to the rest of the story. You see, each Watcher was giving me ideas and encouraging me to help them bring them into reality as I was their connection. I began forwarding their ideas to various galaxies and our world simultaneously." Jones said seriously. Ms. Orin tried to keep a smile on her face, but she was feeling very confused based on everything Jones had explained. "I think you should come in tomorrow, Jones. Go home and get some rest," she said. Jones smiled, "I suppose so." Jones replied walking out the door. Mira came to mind again, "Jones you idiot! Blend in." she said whispering. "There are other Watchers around here who may accidentally expose you. If you're caught again, there will be no help for you." Jones walked down the stairs feeling as if he had to get away from the situation. The security guard stood at the door as she opened it up for Jones. "Come again." the security guard said, smiling. Jones walked further down the street towards his car. The man blowing leaves with a leaf blower stopped and looked at Jones from a distance. He remembered how Jones had danced around in a circle in front of him and

CHAPTER EIGHTEEN – CHASE

then ran away down the street. The man politely waved at Jones to come over as he was about to get in his car. "Hey Mr.!!"." the man said loudly, but politely trying to capture Jones' attention. Jones was too freaked out by his thoughts as he shut the car door. The man waved more frantically and shouted, "Mister! Your wallet from last time!" The leaf blower held the wallet up in the air as Jones saw it from his rear-view mirror.

Jones stopped wanting to get home after realizing what Mira had told him. Rolling down all of the car windows, Jones tried to revel in the fresh air flowing through. He drove towards the mall where he parked by the leaf symbol in the parking structure. "People who work in environmental industries must park here often." Jones thought to himself as a man wearing a black T-shirt with a tree on it walked down the stairs. Jones followed him out into the open space where the coffee shop and the Apple store were located. Jones viewed the crosswalk and wondered why some people were going across it diagonally while others were walking the normal way from corner to corner. He sat there on a bench in front of the coffee shop closing his eyes as the sun beamed down on him. Jones blinked again as the butterfly that he saw on YouTube came back into his mind. 'Minds connect' went through Jones' head as he looked at the world from a new point of view. The traffic lights flipped from green to blue to gray as Jones laid down on the bench. "These damned galactic colors are so hard to read." Jones continued to think to himself. Every time the light hit gray, twice the amount of people walked across the crosswalk. Some of the people started to run as if they were teleporting through to the other side. Jones watched this for a bit. Then he wandered down to where the local free green trolley picked up passengers. The free trolley keeps going around a continuous loop through the shopping district with a stop at the BART station.

Jones sighed as he hopped on, "To no man's land." Jones said out loud. Jones got off at the next green trolley stop and walked around aimlessly trying to make sense of his surroundings. He then wandered down to where the next continuous loop green trolley stop was and got back on. The trolley took off, speeding through downtown towards the BART. The air conditioner blasted down in full on Jones' forehead. A black jacket that looked like a full-body suit covered a Watcher as he slept sitting upright. Jones looked over to his right as men and women stood frozen at the moment. A man tapped Jones on the shoulder, "Got any change my man?" he asked. Jones stepped away from him walking towards the other side of the trolley. A black feathered hat popped out from the crowd as he got in between the two. "Jones back up." said the man in the feathered hat. Jones looked at the man recognizing him. It was the demi-human hunter he had met previously. Jones backed up slowly as the pan-handler ran for it. "I'm known around these parts." he sang out in a blues voice, cackling. Jones looked back over at him, "Known?" Jones asked.

"Yeah, well known my young demi-human!" he cackled again. "Ciex is the name. Sorry about before when I saw you surfing and balancing on the BART. I was very confused. I've been studying ancient scrolls for over three decades." the man smiled. "You seem a little lost there," he said out of curiosity. "Can I help get you home?" he asked. Jones sat there in awe and confusion. Feeling drained he was tempted to walk towards the train tracks to electrocute himself back to having energy. "Yeah, my phone is about to die. I can't get home without it." Jones said, showing the signal at zero as his phone blinked and suddenly shut off. "I'll call you a cab there, boy!" he laughed heartily. "Remember the name is Ciex!" The trolley arrived at the BART station. After a few minutes, a cab driver showed up with pure black curly hair. His eyes were wide as if he had not slept in two to three days. Jones got into the black cab. "Gum? Any side dishes Jones?" the man asked him using his name.

Jones peered around from the corner of the car window as the car sped through the streets. The driver began trying to make conversation. "I've heard your music lately. It is extremely good." the driver said as he looked back at Jones in the mirror. "You should play the songs on the radio, you

CHAPTER EIGHTEEN – CHASE

know. Take a crack at the whole business." The driver shifted his focus back to the road as he swerved around a car, missing it by an inch. "I was a manager, not a musician," Jones replied, not seeming to notice that the driver nearly missed a car. Oddly, the driver offered Jones a piece of gum a second time. "I know Nepharius escaped recently." the driver said, smiling. Jones sat back in his seat and contemplated what he had heard. "Come again?" Jones asked the man who was driving. "I said I know. It makes sense for you to get on stage. It's been rough recently." the driver said. Jones fell back further into his seat. His mind was churning. It was happening again. The world around him was turning back into the galactic universe that Jones had created around him. The Uber arrived at Jones' house. As Jones got out and waved to the gentleman, the mysterious man said, "You will not be seeing me again. Take care." As Jones wandered into the house, Ms. P was standing by the front door. "Where have you been Jones? And where is your car?" she questioned him in a worried tone. She hadn't seen him in weeks and his father had already left. "Where's Dad?" Jones asked curiously.

"He left today and went back home as I'm back from vacation. He reviewed your therapy schedule with me, so I have been worried since you didn't come home. Where's my hug? And more importantly, how are you? Are you hungry?" Jones' mother offered up a meal as Jones headed towards his room. "I already ate a little," Jones said, his stomach swirling. Nepharius was back out in the open. He was already on the way on the seas, now with a crew. What would he steal next? The book of Thoth? The deep temples of the Tar'j'kun? Did it matter? Jones shook his head wondering. After all the worry he put his mother through he didn't want to leave the house for a nighttime walk. After all, if the corporation running the therapy sessions found out about what he was up to there would be a battle for his freedom. Jones loaded up his PC for the first time in what felt like three months. His song stared back at him as he started to make it. "Stop, Stop!" Nepharius said in Jones' mind as the program stopped midway. Jones ignored the sound in his mind as he hit the spacebar on the keyboard to continue the program. "I said stop!!" Nepharius said again as the program stopped itself after glitching out. "I want to finish this song!" Jones shouted out in his mind. Nepharius bulked up and grabbed Jones by the left side of his neck, "I can break you in an instant. But because I like you, you're still in my crew." Nepharius said as Jones sat there feeling the tingling on his neck. "I said 'stop' because we have a job to do. The posters are all over the galaxy. Congratulations Jones! We are wanted men." Jones laughed it off trying not to lose his composure as Nepharius sat down in front of him. "Why war? I don't want war." Jones said.

Nepharius replied, "Why not war? War is fun. War is destruction where no one can keep up." Jones' smile turned into a disagreement, a frown. "War? Fun? There are better ways to have war and fun than to destroy everything in your path. It is easier to destroy than to build Nepharius." Jones said. "Aktu Japo'!" Nepharius said out loud as a command. "In English, please," Jones said, curious about the language he was speaking in. "Listen here you stupid arbiter. You might be a keeper of time, but you are my general! High end from war days of consciousness. Do not dare defy me or I will leave you in the ground in 3,000 years from now!" Nepharius stormed off to the other side slowly fading from Jones' view. "Wait Nepharius… okay, I will at least hear your plan," Jones said in return, sitting on the chair in his room as the world now floated around him."Good! Then in brotherhood, I am sorry for my outburst. I've gathered costumes and show designers. I'm teaching them martial arts. Soon we will be traveling to the old relics in Brazil to take back what's mine. The power to heal others. There was an old monk who sat in a tree only living off berries for two hundred years. He had let go of all and saw it all as it is. By doing so he could heal from whom he touched, the ability to go anywhere. He was unconfined by the skin of society's teeth. I will take this relic and learn it. I am getting close." Nepharius laughed as Jones sat there in fear of what was to come next. "And what will you do when you find this relic?" Jones asked Nepharius.

"As we gather support through stage and movies, I will heal the crowds

CHAPTER EIGHTEEN – CHASE

and take from the others who are after us. We will be full-blown pirates. Have you done your pushups?" Nepharius sat in place questioning Jones. "No, I was captured," Jones replied. Nepharius laughed, "You'd better catch up. I want my men to be as good as lions. Kings of the jungle," he said. Jones smiled, "Okay, this world, right? It's only a piece of our perception?" Nepharius laughed, "You already know." Jones' mind went silent as Jones sat there continuing the song. The play button finally went through as his screen turned dark. Jones felt as if it turned to gold for him to call him that king of the jungle. As each note played his mind saw and felt the vibration. Each piece Jones calmly called to his mind writing out note by note the exact frequencies in which he loved. In a few minutes, he was done with the masterpiece. He was also thinking about therapy. "I almost forgot." Jones got a text from Nepharius. "This movie producer needs music for the movie. You should attempt to make some." texted

Nepharius. Jones thought for a moment about contacting Ottie who had long left Monterey Bay for back home. Jones gave Ottie a call, "Hey buddy, how are you doing?" Jones asked. Ottie picked up, "Dude I'm so glad to hear from you. You disappeared after going crazy. What the hell happened?" he said with genuine happiness and concern. Jones cut straight to the point. "Well, I had a breakdown, therapy and all. I'm still in it. Anyways I called because I remembered you have my laptop. I also found a music deal for making it for a movie." Ottie questioned it, "What? That's cool, Dude. Hook me up. Except, I'm in Ohio again." Ottie said.

Jones smacked his forehead, "You took my laptop to Ohio?" Jones said, raising his voice but remembering that Ottie had gone through a hard time. "Yeah, I'll mail it back to you soon," Ottie replied. Jones sighed, "Anyway, I suppose it's good you have my laptop because from that we will be able to make the song together." Jones said, trying to hide his frustrations. "Yeah, alright. I have to go for now but I will talk to you soon." Ottie hung up the phone as Jones went over the basics of his song he just made over and over. "It sounds pretty good," Jones said to himself as he exported the song. Jones went briefly outside to get some air. He came back into the house and hugged his mother as she sat there reading the newspaper. "There's food in the fridge." Ms. P said as she pointed towards the kitchen. Jones went over to eye the pasta with red sauce and clams. "Yum! Looks pretty good, Mom." Jones said, taking it out of the fridge and heating it up. "So, I overheard the conversation from your bedroom that Ottie took your laptop to Ohio. Will you be getting that back?" Jones's mother questioned him. "Yes, ma. Of course, I want that back." Jones said.

"By the way, Doctor K. called. He said to message him if you had any further questions about the next steps." his mom continued. Jones's eyes were surprised. Was the corporation and IOP Therapist already notified by Nepharius? Mira came into his mind, "Jones, don't…" the connection in his mind dropped out as he picked up the pasta with red sauce with clams. "I'll be sure to send him an email. I have a few." Jones said acting as if nothing had bothered him. "Okay. It's so good to have you back Jones. The doctor said you do not have to take any more of those pills for now." his mother said with relief and genuine love in her voice. Jones already knew this as he had already been faking taking the pills that kept him sane. Jones went back to his bedroom where he laid back down waiting for the time to pass. His mind wandered as if he was waiting for something to happen. "Why? was the only thought going through his mind. Why did I find the adventure I was looking for?" Jones asked himself. Jones drifted off to sleep as the clouds drifted by in his dreams. He landed back on the beach as men pulled wood together. Nepharius stood there as he commanded them to sit on the side waiting for a signal. Nepharius waved to Jones, "This is no time for lackadaisical sleeping on the beach." he said.

Jones laughed, "Oh… uh…" Nepharius walked over to him and held out his hand, "Take it." he said. Jones took it and got up. "Nepharius, have you ever met the Spirit of Music?" Jones asked him curiously, wondering if his experiences had intertwined with Neph's. "Yes, I've been there and done that already. The Spirit of Music is a sweet person," he responded. "A sweet person?" Jones asked, "So you do have a soft side!" Jones said laughing as

CHAPTER EIGHTEEN – CHASE

Jones and Nepharius shared a small moment. Nepharius laughed, "Yeah, but only for good people. I'm tired of this World's games." Nepharius said seriously. Jones handed him another log, this time feeling that it was lighter than the first one. He didn't understand or notice as the boat was slowly being built. "Careful with those logs Jones. These break very easily when handled by our crew." Nepharius said. Jones curiously sat behind Nepharius as he watched others pick up the wood on the beach working in a line. The assembly line was handing each piece of wood moving towards where Nepharius was standing. The white sail, which was half-built, lay on the ground as Jones reviewed the pieces. As Jones was handed an item, he saw one of the crew members smoking. The smoke glowed as it gave off a reflective light. "Huh…" Jones said to himself, speechless of the situation. He walked back over to where the trees were to get a better view. Jones looked up at the sky as the clouds now had a galactic space glow. "I see," Jones said as he rolled back over in the sand as his back felt hot. "Time for you to wake up," Nepharius said as Jones continued dreaming. Jones was starting to sweat under his covers in bed. His sheets were white like the sails of the boat. A carpet that lay on the floor in his bedroom was rolled up like a log. Jones had been moving it in his sleep. "Guess it's time for therapy again," Jones mumbled to himself.

Chapter Nineteen – Mind Chess

The next day Jones' mind felt as if a million tiny pebbles had continuously hit him throughout the night. He sat there thinking through the boat that had been built on the shoreside. Nepharius had crashed it on an island from the escape, so he had Jones repair it with his crew. The sun's rays reflected off the ground as the molecules flew across the air in waves. Jones could see it flowing across the room's rooftop alongside him. He felt as if he was a ghost in society retaining the knowledge as every passerby went through the same patterns over and over. Jones hopped out of bed and went over to the shower getting all of the clothing necessary. He put a warm towel under his eyes to alleviate the headache that pounded in his head. "Gah, this heat is finally working. Goddamn Nepharius always pushing the boundaries of human limitations." Jones said to himself as he looked at his phone. "Get working." Jones read the title of the song while washing his face. "Yeah, Yeah I know." He mumbled to himself out loud as the phone's song title was communicating with him again. His mother knocked on the door. "Jones, it's almost time. Need me to drive you?" Jones replied, "It's fine mom. I can drive again." She backed off as she went back to making breakfast. Jones's mother had become more lenient lately ever since he had been off the pills. Walking outside of the house. He picked up his car keys and opened the trunk. Inside had been the brown felt hat in which Jones thought he had lost. "Returned properly." - The Spirit of Music." The note read as Jones smiled. He plugged in his CD and turned up the new music to the top of the

CHAPTER NINETEEN – MIND CHESS

volume meter, practicing singing for the show that Nepharius would be inviting them to. On the way to the therapy session, a voice asked. "Jones is back?" More voices ran through his mind continuously as if waiting for an answer. "Yes, I'm back." He replied. The council of five rang through his head again. "He's back!" Clapping rang through his head. "I will keep all of my words!" He said looking at the development of the world. "A world where we develop!"

Cheering clapped again as the entire galaxy could feel his momentum. Jones parked his car half in the shadow and half in the sun as a parking space lay under the roof. He put his car keys in his pocket as an old 1954 car shined. The wind blew the leaves around the pole towards the wall where trash had completely lined up. As Jones followed the wind in the parking lot a small whirlwind started right in front of him. He quickly reached out and put his hand in it as the wind quickly died out as fast as Jones put his hand inside of it. The leaves started to form into curved lines as if telling him where to go again. Jones followed the wind further down the wall as a scratcher that had been an untouched lie in the leaves along with a scratcher that had a jackpot on it. He picked it up reading it as another scratcher hit the wall. "Lucks on my side today." Jones read the dates realizing that the scratcher had already passed as he picked up a ten-cent coin from the ground. He started to scratch each one away. The white and green showed that he got a triple win as Jones went further down the wall that separated the Iron Trail from the therapy building. Jones slowly waltzed up the stairway again as he tossed away the two scratchers in the garbage can. Pearl followed right behind him as she tapped Jones on the shoulder, "Hey stranger!" she said looking Jones in the eyes.

"Oh, hey Pearl," Jones said in return, feeling the intensity that something had happened between her and her prince in a wheelchair. "Today's not going as planned, Jones, he's so sweet but I feel so far behind," she said to him as she wore a colorful dress representing her feelings. The deep blue mixed with green showed a happy sadness as the pearls reflected the sun towards Jones's face. The weather had been following Jones all day as his senses picked up again. He could hear the doctors talking upstairs ahead of time as well as the security guard walking downstairs. Jones grabbed his head as if he was in pain without a headache. "I'm sorry, I really need to listen to music right now," Jones said to Pearl to shut out the world's noise so that he could focus on becoming free from the therapy sessions. Jones put on a song that held violins in it as he further continued up the stairs viewing each person's step, reading them along the way as the world felt connected. "You look tired," Pearl said, trying to get through to Jones, ignoring his statement about needing to listen to music. Jones took out one of the ear pods as he turned to her again, "Yes, I can't function without it at this level." He said in return to Pearl as she slowly nodded her head.

"Is that why you're here?" She questioned him as he picked apart every last piece of the building in his mind. The process of Jones's brain sped up again gathering all the data his eyes were consuming. "Yes, I can't think very well at the moment. I'm sorry." He said walking away from Pearl as Jones wandered towards the check-in desk where the same lady had sat with her comfortable running shoes. "Hey, Jones!" She said happily as if she awaited him in the hallway every time before starting her sessions. Jones was completely known by now throughout the Office. "My tendency to talk to everyone is going to get me in trouble one day." He went over to the front of the desk and talked to the lady sitting at the desk. The front desk lady looked at Jones with wide eyes. "What brings you in here today Jones?" He stood for a moment as the room's details came to life. The woman who sat behind him with the broken brace had become younger as Jones saw her movements and past actions leading into her past.

He blinked his eyes a few times quickly, "I need to see Orin." The front desk lady got up slowly as she hit the buzzer. "Okay Jones, go ahead." She said, rolling her eyes. Jones walked as fast as he could towards Orin's room where he felt safe. Safe as if the room was blocked off from the noise that entered his head. "What brings you in today?" She calmly said as Jones's

CHAPTER NINETEEN – MIND CHESS

hat fell slightly to the side. "Cool shirt, the galaxy is one?" She questioned Jones. "Oh. Where did I get this?" He said calming down as his left hand shook. He hid his hand behind him as a song came on, "Relax, no stress." Into his phone, it played. "Well… I was…" he thought for a moment as Orin stared at him with her piercing eyes as she always had done. "I was going to meet a special friend of mine and had driven my car out for an hour. I suppose I didn't understand how or why I started driving to him. You see… I wanted to discover more factories…" Orin looked at Jones, "Factories?" She asked him out of curiosity.

"The universal car, you see it's this idea… that when you look at it, it has everything a person could want but also resonates with everyone, it's yellow because it's sunny and has color-changing abilities. Runs on music and energy power and can well… essentially fly out into outer space." Orin nodded her head as she listened to Jones' quick description of the car. "Tell me how you got to driving?" Orin said as Jones started to get into the story deeper. Jones drove down the road where there was nothing but trees. Following the music and the old cars that caught his attention a house lit up off to the side. He looked for a place to sleep as he had been driving for an hour and a half off the road. "There." He said to himself as a hotel-house lit up. "Here we hide in the shadows for those who are tired." Read the sign as the house stuck out to Jones. He backed his car down into the back of the dirt road and parked next to the old car which had a man also sleeping in it. "Look up." He mumbled to himself. Jones looked up at the stars as the night sky passed.

"What brings you here young man?" Jones didn't think the old man was talking to him. "I'm searching for someone, something more to help me build this." The old man spoke up, "Don't worry about it, get some rest and enjoy the moment." Jones laid back for a moment. He hadn't slept more than in twenty-minute increments, his mind told him to keep going as he kept waking up after only a short amount of time. "You're free to stay for a little, not too long though. A couple is waiting for you." The old man said as he resumed staring up at the stars. Jones didn't understand what he meant as he slowly fell into a short slumber. The sleep debt was catching up to him again. "A couple, huh?" He thought to himself as he continuously focused on the stars. "I can't stay here tonight," Jones said to the old man, unable to rest. The old man cracked a small smile, "I understand, safe journeys." People came out of the hotel right as Jones backed out of his car, "Hey, what are you doing here?" He didn't answer as he left speeding off down the road towards the next place.

After a few hours of driving, Jones arrived as an old car was completely lit up with white Christmas lights. A couple sat in the corner with a dark hat and bones on it. "Watchers," he said to himself as the two people started talking to one another. "Yes, I'm an old member from the CIA." The man said as his partner sat next to him. "Put this wire in, we can make it work." He said as a small antenna was sticking out of a broken-down computer. The woman with blonde hair and one glove reached out through it. "Oh, what the hell. Anyway, he said as he took a seat next to Jones. "Join in and let me take you on a different journey back in time. Movies, music, it's all the same so hop on in for the ride or fall down the rabbit hole. We ended up here on the side of the road because no one really cares what we're doing or where we were. It didn't matter if we shat or pissed ourselves after the CIA threw us to the billiards. At this moment, Jones, it didn't matter. Because all that made sense up until now in this loving beautiful messed-up world was…conjoined together. A sort of peacefulness and if you weren't allowed in that world you weren't let in. That's the world of the watchers so buckle up." Jones sat down next to the couple with a pair of gloves on as she spoke to him about the problems she was having with her current spouse.

"One last book, one god damn last book is all that matters." The agent mumbled to himself as he tried to make sense of the situation he was in with his wife. Jones sat there listening in on their conversation not wanting to let himself go as he clung to his soul. The cold weather started

CHAPTER NINETEEN – MIND CHESS

to creep in as the Christmas lights on the white van stayed lit up in the hotel parking lot. A gray bridge with ridges cut into it stuck out as lights with round heads changed colors as if egging Jones to walk over it. "Hey, it was nice meeting you kid but we've got to go." The man said as the two of them mumbled together trying to figure out their connections. Jones nodded as he went towards where he parked watching the two watchers waddle out of the corner that they were sitting in."The CIA does that, it just gobbles you up and spits you out sometimes." The man said with laughter as his voice faded into the distance. Orin put her hand up as Jones continued the story. "Wait, so you met two old defunct CIA agents? What made you want to travel so bad?" She questioned Jones, curious as to why he was mentioning this to her. Jones nodded as the mint smell filled the room. He could see the wind outside blowing the tree's in waves as he followed the wind reading its every detail. Jones continued, "I wanted to travel because I felt there was a man who could help me build the universal car that I once saw being built. Build it into our current world at this moment in time, considering I saw it being built in that future." Jones said, trying to help Orin understand.

Orin shook her head in dismay, "Jones, I think you need to let this one go. It's getting late in the day. You've already missed half of your therapy session." She said as Jones stopped his story. "Okay." He replied accepting that Orin had simply become his listening crutch. She didn't understand the dangers of the galactic universe or that he had the power to build what he imagined around him. Jones simply had to find the right people. Jones got up out of the black leather seat that smelled all too clean for him as his feet touched the carpet. The bland color stuck out at Jones. "You know, if these walls had color-changing paint when they got water on them it would look awesome and show people what's wet…same with these damn bland carpets". Jones mumbled to himself under his breath as he wandered back down towards the therapy session. Pearl was holding a purple clipboard. As Jones blinked the clipboard turned multiple colors from its original see-through form to where Pearl was tracing a video game with her fingers. The therapist looked at Pearl as Jones blinked again. Her fingers scratched the board as if nothing was happening. "Pearl stop scratching up my boards please." The therapist said as Jones took his seat again next to her. "Pearl, what are you doing? Stop playing video games." Jones whispered as Pearl completely understood and stopped. "It's so boring in this place, Jones. I feel as if I'm going insane by just sitting here." She whined as mint came out of her breath.

"It's time for you to leave therapy soon, you've been in here too long." A voice came from inside Jones's head. "Mira again," Jones said to himself, this time she was wearing a suit that held LED lights on the costume. Each one of the lights dissolved as she ate one. "What does that taste like?" Jones asked. "Like a fresh idea." Mira joked "What does a fresh idea taste like?" Jones said in rebuttal. "Sweet, sour, and everything in between the two." The stench of her breath and perfume blended as she pulled up a seat. "Jones, remember that ship?" She asked him as he recalled his dream of helping Nepharius get through. "That relic holds the power of our collective imagination. Nepharius wants it for himself to make us into brain-dead, in-the-box thinking zombies. The watchers exist to retain that lost creativity." Mira revealed to Jones what it did as the giant eye behind his back turned around to stare at Mira. "I know Nepharius hears all of this. He was going to tell you once you boarded that ship. The car sounds better don't you think?" Mira smirked as her eyes now turned into a pure black with yellow. The galaxy flowing through her iris as she laughed.

"Don't worry, I know you're already thinking about it. Remember? The whole galaxy can hear you as long as that eye is watching you. Jones, do you know how ideas get inspired? Come to life?" Mira asked. Jones slowly shook his head, keeping his head on saying empty thoughts over and over as the eyeball fell half asleep. "Visuals and sound, our universal language. Without even a word the two ideas combined to make better ones spawn more ideas. If that didn't happen anymore what would happen

CHAPTER NINETEEN – MIND CHESS

to the universe?" Mira said, "My dear little musical warrior, arbiter, black hole, and whatever else you've been called. You're simply Jones and you understand so much, yet so little." Jones put his hands on his head in reality as the therapist asked if Jones was okay. Jones didn't respond as he blankly looked over towards Pearl and shrugged. Bey spoke upright as it happened, "I need to go to the restroom." She said distracting the therapist from her questioning as Mira continued to talk to Jones in his mind. "Get on that ship Jones. It is your only way back out into keeping us from eternal stagnation. Your only way to stop it is to start. Hunt for that chip in the real world and keep Nepharius out of the galactic Brazilian temple in the cosmos." Jones shook his head, "yeah?" He said to the therapist as she scratched her head. "Can you...?" she stopped. "Never mind, the exercise is almost done, we'll be moving on to the next one next time. Everyone goes home." The therapist seemed frustrated with the lack of attention she was getting out of the group. Jones smiled and silently left out of the door leaving it perfectly half-opened and half-closed Jones thought to himself that maybe it wasn't chi of two extremities giving him thoughts of wanting others to succeed or fail but rather telling him "if" it was to fail what else would he do? To be prepared for those failures.

Jones laughed to himself, "I am prepared for those failures or successes. As a musical warrior, the world depends on us winning this war." Jones walked down the stairs not wasting any time as he looked over his shoulder to make sure he wasn't being followed. He hopped in his silver car and raced home as fast as he could blasting the EDM music at full. The wind whipped by as people looked at Jones' car walking faster. Jones held out his hand to signal people to clear the way as he ignored the light. People abided and cleared the way even though Jones thought he was playing with their will and moving them by his own hand. His brown felt hat bent back from the front side as he landed right at home. Jones pulled up in the driveway of his house and laid on the sunny grass to try to catch his breath of what had happened. As he closed his eyes, he saw Tober. "Jones! The golden piano! It's almost done!" Tober exclaimed. Jones got on messenger after opening his eyes seeing him appear on his suggested list. He held his phone close to him, "How in the world?" Tober had only been mentioned once and Jones did not have Tober's number. He didn't understand how he was appearing. Jones slowly fell back asleep. "Don't cut me off like that," Tober said standing on the beach. Nepharius was right there as the ship was fully built. "Who is entering our space?" Nepharius questioned.

"This is Tober. He can build us a golden piano. You wanted to perform right?" Jones asked Nepharius thinking quickly on his feet. Nepharius laughed, "Good job Jones on finding us a performance item. This will impress those during the show."Jones looked over at Tober and shrugged. "You promised." Jones pointed as he dipped his feet in the sand. The waves climbed up the beach as Tober took out one of his tools. "I did and I will fulfill your wish," Tober said to Jones. "So how did you get out? Heard you were peeing in your roommate's sink and rotting away." Jones questioned Tober as he looked at the man with a sight of sorrow. His feet looked as if they had been peeled off for over a year. "Well, you helped me get focused. After the place realized I was stable to them the nurse let me out. I came out of the zombie which the people had made me into." Tober laughed. Jones's mother went out to the grass as she saw Jones laying there soaking up what little sun was left. "What are you doing out here, Jones?" Jones woke up as his mother wiped her forehead. She had been gardening all day and smelled of grass and roses. "Soaking up some sun." Jones smiled as he looked back over at his mother who had been sweating. "Sun, huh? Comfortable?" She laughed. Jones laughed back for the first time in a while with his mother. Instead of arguing vigorously, the two were getting along.

"Yeah, it's pretty nice," Jones said as she started to pull out more weeds upfront. "There's food inside if you're hungry," Ms. P said pointing inside at the door. Jones got up and started walking inside as he turned around thanking his mom. "Alright, I'm pretty hungry anyway." He said walking inside as the cane he had previously been using now sat in its rightful place

CHAPTER NINETEEN – MIND CHESS

near the door. "I know I'll need this again someday but not for a while," Jones said to himself. He walked further over to the plate of food and scarfed it down, wasting no time. Jones was determined to get back to the dream, worried about what Nepharius may do when Tober finished the golden piano. Jones went over to his bed and laid down, closing his eyes again. This time, the golden piano already had its legs built. Jones could tell Nepharius was about to make a move as one of his crew members practiced martial arts on the side of the beach. Nepharius had a way of making the universe work in his favor by melding acting in with movies. As Jones had figured out in his mind and world, actors and movie producers were their real personas and in Jones's world, they were hiding in public by acting "normal." Jones had seen Nepharius movie and his lust for war. All those people that Nepharius had hurt in his movie were gone. Jones was unable to contact them by number as he had attempted to do through the Nebulous magazine. Jones walked over to Tober and mouthed to him with his lips rather than his thoughts as Tober hit his hammer over and over on the piano. "Almost done there, boy." He said eating an orange laughing to himself about how simple the solution was to his problem. "What's that, Jones?" Tober said again as Jones tried lip-syncing to Tober "Run" a song title.

As Tober's last hammer struck down he smiled loosely and shook his head. Tober knew he was caught up in the plan. Nepharius flung one of his men over himself which landed right on Tober's body as if the two of them had acted it out and made it an accident. "Tober!" Jones said out loud. Jones lost his cool. "Why would you do that?" Jones walked over to Nepharius. "War? Is this because of war?" Jones raised his voice. Nepharius shook his head slightly, "Tober was trying to harm me. Look at that inscription in the golden piano. It's a lock reversal." Jones looked at the side of the piano which had an inscription built-in it much like the one he saw in the park by the Lafayette building. Jones knew it was part of the plan but didn't think Nepharius would spot it. Jones said nothing as the man got up off of Tober's now cracked and frail body. The crew member took off the inscription turning it to favor Nepharius. "We'll play this as a shield." He said laughing maniacally. "Come on Jones! We have work to do." Jones followed him unwillingly onto the ship as the men lifted the golden piano aboard. "Bury Tober as a thank you note. Tell the show that Tober had been paid and had an unfortunate accident." Nepharius said. Jones wandered over to the side of the ship looking out over the horizon. He broke a sad smile as Jones woke up staring at his room trying to forget what had happened. "Zaya needs to play that, doesn't she? Another key to society's development..." Jones questioned himself.

The room was completely dark as night had fallen. "Remember Jones, the Spirit of Music is always on your side." As the hat was hung back up in Jones's closet. The voice rang through Jones's head as he went to wash his face in the sink. That would be the last time Jones would see Tober. Jones walked over to his fridge grabbing a drink and shaking his head at the thought of what had happened. "It's not real," he mumbled. as his mother watched the T.V. Tober's name appeared in the news as a man who had passed away by going crazy. A car had hit an old man reading the story as the clock hit 9 pm. "It is real..." Jones said to himself. "This is happening." Jones walked away slowly from the T.V. not wanting to accept the situation. He went back to his room to lay down. The next day, Jones woke up unwilling to get out of bed. "You need the discipline to wake up early every day. Look towards the positive Jones." Mira said in his mind. "It seems you still don't believe me. Your mom will ask you for therapy in a few minutes. Watchers are real, this plane is real. Accept it, Jones. Tober is dead!" Her voice echoed loudly throughout Jones's head. Jones sat there, wondering the same question that everyone else did. "What's my worth?" An age-old question posed throughout time. "What does that even mean?" was the next statement that followed out of Jones's mouth. The clocks struck 10 AM. Jones rubbed his eyes feeling beaten by the night before as it had taken all of his thoughts away.

"Jones, you have therapy in an hour." His mother said from the other room

CHAPTER NINETEEN – MIND CHESS

as Jones sat there moping about the loss of Tober. "I'm not going, Mom," Jones replied filled with rage and regret as his mother opened the door. "Yes, you are Jones! I am paying for this!" Jones stuck his nose up in the air. "Paying for what? Some bull-crap statements made by a therapist to distract me from the real problems out there?" Jones stormed over to the fridge as his mother looked at him startled unsure by what he meant by his statement. "What do you mean Jones? Don't say that." She said as she went into her room frustrated. Ms. P got out the shoe box and started polishing her shoes to calm herself down. Jones watched feeling guilty but didn't know how to apologize at the moment. He grabbed water out of the fridge and walked back outside feeling as if he didn't fit in anywhere as the wind blew lightly as if to caress Jones. Jones wiped his eye as the other eye didn't tear up. After going through everything that had happened his strength inside grew heavier. Jones had started to grow distant from the people of the world feeling as if no one was awake to what had been going on around him. Feeling isolated as if it would be up to him to save the world's imagination and progress it forward through developing his ideas from the world around him. "What's wrong, Jones?" A voice passed by his head as it was recognizable. Zaya's calming tone helped Jones recognize it even in his dire situation. "Family issues that's all, I sometimes don't feel understood," Jones said out loud to himself as one of his neighbors looked at him weirdly.

Unable to understand the rants and watching Jones talk to himself line by line. "You alright there, buddy?" The neighbor said from across the street. "Yeah, yeah. I'm fine, cute dog." Jones said in return remembering to blend in as he walked further down the neighborhood. A black terrier stared at Jones from across the road as it barked at him making Jones stare back. "Are you okay?" The dog asked as in Jones's mind, he thought to himself. "Yeah, don't ask right now. Be on your way up." He said communicating telepathically. Zaya tried getting Jones's attention again. "You need me to play that golden piano don't you," Zaya asked Jones in a questionable tone. "It's dangerous though, it could cost you your life," Jones said back as Zaya's image now appeared in Jones's mind. Her yellow and green eyes looked back at him. She no longer looked beat up. Her hair blooming in a beautiful afro undertoned skin. Her face was no longer sagging from the damage previously. In her own right, Zaya was a galactic celebrity. "I know how to defend myself; I'll be fine in this world," Zaya said back to Jones. "You just focus on what you have to do, you know…waking up every day, discipline and stuff. Isn't that and doing the same thing over and over what makes us, well us?" She said with encouragement. Jones stopped walking for a moment as he reached the end of the street. An old lady now walked by with her dog on a leash as this one quietly looked at Jones. The dog stopped in its tracks, refusing to move as the lady pulled on the string. Jones waved at the brown and white husky telling it to move and keep going. "Don't break my cover" he said to himself as the old lady reared her head wondering why Jones kept talking to himself. She turned around as the husky obliged willingly further walking down the street. Jones walked further down the road in the same pathway that he and Ottie had walked. An old fence stood there with a sign that read "old land mines and hole traps present, do not enter." Jones shut his eyes as he walked across the field. He stepped from place to place on each mound using his mind to keep the mines from going off as he avoided each one with each step. Jones could feel the electrical energy going through the ground pointing him through and navigating him past the running trail to the other side.

As Jones walked further past the field an old sign stuck out, "Gardening for free at your own will." read in big green and yellow letters as the smell of oranges sprinkled by. Jones peaked at it but was too shy to wander further in as he walked in towards town. Needing to use the restroom he went in and sat down for a moment washing his face as he noticed the toilet paper was out. "It'd be really damn helpful if there was a small light that blinked on this thing whenever the rolls got empty. People don't check before they use these restrooms." He complained to himself. Jones, already feeling isolated from the rest of the people, didn't care about time as ten minutes

CHAPTER NINETEEN – MIND CHESS

had already passed. A knock on the door startled him. "Come on man!" A voice shouted from the outside. "I need to use it." Jones got up washing his hands acting as if nothing had happened. "Yeah, Sorry, coming out in a moment." Jones turned on the sink to wash his hands as he unlocked the door watching the other man speed by. "A holder to place our phones before we clean up on one of these damn side places would be good too," Jones said to himself, annoyed, as he talked to himself aloud. "Phones are always dropping I swear…" he mumbled walking further into town as he walked towards the park in the middle of the area. Jones started singing as the sunset slowly crept on him. He sat on the bench and looked at the middle of the park where rain had fallen on the grass. Jones started to move in the grass as if he were skiing in the snow, doing ice-skating moves in the park to a song he played on his phone. A woman walking with her kid laughed at Jones off to the side and backed off walking away as she wondered why a man was flipping in the park. Jones had been practicing in preparation for Nepharius's show as the upbeat song loving with electricity played. Sliding across the grass Jones wobbled and fell staring at the sky laughing to himself as the park emptied. For a moment he sat there staring at the sky. The Spirit of Music entered his head as the wetness seeped through Jones's clothing.

"The orchestra is still our world, Jones. Galactic space will always need your help. Our help as we watch over it." The man turned into his blue octopus' self out of his male form still wearing the felt brown hat. He hugged Jones as the stars shine again. "When Nepharius strikes again, we'll strike back. I know you feel alone in this, but no one is ever struggling alone. None of the watchers are ever alone." Jones nodded, smiling at the support that the Spirit of Music had given him. He stood up and started walking back towards his house hoping that his mother had calmed down. Jones was ready to go back to therapy tomorrow to tell Orin what was happening and what he had seen. The night was silent as the music played into Jones's ear to keep him walking forward back towards his home. The road was now in complete silence as no wind, no sound other than the crickets chirped into the background. Jones smiled like an idiot as he got home.His mother made a grilled cheese sandwich and placed it on the table as Jones opened up one of the cabinets looking for bread and vinegar. "Jones, are you hungry?" She offered as the sandwich sat there late at night. "No, not really," Jones replied to his mother as he went straight for his room. "I'm going to take this bread and go to my room to relax," Jones announced as the smell of grilled cheese made his stomach rumble. He laid down on his bed staring at the ceiling "feeling broke Jones?" Mira rang out through his head.

"You know all those watchers have been giving you discounts because two dollars converts to two hundred in galactic money." She laughed. "Why else do you think watchers only ask for spare change?" Jones yawned to himself, "You didn't tell me this sooner because?" Mira smirked. "I didn't want you arguing with people who weren't connected to galactic space." Jones sighed as he pulled a pillow over his head. "Mira, what do you need? I'm busy." Jones said as Mira chuckled, "You can't lie to me, Jones. I can literally see you. Are you prepared to stop Nepharius?" Mira asked once as he put a pillow over his head. "Tober…" he said to himself in remorse. "Yeah. Let's get revenge on that son of a bitch who messed up my life. Who threw me in that damned ward of a jail! Who's there trying to take over with corporations for his own damned relic." Jones replied not leaving any room to hide his anger. "Okay if you're ready to do this the right way Jones you'll have to be prepared to go back into a lack of sleep. Your communication, in reality, will go down and you'll forget where you left your items. You'll get confused and may not even know who you are at times. The world of the watchers is a hidden one as you've experienced. The only way to take down Nepharius is to have a musician play on that golden piano in an arpeggio as he tries for the relic from. It will be up to you to decide what to do when that time comes, Jones." Mira looked at Jones with a stern face. "Humanity's best savior of humanity is with you Jones. You may have to spend time resetting your mind again after this… back there." Mira gave a wicked smile with a bit of sadness in her tone as

CHAPTER NINETEEN – MIND CHESS

she tossed him an idea.

"Eat one if you want." Jones took it as he flipped a water bottle in his room over and over crushing it down to size in his hand. "Why would I want to eat this Mira?" He asked her in return. Mira laughed, "For the experience." The idea swirled in Jones's hand as he tucked it away in his pocket while his eyes were closed. The water bottle lies on the wooden floor crushed into a pretzel as water lies there inside. Rain began to pour as Jones looked outside. Puddles of water started to gather towards one another as he imagined himself dodging each rain droplet on the ground. The weather was within Jones's eye, within his control as the galaxy reflected in his eyes. Electric blue energy surged back through Jones's body as he fell back into his blanket. "No sleep huh? Back to sleep debt…? Can I do that?" He questioned himself and his capabilities. Jones had been gaining confidence through his entire journey of meeting and talking to these people. His mind was ready to go to war with Nepharius who so desperately had wanted his assistance. "Nepharius, I'm coming for you. You damned son of a-" Jones stopped his anger from arising as he laid down keeping his eyes open. Reading on his cellphone and attempting to keep himself awake as his senses came alive. "You better be right Mira…" Jones stated to himself as he drifted back off towards sleep until morning. "I am," Mira replied drifting off. "Remember the deer soldiers near your house? They will escort you." She said as the bushes outdoors shook. Jones faded into black as fast as he woke up in the morning taking naps in between each moment. Jones put on his brown felt hat and walked outside to look at the roof. A ship was pointing east along with the wind telling Jones which way he would be heading.

"You're going east, huh?" Jones said to himself going back in the house to grab his black and gray jacket that he had bought in Monterey Bay. "Good morning." His mother said from the kitchen as Jones got ready to go out the door. "I'm going over to a friend! I won't be home for a while!" He said as she looked back over at him. "Love you, mom." He said with a hint of nervousness. "Love you too, sweetie! When will you be home?" She asked him. "I'm not sure. I'll be home soon." He said as he smiled at her. Jones went out the door fully dressed and cleaned up as the wind and water from last night's rain would now be his indicator. Jones watched the wind go through the trees as he followed the direction with his head before the wind hit his body. Jones would be using everything he had previously learned to track down Nepharius's connection simultaneously in the world. As Jones got into his car, he put on a song titled "Stay away." blasting it down the street to make sure watchers and onlookers would make way for Jones to get through the traffic. "Lack of communication" was pre-loaded in case of the potential watcher who he felt would become aggressive. Now that Jones had lived in the world, he was prepared ahead of time to combat the problems thrown his way. "I'm Jones T. Harver, dammit! I will save our imaginations and this world if it's the last thing I do!" He yelled to himself as the windows slowly went down. "You're an actor, stuck forever acting for yourself in this world Jones." Nepharius's voice rang through his head. "In my movie, you are acting. Like the other actors who hide on the big screen! Hide from their true freedom where others can only watch!"

Jones yelled back, "Shut Up you murderer! You know so little of our world even with so much knowledge! The more you know the less you know, don't you understand a thing?" Jones said, trying to reason. Nefarious laughed, "I taught you. You belong to me!" Jones replied in his mind as a car drove by. "No. I belong to me. This is my mind, my world living on it with others. No one, not even you rule it." Jones took a breath and reoriented himself as the wind blew him towards the "Ships R Us" store. As soon as Jones arrived at the "Ships R Us" store, he parked his car right where the wind blew. A man stood out front welcoming Jones in with a glare."Anything you like it's yours but for a small fee." The man slowly approached him holding out his hand as if to point Jones in the right direction. "Ciex?" Jones said to himself, noticing the blue clip and black feathered hat sticking out from the man's head. "That's right Jones! You

CHAPTER NINETEEN – MIND CHESS

found me again!" He said ecstatically. Jones smiled in return. "It's great to see you!"

The ship store in bright blue words stuck out to him. "Great to see me huh?" The demi hunter said. "Well…listen, the reason I'm here is that you're going to need a ship. One to return off the island after you land with Nepharius. Jones lowered his tone. "Nepharius is on to me you know." Jones surveyed the shop viewing the old wood that lies up top. The smell of coconut and furnish filled the air as sea salt crept into the old store. Gray books of old-time and scripture poked out from up top of the shelf. "What are all of these?" Jones asked the demi-human hunter as he wandered around to the backside of the store."These? These are all scriptures of encounters with those like yourself. Similar experiences to the ones you were having." The feather hat twitched back and forth as Jones grabbed a small piece of wood from the shelf. "Woah, careful!" Jones jumped backward at the man's words. "What is it?" Jones said curiously, studying its beauty. "This wood is special cherry wood meant to withstand any sort of weather. It's imbued with the same shield that Nepharius had put around you."

Jones had forgotten that there was a protective shield around him. His memory sprung up as he was reminded of when he walked down the street. A car almost hit Jones off the sidewalk but then realigned randomly to the road. The car sped off down the street as if nothing had happened that entire time. "So that's why…" Jones said as the feather hat turned again to the right. "Yes Jones, that's why you have been protected all of these times from those who had the intent to hurt you. Make no mistake Jones, Nepharius is a bad man." Jones put up his hand to stop the demi-human hunter from continuing. "Will this piece of wood help me track Nepharius through the weather?" Jones asked as he sat down on an ashen chair crossing his legs. "Jones, this piece of wood will bring you on the light water as the ship glides to its destination. You will be as free as the seagulls who claim the wind on a sunny migration day."Another piece of wood was thrown Jones way. "Take this for backup." The demi-hunter pointed at an old gold clock on the ceiling as it melted off the roof slightly. The time slowed down almost to a stop. "I heard Jones you had an experience, a tassel with your mother at one point. Is that right?"

Jones looked at the Demi-human hunter and laughed. "More than once. It's a constant bicker." Jones said in return. "One time you got so angry while she was sitting in the car you yelled at the top of your lungs. Remember?" The demi-human hunter sighed as Jones nodded his head. "Yeah, I remember, so what?" Jones replied, growing impatient with the situation."At that time, you froze time. For a split second. I'm sure you remember walking around the car as your mother didn't respond with her finger up. You yelled "Stop." As the demi hunter paced the room he eyeballed Jones picking up a small snow globe. "As an arbiter, you are a keeper of time Jones. Why do you think you don't age fast?" The Demi-hunter questioned Jones "Do you even need this lecture? I'm sure you know." Jones slowly took a step back wondering how he had known all his shortcomings. "Listen, give me the wood and that's all I need." Jones requested. The black-feathered hat now was taken off as the man's golden hair flowed out towards the ground. "As you wish." The Demi-hunter rang up Jones. "12.34 galactic quar." This was the first time Jones had heard the word. "Croxi..." Jones repeated. "That in American money?" Jones said to the demi-human hunter who was now behind the cashier. "Two dollars and forty-five cents." He replied, annoyed at Jones's question. Jones took the cherry wooden pieces and put them in his pockets as he went over towards the back of the shipyard. Over there sat a small boat with a similar color to the cherry wood ship that Jones was given. The demi-human hunter came up behind Jones looking out at the open sea. "It's a beauty isn't it?" He said as the ship swayed lightly in the ocean.

SS. Departure was written on the side of the boat as Jones burned the image into his mind.

Jones nodded lightly, "Yeah. It's bright and well taken care of. I have to go

CHAPTER NINETEEN – MIND CHESS

now. There's therapy still waiting for me." Jones said to the demi-human hunter as the man towered over him. "Safe travels kid' oh yee will is one." Jones turned back towards the door and walked out of the Ship store back towards his car. Once dirty, Jones's car shined as if it was brand new. He drowned out the sound around him by continuously listening to soft music loudly as he held a cherry wood piece in his pocket. "It's the history that drives us," Jones said to himself quietly. Arriving back home in the afternoon no one was there. Time had returned to normal around the household for Jones as his mother was no longer worried about his breaks. Jones sat on his bed with the wooden piece thinking about the decision he would have to make on Mira's orders. "All I wanted to do was build this car for the world..." Jones mentioned to himself feeling discouraged. He set aside his jacket and cherrywood piece attempting not to feel isolated from the rest of the world. Jones got into his car and headed towards his therapy appointment getting ready to speak to Orin again. There were only two days left to explain to Orin how he felt in his much-needed freedom. Jones ate an orange slowly as the juice spilled out over the countertop. The patterns of the orange pointed towards the door as if telling him to hurry up or else he was going to be late. Jones threw on his clothing and felt-tipped brown hat aiming towards the white door that had Greek designs out front. The history built into buildings and households intrigued Jones as he noticed owls written on houses' mailboxes. One mailbox had a general as Jones thought to himself, "This is how mail must have been delivered in the old days. It had to have been. He ran back towards the car. After a few minutes of driving, he reached the therapy building where Jones spent no time talking to anyone except the front desk person. Pearl and Bey had been completely released.

All that remained were magazines at the front desk. "Orin can see you now." The front desk lady buzzed Jones in as he walked into her office. "How are you feeling Jones?" She asked him as Jones sat down well dressed. "Much better," Jones said in return. Orin looked at Jones, noticing that his clothing wasn't tattered and that he was well cleaned up. "You look good

Jones! Like you've fully recovered." Jones scratched his head embarrassed at the statement and thought that he could have been "crazy." "Thank you, Orin," Jones said in return, ready to continue his story. "Jones, tell me more about your experience?" Orin asked him. "Well, you see…" Jones started back the story of his drive home after the meeting with two agents and started to explain his love and need for music to help him fall asleep. "After I met the two agents, I drove back home from there as I was lacking sleep." Orin nodded her head. "What was the song?"

Jones pulled out his phone and showed her. "This song helped me sleep along with this channel." He mentioned to her that Jones showed the differences. "This helped me be able to rewire myself a little," Jones said. Orin smiled, "I don't see a reason for you to continue therapy here. That's a good solution." Orin mentioned as she got on her computer to take notes. "Still, continue your story," Orin said, lightly tapping on the keyboard. Jones nodded, "After I got home, I realized that the term being grounded kept being tossed around. As if we weren't grounded our consciousness would end up somewhere else. After I came to, I found myself wondering what my next steps would be. That's how I ended up here…" Orin turned to Jones surveying over him a moment deciding to see if he was better or not. "Come in tomorrow Jones. Seems you are fully back to your good old self. I'd like to see you one last time." Orin suggested. "Try staying out of trouble from now on." Jones nodded slowly as he got up towards the door. "Small pizza party is down the hallway to talk about problems and solutions," Orin mentioned. Jones replied swiftly, "I'll pass this time. Thank you."

As he slowly shut the door walking out of the building and back down the steps. The normalcy of the world bothered Jones still, Nepharius was out there wreaking havoc. Jones would be free to stop Nepharius soon as the finish line was so close Jones could visualize it. "It is impossible to learn all things. That is why we know more, that is why the more we know the less we know." Jones said to himself recalling the statements previously passed

CHAPTER NINETEEN – MIND CHESS

down to him through what seemed to be millions of years. Jones sat down on the bench near the Safeway watching the clouds go by as he dozed off. "You. Jones, to the starboard now!" Nepharius's voice rang out as Jones found himself on the ship floating rapidly down a current. Water crashed into the ship as one of the crew members slid down to the opposite side of the ship."We are almost to Brazil, Jones," Nepharius said as he laughed at the sight of danger. Jones took hold of the ropes making sure they were tied. His shoe soaking up a small puddle in the Safeway bench from a minor spill. "Right," Jones said to himself, the cherrywood. Jones woke up with his foot wet as he raced towards the car driving home towards his room where the cherry wood lies that the demi-human hunter had given to him. He grabbed it and fell back asleep in his bed gripping the item. As Jones fell backward into the ship's cabin it became lighter. The waves heavy of rocking calmed down while the storm hit the boat. "I see you've picked up some featherlight," Nepharius said as the golden piano had been moved to the cabin. "I'm not sure where you got that Jones but you've saved us some trouble."

Nepharius took it into his hands as he moved his crew further towards navigating out of the storm. "Soon, imagination will be ours," Nepharius stated. Jones shut his eyes in his dream attempting to wake up as the speed of the boat picked up. As the cabin shook, he was able to open his eyes. He woke up again from his dream. The clock hit 5:00 PM as his mother got home. "Jones, your classes are starting again soon." She mentioned putting the groceries on the counter. "Did your laundry too." She said as the tone of her voice drifted off. Jones replied, "Thanks mon, I'll look into it." Feeling exhausted he went over to the computer to search for classes where the cherrywood now lies on the desk next to his hats. A list of teachers popped up for his final semester as he looked at times later in the day. "I'm going to finish school and get through this," Jones said to himself promising the completion of his opportunity towards a degree. As Jones registered for his final courses on the computer, he got a text. "Yo, how have you been my man?" Tennor had reached out along with

Bernz. "Every night is a journey, isn't it? You stupid fucker, come hang out we miss you." Jones thought about it contemplating the world around him as he looked down at messengers getting distracted by the videos that were popping up on his phone. As if he was being challenged again, actors and professionals alike were calling out to Jones doing flips and hanging off buildings, swimming miles on end. "I told you, Jones. Like a lion." Nepharius voice rang through his head. "Everything has a time and a place. Some people will wish the worst and best, some people will think in "If then me, and others like me, choose destruction and war. You know why Jones?"

Jones put the phone down as another text from Tennor went through. "Hey, stupid! Respond!" Jones listened to Nepharius speak again, "Because people want what's easier. Destruction is easier." Nepharius looked over in disappointment as the calm seas raced slowly pushed the boat along. "remember Jones, see everything for what it is." Jones didn't reply, letting Nepharius fade into the background. All he wanted to do was have Nepharius disappear. The feeling of betrayal grew stronger within as he clenched his fist. Jones calmed down texting Tennor back, "I'm all for it man. Is Bernz there?" Jones asked out of curiosity. "I don't know bro, ask his stupid ass to come," Tennor replied. Jones texted Bernz as well, getting a reply right back as the few of them set a meeting time at the bar. "I'm going to China. Over there I can be a teacher, get a scripture. Tired of being here." Tennor texted again as Jones thought about traveling again. "You know we're all always traveling anyway." Jones texted back thinking about how he was idle on Nepharius's ship. His consciousness floating through the galaxy now disconnected from his own body due to the therapy sessions that Jones was forced to hold. Not able to sit still anymore and starting to lack sleep again to reconnect his consciousness with reality. Jones went outside to catch the only thing he had to recharge his body. The sun shined down brightly as he walked outside in his pajamas lying on the grass again. His sanctuary among others. Jones had already forgotten his toothbrush amidst the chaos of thoughts that had been running through his head. As

CHAPTER NINETEEN – MIND CHESS

Mira had told Jones what would happen if he chose to hunt Nepharius there would be consequences on his own body. Jones's senses exceeded the normal expectations again hearing birds among construction as the world spun around him. Unable to garner proper REM sleep as he lay there in the sun. The clock now struck 3:00 PM as time went by. He was supposed to meet Tennor around 5:00 PM. Lately, his phone had not received spam emails in the same fashion. He looked down into his phone waiting for a simple response but received no reply from the masses. Jones was ousted, on his own in the galaxy away from the celebrity life and now virtually isolated in his own world. Going back inside of the house Jones put on some proper clothing and headed straight for the door to take a walk down the street. Jones's mind was scattered, so scattered that he couldn't decide even when to properly sleep yet alone which task to do. As his mind grew less and less focused on the world around him while trying to force himself to do more tasks he walked into town.

"I need to find out what I am. I need to find out what it means to be an arbiter." Jones said to himself remembering what Nepharius had said about comic books and movies in today's society. As he got closer to town, he started singing to himself to calm his nerves and focus on the short walk ahead. Jones had never bothered to walk into his local library before. As he arrived, steps in Lafayette led to a statue stacked high as a representation of books tilting over. Each piece of the sculpture looked as if it had a meaning built with time. Jones continued up the steps towards the doorway where the automatic doors slid open. People were there reading all types as the library had books stacked to the top on each shelf. Information junkies scratching their heads as each one comfortably lies in each place. "Do you need help, sir?" A woman said from behind Jones as he sat in the library for a moment thinking. "Yes, do you have a book on arbiters and what movie franchises are based on?" Jones asked as the librarian looked at Jones with a "what in the world." look. "Yes, we have three, I think… Do you know the title?" Jones pulled up his text messages scrolling back to where Nepharius had communicated the messages. "Uh… well…I uh."

Jones stuttered. "Do you have a library card, sir?" She followed up politely. Jones shook his head, "Unfortunately no." He said in return. "The library card is free for you! Be sure to return the book if you check it out." She smiled.

Jones remembered the title, "A Guideline: Arbiter Times." He told the woman as she searched for the book. "We have one copy." She replied swiftly pulling it up on the computer as the comfortable colored carpet stuck out at Jones."When was the last time it was checked out?" Jones asked curiously. The librarian woman replied, "Three hundred years ago...? That can't be right." She said curiously. "Anyway, the book is hardcover and brand new. It must be a computer malfunction. Sometimes things get shaky around here." She replied. Jones was no stranger by now of odd happenings going on around him every time he had a task. Watchers had a disruptive personality, being one in the world of the galaxy himself he too had weird messages. "I see. It's no problem, can you show me where a "Guideline to the Arbiter the Times" book is?" Jones said in return. She spoke to him lightly. "Yes but... I'll need a ladder. Sit right in one of those chairs and make yourself at home while you wait, sir." Jones did exactly that as he went over to the chair in the corner. The black and brown chairs had an inviting feel to them in which readers and information sharing alike became a sanctuary. An archive of sorts in which anyone could spend their time figuring out the history of life or losing themselves in their fantasy worlds. Jones looked around as people of all different life forms walked through the library. Some of them being watchers who he could tell glanced at him sitting there from time to time.

"Here you are, sir." The librarian lady handed Jones the book. "That's an interesting read, I've not read it myself yet but it seems it was a best seller for its time." She mentioned it briefly as Jones said there pondering what the librarian had said. "Were best sellers even around three hundred years ago?" Jones questioned the idea. "Well anyways..." he opened up the book to read down the first page. "Arbiters, the keepers of time and the

CHAPTER NINETEEN – MIND CHESS

regulators of the galaxy. This species is known to be able to change will on hand as well as rewrite history as one sees fit. Arbiters do not age but can whittle by tricking one's own will into telling themselves that they will grow old. My name is Nepharius N. ——- "Jones stopped reading for a moment as Nepharius last name was scratched out in the book. Due to Jones feeling tired and scatterbrained he started to doze off within the first page. "Arbiters will take the lead where necessary and make sounds based on video games. Usually, these species are docile creatures as my own experience with them, one as my general at the time had battled the K'thuk'tansin. In the old war of the past. Young arbiters do not know they can temporarily stop time as their will must be stronger than the opponent. Scriptures from these species can be found in old buildings and history written into the world that many of us treasure. If you run into the arbiter race contact only those that stand before you for there is eternal power in one's energy life form. The arbiter's force is not to attack but simply to moderate. These species do not run on ships.

Arbiters run on time…" the first page showed the anatomy of an arbiter dressed much like a human. Jones drifted off to sleep on the chair as the noise around him faded into the distance. "Jones T. Harver was it?" Nepharius said as Jones found himself on the ocean again as fish jumped around the boat, the crew snacked on their catches. Jones nodded still refusing to reply to Nepharius afraid of what he might find. "You are me, Jones, I've immortalized you with my words. My imagination in that book you're reading." Jones shook his head, "Impossible. You did not create me." Jones talked back to Nepharius for the first time since Tober's death."That book. You knew ahead of time. How?" Jones asked Nepharius as he sat there with a fishing rod.

"I know you seek revenge, Jones. You won't win this. Our body is our temple and our mind is a sanctuary. I am already in most people's thoughts. That is what these words are written into eternity to do." Nepharius spoke to Jones calmly as Jones expected him to get up and fight. He didn't, he sat there looking out over the water. "I knew this would happen because one in tune with their senses can feel what's going to happen by one's thoughts. Your thoughts become reality with minor beliefs. Do you know why music is the universal language? Your friend Ottie explained it." Nepharius said questioning Jones. "The algorithm predicts emotion and the future through math and vibration. You as a black-holed historian of all people should understand this concept the most. As my old-time general, modern-day red hundreds. Magic existed, a world of the golden age was a real place and soon we will be on top again." Jones couldn't accept what he was hearing. "No! This is modern-day. I refuse to accept in this informational age that the golden age isn't already here! We are rediscovering ourselves again!" Jones didn't understand why he said what he said to Nepharius as the wind lightly blew.

Both Jones and Nepharius looked the same way as a small whale swam towards the boat. "Not all is bad, Jones. I do not intend to destroy everyone. Although, I am not a saint interested in helping either. I have already done that and had repercussions for it. Do you understand why I said to experience your journey as I have been watching you?" Nepharius asked again as Jones sat there in distraught. "To show you, the neglect of human nature. To show you the watchers that no one cares about. To show you that one's first self before others is the only way the world works within all the worlds. Why are ideas all including earth?" Jones shook his head again, "because... all the stories come from all the species coinciding here on earth..." Jones said. "Correct, we seek other worlds because we already know we're all here in tune with one another. All of those watchers are different species of the same dating back to your infinity of time." Nepharius said softly feeling remorse as the whale calmly looked at the both of them. Nepharius's eyes moved upwards, willing the whale away. "Now you will wake up." The librarian shook Jones twice. "Sir, we are closing"

Jones woke up. "Let me rent this book. I know you are closing but issue me

CHAPTER NINETEEN – MIND CHESS

a card." Jones asked the librarian half mumbling as he conversed. "Okay, quickly then," the librarian obliged. The librarian went up to the front desk and checked out the book after issuing a small blue card. "Special Archives." ended up being written on the card as Jones took the book. "Be sure to return it to us in good condition." She smiled as Jones walked out of the door of the library down the steps towards his house. Jones went down the steps with the book in his hand happy that he had successfully found what he was looking for. Despite his brain going through a scattered momentum of failure Jones had some sense of what he was trying to accomplish. As the ship grew continuously closer to the Brazilian shore, he would have to figure out more about the arbiter life from his past. His humanized form took complete control over his soul as he looked for a galactic connection. "No ships to outer space, no connection to the old times." Any piece of history Jones saw as a clue had paved the way to making Jones feel further and further away from his potential findings. As Jones walked down each step thinking his every thought, he began to further dive into figuring out how to not corner himself again. "Last time I broke because I set rules, I had to follow its to the very core," Jones said to himself as he started to walk down the street. "Red meant to stay away, yellow meant okay, green meant life, blue meant re-energize. I forgot these colors could have more to them than just their extremities." Jones continued as men and women looked at him pointing or avoiding him as he talked to himself. Trying to rebuild society's imagination from scratch was no easy task.

People didn't realize what was going on as the tree's stuck out to him. Due to Jones's senses going out of whack again each molecule on a branch or stem popped out towards him even more than it originally had. "Perception, Jones. It is all simply perception," Sao said. "Why didn't you call on me? Do you know? The guy dressed in red, messing with my template man. You let yourself get captured. I could have helped then." The voice seeped into Jones's head before he looked down at his phone. Sao sent a text message to Jones, "Where are you now? Let's meet up, see if our templates match and all." Jones reluctantly texted back, "Later, I am meeting up with my friend at a bar." Jones replied quickly putting away his phone as he realized it was almost time for the meetup. He hopped in his car and drove home. Five minutes later Jones had opened the door, threw the book on the bed, and headed back out again. He forgot to close the door on the way out as the warm puttering of the car was still running outside. Dressed in slippers and pants that felt slightly too big for Jones he started driving towards the bar. "This is Bernz, where are you?" Jones got a text message as Bernz had also decided to go to the bar to meet up with Tennor.

Tennor had a way of wearing the same clothes every time Jones saw him. He was always consistently sitting there ranting and raving about how Walnut Creek was a terrible area and he wished to leave for China. Tennor spoke up, "Walnut Creek is always filled with entitled people, old money, and this sense of fake humanity. This perfect bubble where hardly anything ever happens without even the slightest sense of community for the isolated. At least in China, there's the struggle showing firsthand. I can't even hold a good conversation anymore." "I think Walnut Creek's pretty awesome. I've had a lot of good conversations." Bernz chimed in as Jones walked through the door to sit down. "Hey, there's the fucker!" Tennor laughed as he patted Jones on the back. "Take a seat, grab a beer." He offered as Jones did exactly that. Jones was set on trying to relax away from Nepharius and the galactic world. Knowing that the war between the two would be the last time resonated in Jones's head. "This may be the last time I have a decent drink for a while," Jones said quietly as Bernz and Tennor looked at each other. "Yeah, and the first of tonight," Tennor replied, getting Bernz to also laugh. The two of them started to talk. "Hey remember that man with the motorcycle helmet?" Tennor commented, "Yeah, he was talking about some military buy operation. Buy a tank and a house illegally and resell it for five million." He laughed.

Bernz replied, "Dude was kind of crazy. Said he could only do it twice or something before someone would catch on." Bernz and Tennor smiled as

CHAPTER NINETEEN – MIND CHESS

the two of them continued to joke about the crazy man's comments on the street. Jones couldn't help but feel a sweet relation to the tone that described Jones as if he were in the same position. "Man, it's alright, the dude is having a hard time." Jones chimed in sipping down the beer that the bartender had put in front of him. A tip was left on the countertop. "This bar would be great with a sliding beer top," Jones said in return. "I mean, put down the beer and it slides across. The bartender would never have to move." Jones continued. "Yeah put that in your great ideas booklist." Tennor cracked up. "You're a funny guy Jones. Come with me to China to teach. It's an English curriculum. I'll get you in." Tennor egged Jones on. Jones waved away Tennor's idea uninterested in teaching English and traveling. "Nah man, I know you'll be leaving soon so good luck," Jones said politely as Tennor downed another beer. Bernz sat there listening as he squeezed some lemon into his beer. "Zesty." He said with one word making a triple finger. Jones sat there as the bar chairs slowly dissipated as his focus shifted "Here since.1904." He read quietly to himself. History was written everywhere within the buildings he had gone to; the buildings Jones had read. Monuments tended to pique his interest as he got up off the chair.

"Yo, where are you going?" Tennor called out briefly. "Outside for a quick smoke, care to join?" Jones said, trying to be witty. For a moment as the bar spun Jones forgot where he was. "Yeah, alright. Bernz?" Tennor turned towards Bernz as he held up a small joint. "Yeah, all this sounds good. Bar food to go with it!" Bernz replied in succession. Jones walked outside as the three of them lit up the Joint. "So, Jones, what are you going to do now?" Tennor asked him staring at the bar worried about his drink as if it would be taken away. Jones smiled as he took a puff of the joint. "I'm not sure maybe find a job or a new hobby I guess, go back to school and all of that," Jones replied as Bernz stood there listening in again. "Yeah? School for Kool kids?" Tennor asked trying to get a sense of the grinding mentality that Jones had developed. "Nothing wrong with wanting to do something, get out and do something though," Tennor said as he drifted off into his world staring up at the sky. "Kinda cold out here. I'm going to head home". Tennor said walking back in the bar as he paid for it. Bernz sat outside on the wooden post for a second turning to Jones, "Ottie was pretty funny huh?" Jones wondered for a moment why Bernz said so, "Yeah, he has my laptop though." Jones said. "Kinda need that back before school."

Bernz 's eyes moved up briefly as he was taken by surprise. "Dude, 311 in the quad buddies. C'mon." Bernz replied. Jones shook his hand waving at Bernz signaling for the conversation to stop. "Yeah yeah, it's alright." He said as the bar now felt dimly lit like the lights were changing automatically as the sun was going down. "I have to get home," Jones said to Bernz, shaking his head in dismay. "Alright," Bernz replied as he put out the joint that had been passed around between the three of them. Jones went over towards his car and sat down thinking about the short drive home. "I have to complete these courses," Jones said to himself. As the door opened the silence of the night crept up on Jones. Plants and squirrels alike were tuned to his energy staring him down as each footstep made a light sound. The hunger in Jones crept upon him as he went over to the fridge to snag a snack. The whole world around Jones felt surreal yet distant as the sound of his footsteps was all he was hearing. As he craved food, he walked into his room listening to the deer and bush creatures. "Jones, how is it?" A deer spoke from the bush outside of his window as he sat there on his bedside. "Well, it goes." He replied in return as Jones sat down trying to accept the reality that he was communicating with a squirrel. The squirrel looked back at Jones through the window with an acorn in its hand."You know in three years people might build a trash can in a drive-through at fast-food restaurants."

The squirrel looked back at Jones chirping as he thought about his friend Ike. Him and Ottie were supposed to go over to Ike's house to make more music. Only Ottie had already overstayed his welcome which didn't allow for studio time between the three of them. Ottie had met Ike once

CHAPTER NINETEEN – MIND CHESS

before attempting to get along before Jones learned of the hidden galactic world around them but had argued previously. As the squirrel sat, Jones looked back at him. "I need to go to Ike's. I need to tell my friends that the few of them are musical warriors, protectors of this world." The squirrel smiled, "Yes, Nepharius is out there and almost to Brazil. You will need your camaraderie. However, remember Jones that the CIA may put you back into the wards." The universe reminded Jones about his downfalls and flaws at every turn as he lay there on his bed thinking about all that he had accomplished previously. He sat there drawing out a map of all the previous connections Jones had met throughout his journey. As the map stuck out to him, he realized how known and powerful the industry was. How much he could accomplish by reaching out to people. On the back, Jones started writing the biggest world issues and possible solutions to them as he rolled it up and put it in a drawer. In case of any further problems he took a picture of the map and uploaded it into messenger to be sure that the time would not be lost. "Jones, the rare materials used in most of the technology are coming together." Nepharius went through his mind again as the squirrel ran away squeaking into the distance of the nighttime.

Animals were some of the safest ways that Jones was able to communicate without Nepharius able to interfere in the battle. Although the two of them were subconsciously on the ship together, Mira had blocked out Nepharius's will when the eye was damaged. Jones saw the moon through his roof now shining down on him as he forgot his slipper near the bedside. By now Jones focused on the world around him was little to none. He was unable to properly sleep again as a text came through from Ike. "Jones, I have something new for our baseline! Listen to this guitar wobble!" Ike messaged him ecstatically. "I need to tell you something important, "Jones replied to Ike, hoping to gather support against Nepharius. "I'm a musical warrior and an Arbiter." Jones texted Ike. "What are you talking about Jones? Come down and tell me in person tomorrow." Ike sent out another message with a laughing monkey emoji. "Seriously, I have a map of how everything's connected through vibrations and music. It all makes sense." Jones texted back as he rolled up the questions and the map on the shelf that he had gathered from the world experts around him. "Alright Jones, I don't get it but explain it to me." Ike said, "I'm having a dab bro." Ike texted back, "Don't kill my vibe bro. You're kind of negative right now or too hyper." Ike texted again. Jones replied "sorry." As he went over and closed the window. "Positive mindset, Jones," Jones whispered to himself as he sat on the bed contemplating his next move.

Had the CIA gotten ahold of Jones's data would the conglomeration mixed with the wards be on his side? Jones couldn't tell, he knew he had to keep this a secret from the rest of the world until he could fully decipher the way the energy flows between people. "Consciousness, a construct?" Jones's mind wandered as he grew more scatterbrained trying to drift off to sleep. "Shut up." The people of the galaxy said as blocks and filters were completely removed. Jones got out of bed holding onto his ears as the crickets grew louder. He grabbed his headphones and phone to attempt to play music directly into his ear. A song popped up on his phone and started playing before he could get the other headphones in. "I will always be here for you." played slowly as it skipped then to another song title, "In your calm soul." Jones listened as his brain calmed down. "Thanks, Spirit of Music." He said to himself trying to focus on the next day ahead. Explaining this situation to Ike would take much of the energy Jones had and Jones didn't have a lot. Jones was able to drift off to sleep lacking REM sleep as the sun had already been coming up the next day. "Jones! Jones! Wake up! It's already 1:00 PM." His mother shook him awake as a headphone piece fell out of Jones's ear.

"Yeah? Oh, shoot! I'm supposed to be at Ike's." He said to her. "Yeah, you're also supposed to talk to Orin." She said sternly. "That's tomorrow," Jones replied as he pointed to the calendar. "Oh, you're right this time." His mother replied. "Made you some breakfast!" She said happily. His mother was in a good mood as she had worked in the garden. The tomatoes were

CHAPTER NINETEEN – MIND CHESS

starting to bloom as summer had come around. His mother went back towards the kitchen as Jones got out of bed. Making even the simplest of movements was starting to become a chore. Jones went into the restroom and took off his shirt as he reached over for the toothbrush. He forgot to take off his shoes as he couldn't decide if he would be taking off his shoes first or brushing his teeth. Jones looked in the mirror as he placed his phone down randomly on the restroom sink. "Fuck it." He said to himself grabbing the toothbrush and the toothpaste and jumping in the shower leaving his boxers on. "Boxers that dry right away would be great…bathing suits exist for this don't they?" He bantered to himself as another idea built off of an idea raced through his head. After a few short minutes Jones was ready to go and hopped out of the shower. He texted Ike, "I'm on my way." Jones went into his room grabbing his hat and went out of the door towards his car. He popped in the CD and turned it up as loud as he could, feeling completely inspired. Not knowing what the weather was like Jones headed off towards Ike to explain his findings of the way the world was connected through music. Loading up Waze the road warriors were ready to go. "Need us?" Said the text this time as Jones gained the support of the galaxy back on his side. "No." He clicked off as he drove at high speed towards Ike's.

After an hour of driving, Jones arrived towards Ike's parking lot as a man stood outside walking his dog in circles. Jones ignored the man as he looked for parking. An old restaurant stood out where the two of them used to consistently listen to music together. A sign read, "Mill Valley." On the side of the road as Jones parked in the very left corner of the parking space. "Ike, I'm here." Jones texted as he parked the car. The entire lot seemed empty as if welcoming him there for the special occasion. "Come up bro!" Ike said as Jones got out of the car running past the garbage can up the stairs towards the top where Ike's door was already cracked. "Open up a window! It's damn stuffy!" Ike's mother complained as the weather grew sunnier. "Why don't you two go outside and get some exercise, you two spend too much time here. Ike goes outside." Ike walked into the living room in the apartment as he waved towards Jones ignoring his mother. "Hey, Jones! How are you, Bro?" Ike said, welcoming Jones in. "Tell me about this…map thing?" He asked. "Universal maps bro" Yee." Ike joked about as he invited him further in. "Can't wait to show you some new music," Ike said. "Yeah man, we'll talk and make some," Jones replied as the two of them went to Ike's studio where jungle props and flowers hung off the desk. Ike's speakers faced the wall as he sat there smoking a dab. As Jones reached for his phone in his pocket Ike put the water on the back. Jones spun around tripping over a small painting board as the toothbrushes with paint on them spilled out onto Ike's canvas. Jones tried to catch himself as a glass of water spilled on his phone.

"Shit," Jones said as he pressed his phone one time. As the phone got water damage from the cup that spilled, he held the button. "One press instead of two huh? Or get rid of this shit altogether." He cursed at himself for being careless. The paint slowly started to form into a river of color that mixed. "Woah dude, you alright?" Ike said as he sat there smoking another dab. "You know that stuff will ruin your brain, Ike. Weeds okay but if you keep hitting dabs along with that DMT you're going to go ape. I'll tell you now." Jones sat for a moment before wiping his phone and pant leg off. Ike turned to him. "Map bro." He said looking at Jones. "We're musical warriors… you see Ike." Jones held his phone this time instead of double-tapping it. "Music is connected to everything. It's the universal language. Here's how the full earth system looks. As Jones showed Ike the map Ike's eyes grew wide. "Bro! That's amazing. It's like looking at the entire world. Have you ever heard of that water specialist on YouTube? How water reacts to the geometry through shapes, the Fibonacci sequence in detail, and all of that?" Ike questioned Jones as he sat there, "Got a hairdryer or a tissue that can re-heat itself?" Jones asked Ike joking around as he sat there seeing the painting now morph from a river to a blob.

Ike reached down and started painting Jones's map in color making sense of the arrows as Jones sat there explaining the details to Ike. "It's a good

CHAPTER NINETEEN – MIND CHESS

thing I've been painting for a very long time," Ike said laughing. Jones asked again, "I need to dry myself off again man." Jones said. "Yeah, you do," Ike replied. "I've got a towel in the restroom. Let's go for a walk." Ike suggested as Jones got up to clean himself off in the restroom. "Let's get some food after a walk," Ike said. "Yeah alright," Jones replied as Ike got up. "We're going for a walk," Ike said to his mom shouting from his room. "One dab before we go?" Dabs away!" Ike said laughing. Jones decided to take one too. The two of them headed for the door as the wind blew lightly. "Later tonight let's make a song," Ike suggested to Jones as he sat there thinking. "Alright, you see the way the energy flows, right?" Jones asked Ike. "Well yeah, the earth's heartbeat is like 2.35hz or something. Binaural beats are like mother earth breathing with you." Ike said as the two of them walked down the pathway towards the forest trail that seemed to extend on for a long time.

"Yeah… I mean we're like a hidden utopia that keeps creating and progressing the world forward huh?" Jones asked Ike. Ike agreed as he nodded himself. Jones briefly blinked as Ike pointed across the forest trail. "This way. Let's keep walking… man my mom doesn't understand a thing. She keeps saying that I need help." Ike complained, "Everything you're telling me makes complete sense. I try to tell her and she tells me I need to go away to a ward for a while. Call my aunt and stuff." Ike said relating to Jones. Jones stood there for a moment as the trees seemed to close in. "Bro you have to know how to blend in. Haven't you learned by now? People aren't open-minded. If you're talking about such complex problems you get ridiculed for trying to understand them. People are scared of truth and change. If these people are crazy enough… close enough they get put back into the same old bullshit." Jones said thinking about the arbiter book and Nepharius. Ike walked along with Jones. "Damn bro. That was a pretty sick statement." As the two of them reached the end of the trail they turned and walked back towards Ike's house. The two of them walked up the stairs as Ike told Jones to sit in the chair. "Yo, it's like 7:00 PM. We should start making something." Jones encouraged Ike as he sat there staring at the computer screen. Slowly night fell as Ike loaded up the DAW. "Bro, we're some of the best producers out there I swear." Jones nodded his head in agreement.

"I don't know but we aren't bad," Jones said, knowing that the galaxy was possibly listening. As Ike went to get ice cream from the fridge along with other various food Jones started on the project. "What should we make?" Jones yelled from Ike's room as he could hear a small argument between Ike and his mom. "Whatever we want, orchestral, bass-heavy, video game mixture with our favorite sounds," Ike said from the kitchen. Jones agreed as the screen started to turn gold. "Yeah… we're going to praise the galaxy as this screen turns to gold," Jones said to himself thinking that the screen turning gold was a calling as it was simply a program on the computer to dim it from hurting one's eyes. Ike walked back with ice cream and popcorn as Jones ended up going in on the program. "Something tribal would be cool," Ike said as Jones started scouring the internet for answers. "You know popcorn ice cream would taste amazing," Jones replied. "Salty sweet?" Ike replied half chuckling. "Throw in that tribal yell from YouTube man." He said as he was slowly falling asleep on his bed. As Jones started to build around the vocal on the DAW he believed that this song would translate to the galaxy where people would be dancing to it everywhere the song was sent out. Jones smiled as he started tossing in drum loops among different drum beats. "I swear we are gods," Ike said.

Jones replied laughing, "We're all gods, here to create. Mini gods of our perception because most of this world is all about perception. Built on that and all." Jones said, looking at Ike for a moment. "I mean don't you think that Gods were just written by us, by the human species who closed their eyes trying to break free into our subconscious?" Jones questioned Ike. Jones continued before noticing Ike fell asleep with ice cream on one side of the bed in a bowl melting away and a half-empty popcorn in the other filled with salt and butter. "Like, yeah mathematically it all makes sense. Symmetry and all that. Geometry to read and build stuff. Still though,

CHAPTER NINETEEN – MIND CHESS

maybe we were making connections that weren't there. Feeding ourselves something to believe in because it was more fun that way. More fun than accepting the truth that we wrote the idea of god into existence from our minds. That's why we're all gods, not god's creation or some shit. We're all creators!" He looked at Ike expecting a reply getting nothing in return. Jones sighed and went back to the program to finish the track as he slowly drifted off to sleep in the chair. An hour later Ike tried to talk to Jones not noticing he had already fallen asleep. "Yo, Jones. I'm going to talk about this with Drew." Ike said. Jones gave a slight nod listening to the song he was created in existence. "I mean put it up on the internet as a talk," Ike said. Jones laughed. "Yeah and end up with the CIA or something after us. I don't think so…Hey, even if our song sounds sub-par here, in the future these works will sound way better huh?" Jones said to Ike referring to the galaxy, their future coming off like ten times better. Ike took it literally, "Practice makes perfect." He said as he started to pass out as well. Jones hung up his headphones as he looked at the golden screen turned back normal. The sun had already come back up as Jones yawned, falling onto the other side of Ike's bed. "Night bro," Jones said. "Night yeah," Ike said in return.

Chapter Twenty – Warrior Radio

The next morning Jones woke up as Ike was already on the computer listening to the song that Jones had made. "These drums are pretty crazy," Ike said he was impressed with the unfinished work. "Like writing our names into history." he continued as he ate the cereal with headphones on. Jones rubbed his eyes as he slept okay for the first time in a while. "Yeah, man," Jones replied. "Hey, I'm going to head home." He said to Ike as Ike turned toward Jones. "I set up a small radio station on the 'net to talk about what you said." Ike mentioned." Drew wanted to talk about all of it." Jones waved towards Ike in return as he put on his shoes. "Sounds good bro," Jones said as he slowly opened the door and left the hose heading down towards his car. Jones had to attend his last day of therapy with Orin, it was a check-out day for him and he had proven his stability. Hopping in the car he put on music to soothe his mind into staying steady against any potential galactic messages that were trying to get through to him. The CIA was still tapped into Jones's phone as he left Ike's house not realizing that the information would put Ike in holding as well. As soon as Jones had left Jones received a text message on his phone from Ike's mom saying that Ike needed help and would be admitted the next day. Drew texted Jones in return. "What the hell is going on dude? I got a knock on my door from the police." Jones received the text as he looked down. "Stop doing the radio show bro," Jones said in return to Drew. "No shit," Drew replied quickly. "Listen, I don't know what's going on but whatever you're on to stop throwing it out there. It's

CHAPTER TWENTY – WARRIOR RADIO

true." Drew texted back worried.

"Keep it to yourselves," Jones spoke in return as he continuously drove with one hand on his phone and the other on the wheel. Jones thought for a moment about where Nepharius was going now. Jones turned up the music in his car to zone out on his drive home. As he walked into the white door looking at the retired cane to the side of the house Jones went over to the refrigerator. Cheese sticks lie on the corner as a juice squeeze half-opened fizzled by the rest of the food. "You're going to be late for your last meeting with Orin." His mother shouted from her office space as the table lay in a messy space with documents collected from Jones escapades. "Alright!" he said thinking about the day as school was inching closer for each class that he would have to complete. Jones took one of the juice-squeezes out of the fridge as he went out of the door and hopped back into his car. Still tired from the night before he drove towards the clinic where Orin was. The semi-tall building glistened in the sun as the windows seemed oddly clean. This would be the last time Jones would be looking at the building for a while. As he pulled up, he parked over by the parking garage in the mall that lies across from the building. Jones could see the security guard in the window keeping a close eye on all the people that were going in and out. He remembered the times he had with Pearl and Bey as he slowly crossed the street getting over to the other side of the walkway.

"These white paint strips should just come up when someone is walking across them to fully stop traffic and cars from running over people." Jones spoke to himself, "No then it would hurt others. That can't be right. Is that not what traffic laws are for?" He said as he looked around the world slowly approaching the building. The security guard opened the door for him as he wandered on in. This time the elevator stood out as Jones pressed the button waiting on the ground floor. The elevator wouldn't respond to Jones every time he pushed the button as if it was telling him to take the stairs. "Oh, it's broken." A random passerby said to Jones as he came down the stairs. As Jones closed his eyes briefly and reopened them a broken sign that he hadn't noticed now appeared on the side. "Oh, thanks," Jones said walking up the stairs towards the front desk lady. This time no one was sitting in the chairs. "We've been expecting you," She said in reply to Jones as he walked in through the wooden door that felt like it had a heavy presence behind it every time Jones laid eyes on it. "Jones! Good to see you!" Orin said from her office as he sat down to talk to her. "Yeah, good to see you too." He said trying to make small talk as she smiled at him with a warm welcome. "Today's your last day. Do you have any questions for me?" She said not wasting any time wanting to move the day along. "You know you could be a huge advocate for health. I mean that song you suggested really helped. It now has millions of plays worldwide..." she slowed down as Jones held up his hand. "I wanted to tell you another quick story of how I was in the city..." He sat in the chair moving it to match hers exactly across as she studied his every action.

"You see... When I got back from the driving escapade after talking to the agents I went back out into the city for more information. My phone was at less than two percent but wouldn't seem to die. It would consistently go off towards forty-two back towards one percent." Jones kept talking as Orin listened intently, not speaking as she always did try to make sense of the stories and chain of events that he was talking about. As Jones got off the Bart, he wandered over to the pier thirty-nine which stuck out in bright blue and red lights. "Do you have a charger sir?" he asked the security guard sitting by a building in the middle of the night. The security guard shook his head as he wandered towards the back of the docking building where he had purchased a coffee earlier that day. A little plug stuck out from the wall where Jones fished in his pocket for a prong that he had been carrying with him in case anything had happened. "A charger," Jones said to himself plugging it into the wall as he listened to the nighttime city ring about. Two nights before he had given bananas to the random passersby who had recognized him on the BART. As Jones thought about the other men who took the meat out of a butcher shop

CHAPTER TWENTY – WARRIOR RADIO

singing sweet songs, he perched himself up on the wall. As Jones listened in the night, he heard the crosswalk stop lights all going off at the same time. The sound carried off through the city as if the sound of gunshots were being fired.

"Must be Mafia night." He mumbled as he slowly started to fall asleep in the cold. Every few seconds the sound carried further and further towards him as he could hear screams of those in the far distance. Jones shivered at the thought of Mafia night as he started bringing it into existence with his thoughts. "No, we can't have people running rampant randomly in the streets like this." He said to himself as he curled up towards the wall waiting for his phone to charge so that he could get home off the BART. Jones's sense of direction had been so tainted that he couldn't decipher where he was. In the dead of the night where not even the water seemed to travel the light walkways making their buzzer sounds echoed throughout each alleyway and intersection. "Wait. Jones…" Orin mentioned as Jones continued his story. "So as part of your episode, you were making connections to sound?" She questioned him as Jones sat there pondering for a moment. "Well Orin, I was looking at brands and buildings and seeing them for what they were. If I saw a store that said mad cows, I assumed that the store was experienced in finding mad cows," he said in reply. "I suppose the sound as it traveled through the city made sense. I mean hearing thousands of lights not saying wait but rather clicking into my ear certainly didn't help." Jones finished his statement trying to laugh it off as Orin sat there confused. "What does this have to do with the car?" She asked him to try to understand Jones' connections towards the agents. "I figured if I could gain a little support maybe someone would help me find someone worthwhile."

Jones sat back in the black chair relaxing his pose as she looked at him. "Okay continue, so how did you get home?" she questioned Jones again following his movements closely. "Well…as my phone charged up, I was able to walk towards the BART station across the pier line catching it home.

I felt so afraid of those sounds and what might be out there I didn't want to explore the city further. I wanted to be in a warm bed away from it all." he said She sat there in the chair contemplating his stability again. "I see. Today is your last day, so I'm going to let you go. Doctor K. is retiring and has already put in his paperwork. Do you want to say goodbye?" She said to Jones. He sat there in the chair. "No, not really…" Jones said, looking about the room for clues to Orin's connections. The striking cleanroom stuck in Jones's mind as he thought about the experience and details he was giving Orin. Jones got up, "I could use a cup of water, please." He mentioned walking towards the door.

"Okay, feel free but come right back. Our session isn't quite up yet." Orin said in a warming voice ready to call for help at any necessity. She had realized that Jones had figured out their plan on studying the people that would come into their workplace. "Code x0" was written on the computer as Jones opened the door walking down the hallway for the cup of water. "Oh, that's right…the music thing." Jones said to himself as he went down the hallways towards where the water sat in another room. Orin had heard him speak under his voice as he brought the water back in and shut the door. "Yeah, every time I hit interest in my messenger more people showed up than usual. Like they knew because I would be there it would be going off." Jones said in return to Orin as she sat back relaxing in her chair no longer worried about the possibility of Jones. With that statement, Jones alleviated Orin's concerns on if he was on to their studies. "I think it's time for you to go home" Orin was looking at her watch at a clear loss of interest in the conversation.

Jones got up out of the chair taking one last look at Orin before walking out the wooden door towards the world that sat in front of him. "Okay. It's me and you now, Nepharius. We are the only ones left." Jones said quietly to himself as the door opened for him on the way out. Each step connected to the other as the sounds echoed off the walls. Jones was playing with them as if the steps were musical instruments. He headed towards the

CHAPTER TWENTY – WARRIOR RADIO

door where his freedom ultimately lies. The freedom that Jones had been aiming for since he had been thrown into therapy. As the clouds slowly move, Jones contemplates his actions. He walked over to a fountain where other people were skateboarding as he sat down looking at the sky. Jones loaded up a map as it sat still unmarked as a place."Jones T. Harver's spot." came up as an option as Jones gave the fountain a name. "Yeah…" he said to himself slowly drifting off to sleep with the water rushing nearby. "Hey up, slime dogs!" Nepharius yelled at his crew tossing against the waves. "Brazil is within sight!" He shouted as the golden piano rocked again within the captain's quarters.

"Jones! Where are the ropes for the sail?" Nepharius yelled at the top of his lungs as the salt and smell of fish went through the air. "Here!" Jones said in return shouting back. "You know you could retire and make movies!" Jones said to Nepharius. "You don't have to try to control our imaginations!" Jones said again trying to sway Nepharius into letting down his grudge. Nepharius stood there and flashed an evil smile. "Humanity does not deserve the ability to progress. The truancy, greed, and unkindness that follows between people have made me realize how unworthy they are. Look forward to Brazil, Jones. Do you see this place? How free-formed and beautiful it is? Untouched mostly by the humans who live here." Jones saw the view of the island now in place from a distant view. The destination of a great structure stood on the mid-point carved out within faces of anguish. The stone structure covered the rest of the forefront of the island as trees and odd plants surrounded the beach end. "We are docking here. It is time you go to the cabin." Nepharius said to Jones not hearing a word he had to say as he moved him into the back room.

Nepharius locked the door as Jones sat in the corner with the golden piano. As he slid down against the wood feeling nothing but darkness and waves, he felt a small knock on the right side of the ship. "Jones." A whisper came from the right side. "Pssst. Jones!" The voice said again as Jones rapidly looked around the room trying to figure out if it was one of

Nepharius's crew members or a sound created by the sea. "Damnit, Jones! I'm over here!" She yelled a little louder now realizing the crew outside was preoccupied with the sails. It was Zaya, she had snuck up on the ship and followed Jones from behind. "Jones I'm telling you; I would protect and play for you." She said as Jones couldn't believe Zaya was there. "Why are you here, Zaya? You can't be, you know you will die." Jones said as the ship precariously rocked back and forth. Zaya giggles, "Yeah, well that idea-eating crazy woman told me to come aboard. She told me everything that was at stake here."

Jones thought to himself of who it could be. "Mira," he said to himself, recalling the words she had told him previously. Jones laughed to himself and then sighed. "Do you know how to play this thing?" Jones asked Zaya as she sat there in her red frilled dress. "I might know a piano score or two." She said back to Jones smiling as she opened the keyboard. Each key was nicely designed with a silver lining in between the gold. On the front of the cover is written-Tober's work. As Jones moved his hand around the cherrywood leggings he read out loud what had been written. "To my dear curator Jones. Without you we would not be free" enshrined on the back was a smiling face with a hammer on it. "That's cute." Zaya teased as she ran her hands across the keyboard.

"Really cute." She said tempted to play a note off the keyboard. "No, not yet," Jones said to Zaya as he went across to the other side of the cabin to sit back down. "Why does Nepharius want to steal the world's imagination for himself?" Zaya asked Jones as he sat there contemplating the question. "Nepharius wants to control us. Aren't you stardust from mars?" He brought it up as Zaya sat there. "Yeah, I am from Mars. It's part of my long-standing DNA." She laughed rolling over to the side as the ship rocked again. "Nepharius wants control because he doesn't believe that the world is deserving of itself. Movies and his own fame were not enough to fulfill his soul. So, he kept on going." Jones mentioned to Zaya as she rolled over with the boat. "So, we shall fight, shall we?" Zaya replies as she giggled.

CHAPTER TWENTY – WARRIOR RADIO

"I may be smaller than you Jones but I am enough to make a dent." She replied as she patted Jones on the back.

"Such will be the life of us," Jones said in return as the boat hit the sand. "You better go back into hiding," Jones warned Zaya as she went back towards the unseen spot in the cabin. Two of Nepharius's crew members opened the door taking the piano out and putting it on the beach as Jones was told to move forward. "See the journey that we have come to Brazil for," Nepharius said admiring the sun mixed with the beautiful ladies and men by the trees. Jones stopped off the ship and woke up as his phone buzzed at him continuously. "You have ten missed calls." Read off from the front of Jones's phone as Ottie had tried to reach Jones. He rolled back over by the fountain. "Shit, my phone's not working properly," Jones said to himself as he got up and started walking to the repair shop. Rubbing his eyelids Jones opened the door and walked back in. The same place where he had sung earlier. "How may we help you?" A man stood at the doorway inviting him in. "Well, my phone's not working right." He said to the man. "What's wrong with it?" The helper said back in return. Jones replied, trying to make sense of what he could. "The phone keeps freezing up and I can't upload much." The helper smiled. "I'll have this fixed up for you in a moment."

Jones thanked the man, "It'd be cool if I could filter my whole phone in different colors." Jones said to the helper as the helper laughed in return. "We'll see what we can do." After a few hours of waiting around the store, the helper gave Jones the phone back. "Be sure you update your phone within the next two hours." The helper suggested. Jones nodded his head and obliged. As he walked out the front door to update his phone, he almost dropped it. "A watcher." He said to himself. A purple filter option was now available on his phone. Jones laughed to himself privately as he walked up the stairs back towards where he parked his car. As he opened his door, he called Ottie back. "What's up?!" Jones said Ottie replied, "Hey man I'm going to mail your laptop back now." He said in return as Jones started driving towards his house. Jones replied to Ottie, "Alright man I can do a lot with that." As he drove towards his house. "You know Ottie, sometimes the cool thing about meeting people on the street is they will sometimes refer you to help you climb the ladder if the people see you're genuine," Jones said referring to the watchers that had reached out in his messenger. Watchers were always trying to one-up one another putting each other in the game. "Yeah bro, there was a guy last week who offered me a good job. It's pizza delivery so it's not much but I can dig it."

As Jones finished his sentence with Ottie a construction worker looked directly at Jones as if he heard the conversation. Jones turned the corner, arriving home within a few minutes. "I have to get out of here. I'll leave soon." He said to himself as he read the class listing. "School starts tomorrow. I better be prepared for my final semester." Jones said to himself as he had paid his tuition fees. Jones put on his glasses for the first time since he had gone to consistent therapy. A small scratch on them showed up from a moment when he had dropped the glasses on the sidewalk. "Hmm..." he said to himself looking around at them. As the light hit his glasses at an angle, he noticed it spread out and continued even further from a concave point of view. "I wonder why we don't do this in shows that often?" He said to himself, "or on the back of cars?" The blanket statements kept Jones's mind calm from the stress over what was happening in the galaxy. He recalled a man walking across the street waving to everyone as if everyone was watching him, ready to battle and dance outside of his element. "Hey, Jones! Heard you were out recently." A text came to his phone.

"Come hang out at our house show. Happens once a year in our backyard. You might enjoy it." Jones read the text message out loud to himself as it went up in pairs of three into his glasses. He took his glasses off to respond. "Hey man, sounds like a place I want to be," Jones responded as the night fell on him. "This time it's during the day. I've been the one sending your show emails by the way. It's time we met." Now Jones couldn't reject

CHAPTER TWENTY – WARRIOR RADIO

the offer for the party. He sat down again on his bed as thoughts floated through his head. "If you don't stop overthinking everything, you're going to crash again." He recognized the voice this time, "Mira? Where are we? How's Zaya?" Jones said confused between the world outside and his own. "I'm here to keep you stable." Mira said, "You're in your room falling asleep. The other part of you is with Nepharius in the Amazon rainforest. I see you have yet to go into sleep debt again." Mira scolded Jones for a moment while Jones sat there in his room mumbling to himself. Remember what I told you. You cannot sleep or you will be disconnected. I see you've already forgotten some of your items which is a sign you're headed in the right direction. The only way to beat Nepharius is to conjoin." Mira lightened up as she floated backward now above Jones's head in his room. "For now, even with your eyes closed this will be the place instead of the bar. Don't sit on the red chairs or you will wake up." Mira warns as two red chairs and blue ones are lined up by Jones' computer. "Zaya is okay then?" Jones questioned Mira.

"Yes, we have tabs on her life. Although I can't see her directly there is a way through my phone that shows me her form. Even from here where the signal is being sent. All I needed to do was triangulate my phone to make it holographic. Mira laughed. "These ideas taste great. Come up with more." Mira said. Jones rolled his eyes, "Stop stealing my ideas." He said as she chewed on the next necklace piece having it dissipate into her belly. "Listen, it's time for you to wake up soon. You have a party to attend. Your world is going to become your own movie and you are the star of Nepharius's. We are all actors playing but a small part in this." Mira warned Jones as he looked over at the red chair. The purple one sparkled as Jones got up cleaning it off briefly. He was ready to put his hand on it. "Good luck out there. These ideas are in your hands. I will help where I can but Nepharius has tabs on me. Sadly, I cannot join you and watch over both sides of your consciousness." Mira pushed Jones, shoving him into the red chair without warning. Jones woke up sweating as he peeked around his room. The sun had already come up as he received another text. "Come help us sweep my man, we're having a day party today!" The text said. "Be there by 2:00 PM!" Jones read it but did not reply as he knew he was already being watched. He reached towards his hat which lay on the corner of the bedside.

Jones went over to the animal beats shirt to put it on along with the brown felt hat. Looking at himself in the mirror he recalled the clock tower in town. "Maybe I can get some sort of connection if I check out the clock tower in Walnut Creek. There's two of them after all." Jones said to himself recalling the hallways that lie before him. As he wore his glasses Jones went outside waiting for the uber to pick him up. "Your Uber has almost arrived. Would you like a rented one or an X for extra money?" An extra option popped out at him showing a driver with a steering wheel. "Deluxe" was written on the right side of it as Jones clicked it. "To Walnut Creek… for now," Jones said to himself as the uber pulled right up to his house. "Oh, you again," Jones said, as the man with glasses peeked out the window. "Yeah, hop on in." The guy said from the taxi service. The old war vet who talked to Jones about his paintings started to ramble on about what he had seen. "Hop in, I'll show you." The old war vet said as Jones went over to the taxi. "Do you want some pretzels or water?" He offered as Jones sat up front looking at the cooler in the front seat. "Sure, I'll take one," Jones said in return as the man pulled up his glasses a little. "Alright, sounds good." The Vet headed towards Walnut Creek driving slowly from Jones's house. In a few short minutes without Jones even noticing during the ride Jones arrived right at the clock tower. He blinked as the door opened and gave the man a $20 tip.

"That's for the last time, thanks, man!" Jones said as the veteran waved, flooring the gas. Jones walked up towards the stairs towards the top of the clock tower. At 1:00 PM, the entire clock tower was orange mixed with gold as the hand struck closer to 1:00 PM. Jones blinked, Nepharius appeared on the island within the forest talking to tribal folk. Down the street, a man was playing music out of a speaker. "Yeah with this…" Jones

CHAPTER TWENTY – WARRIOR RADIO

said to himself as the music transferred back to Brazil in the jungle that Nepharius lie. "You won't best me here Jones!" Nepharius said Jones replied, "Oh that's what you think!" Jones lunged forward jumping off one tree to another. As Jones closed his eyes and climbed the steps of the clock, he tripped over a glass bottle. A rock lies in the jungle next to Nepharius as Jones rolled over himself ending up in a pile of grass. Jones propelled himself forward as Nepharius threw out a right-handed punch which nailed Jones right in the chin. "I could crush you," Nepharius said to Jones as he reached out grabbing Jones's shoulder. "I could really crush you Harver." Jones screamed out in pain as Nepharius started to squeeze harder on Jones's shoulder. As one of the bones popped, he reached back towards Nepharius and dislocated his shoulder. "I'm going to win our imaginations back, Nepharius! You'll see!" Jones got up with one hand as Nepharius charged him. All this while Jones sat in the clock up top rolling in water tripping over cracks in the ground. As he fell to the ground Jones took a few breaths sitting by the wall of the clock tower. Nepharius stood over him as Jones blinked a few times trying to reorganize his thoughts. "You see now? You can't defeat me!" Nepharius said as he now appeared in front of Jones at the clock tower at the same time the other part of him was in the forest. "I told you, join me. You were always in my crew."

The signs changed colors as QR scan codes now appeared under them from the view of the clock tower. The once busy streets of Walnut Creek were now deserted as both of the towers aligned. "This world is all connected, something you wouldn't understand." Nepharius ranted on as he smacked Jones again. "We may be weak on our own but even you can't stop us!" Jones said back to Nepharius. He laughed. "You can't overcome fate unless you're so unpredictable fate itself can't keep up." Nepharius grabbed Jones, dragging him across the dirt as Jones's eyes were closed in the clock tower. A security guard ran up the stairs. "Hey! What's going on here?" Jones quickly brushed himself off acting as if nothing happened. His face was bruised and his jeans ripped. "What happened?" The security guard asked. Jones stood there frozen. "I fell." He said. Nepharius put Jones down in the dirt. "Stand up and walk yourself." Nepharius voice echoed through Jones's head as he headed towards the stairs of the clock tower at the same time as the village in the forest. "We will rest here for now," Nepharius said as he pointed towards the day campfire sitting down in the village. "Na'aktum shemadda," Nepharius said as a leader came up to him. "Who is that?" The leader said as he pointed to Jones. "An old crew member," Nepharius said as the leader raised his head.

"Everyone has a story, every fleeting moment you are in the forest. Or if you are in a car. We see thousands of people a day without a second thought. Where do you think those thoughts go?" The leader looked at Nepharius and Jones. "These thoughts come to us." The leader nodded his head. "I hear you're looking for our prized possession is that so?" Nepharius nodded. "Yes, you are correct. Maku'ustu Nandrem." Jones watched Nepharius and the leader talk back and forth. He woke up to find himself stuck in-between vision. He stumbled with one eye closed down the clock tower towards his car. The lack of sleep had slowed Jones's footsteps down to a minimal speed. "I have to get home." He said to himself. "I have a party to get together." Jones got into his silver Jetta and started his drive counting the merge of cars every seven seconds where an opening lie. He started to pay attention to the patterns of the wheels of the drivers knowing what the people would do before even changing lanes. Jones stopped on the gas as classical music played in the background reigniting pieces of his brain that were lost to sleep. As he was able to focus, swerving in and out of traffic those fifteen minutes felt like an insanely short five. Jones ran into the house to shower not wanting to be seen by his mother who sat on the couch. As he hopped in the shower his feet started to heal up, his cut got better like the first time that Jones had stepped on the glass bottle out near the pier. Jones closed his eyes again.

"Jones, is it?" The leader entered his mind as he could hear short conversations between Nepharius and the village. Jones quietly held his head as he yelled in his mind for the galactic space to get out of his. Taking

CHAPTER TWENTY – WARRIOR RADIO

the shampoo, he washed quickly and got dressed heading for the door. Jo's legs only had a small unnoticeable bruise on the left side. Dressed in his white animal beats T-Shirt and the brown felt hat Jones drove out towards Oakland where the gathering was. A fence lay on the right side where lots of people lined up at the door. The clock hit 3:00 PM as very few people were there. The fence had graffiti on it with multiple cartoon characters written on it. As Jones pulled up to the front gate, a man stood with a hat and a phone in his pocket. Music was already blaring in the background over his yard. "Need anything? Soda? Water?" The man asked right from the start. Jones could feel the aura bursting out from the place as he stood there surveying the area. "Not right now, anything I can do to help?" Jones said, looking at the yard filled with leaves. Cement with a sandbox in the middle of it stuck out as mini palm trees protruded from the ground. "Here, we need to sweep it out before people show up." The man said as he tossed him a broom. The man was also wearing a felt hat similar to Jones's. "How many people are showing up?" Jones asked in return.

"Well now that you're here." The mysterious man said in return, "A few hundred." Jones' eyes widened as he realized who he had been talking to. "The emails, you're the one who wanted to talk," Jones said in return. "Keep sweeping kid." The mysterious man's tone changed briefly as Jones swept each of the leaves using the power of his wind to move them into the corner. In the back, a little booth to collect five dollars from people on donation stood up as a barbecue sat in the back. "Yeah, they'll be here soon." The man said. Jones looked around the yard taking in the palm tree hit at the front of it next to three seats on both sides for people to sit on. "A day party, huh?" Jones said to himself as he continued to sweep. "It's Taz." The man said revealing only his first name as Jones finished sweeping the dirt and the leaves around the house. "Nice to meet you more officially. I'm part of Nepharius's crew." Taz said as a warning shot to Jones to keep his composure throughout the party. Jones quietly shook the man's hand. "I'm the organizer. Most of those emails that went out to you were from people I had reached out to for the interviews. Nepharius told me he had a new crew member on his team." Jones wondered for a moment. Taz didn't receive word from Nepharius that Jones was now their enemy.

"Make yourself at home," Taz said to Jones as the first person walked in. "Hey, Taz!" The man waved wearing a sun hat that changed colors as the day went on. Jones blinked as he went over to the chair feeling tired from the lack of sleep he had gotten. The galaxy swirled within the hat as the oils reflected off the sun. Taz turned around to wave back as misted water droplets spilled onto the hat changing colors. The smell of burgers now filled the air as a line slowly gathered. "Jones, I want you to enjoy yourself for now," Taz said. "Then we'll talk later when the party's over." Jones nodded his head as more of the pirates filtered in of different races and classes. "Space pirates are all here, huh?" Jones said to himself, keeping calm. "I suppose I should make friends." He thought to himself carefully trying to focus on the music so that others couldn't hear his thoughts. "Nice to meet you. I'm Nox." A man said with long dreaded hair. "Heard the arbiter was in town. That true?" Nox said, looking right at Jones. The man's dreads went halfway down his back as his art showed on his shirt. A sword and a one-eyed man were self-painted onto it. "Nepharius is hot on the radar right now. Heard he's close to getting it." Jones replied swiftly. "Yeah, we're really close to regaining control." Nox laughed, showing a big grin as he grabbed Jones. "Have a beer, yo." The man called one over as he opened it up, handing it over to Jones. "A-Alright." Jones stuttered for a moment feeling the power behind the man's arm. He backed away holding the beer as the yard was now full.

"When did this place fill up?" Jones said to himself as he was about to walk forward. Taz stood in front of him. "Thanks for helping with the sweeping," he said. "Look Jones, most of us need beer or weed to get out of our realms. Do you know why you're so important?" Jones shook his head, "I've read some of the arbiter books," he replied to Taz. Taz held up his hand, cutting Jones off from speaking further. "You're able to connect without the need of those. Your mind and self are that powerful. You

CHAPTER TWENTY – WARRIOR RADIO

get it?" Taz said. Jones nodded, "Loud and clear." Taz replied, "Good. People got here because you were so focused on the conversation you didn't notice. Although some of these guys and gals are pretty quick." Taz said as Jones noticed them moving around at immeasurable speeds. Each one of them talked to one another. "You see? My playground, my rules." Taz said as Jones finished his beer. "Enjoy the burger." Jones wandered through the crowd eating the burger as one of Jones' friends sat on the three chairs. "Sar? Haven't seen you in a while man!" Jones said. Sar waved at him, "Hey! Come take a seat. I knew Taz from the club a while ago." Sar replied cluelessly to what was going on. Jones sat down by the front as a person dressed up in American flag clothing started dancing. Slowly a crowd formed around in a circle as Jones watched. Taz called Jones over to get into the circle, "Breakdance at all?" Taz questioned, as he pushed Jones in.

Jones stood there for a moment watching as the man in front of him moved in perfect sync kicking and dancing. The crowd clapped their hands and cheered as Jones then got down attempting to breakdance. As he rolled over on his brown felt hat Jones floundered around. The crowd laughed as Jones fell. He got back up and brushed himself off. "Not so easy huh?" The man in the circle said as Jones nodded. "I'm feeling winded, I'll watch," Jones said, stepping out of the circle as hundreds of people were now dancing around. Jones realized if Taz caught wind that Nepharius was after him Jones would be in trouble. He covered up his bruises the best he could to avoid confrontation. "So, Jones!" Sar said, calling him back up towards the stage chairs where he shared a beer. "Where have you been?" Sar wore a basic hat as he smiled enjoying the sun that beamed down on the chair. "I'm glad you're here," Jones said to Sar, able to blend in with the crowd against Taz. Jones could use this to his advantage as he sipped the beer. "Yeah, I want to simply get home safe," Jones said to Sar. "Been out and about a little too much lately." The crowd continued to dance and cheer as the DJ put on variations of house music. "Great party though!" Jones said to Sar, giving out a small yell of satisfaction.

Jones danced around as he conversed with the people at the party. The sun slowly went down. The people looked at Jones happily as he blended in. Taz Leander over to Sar, "Your friends alright, kind of crazy though." He said watching Jones dance in variations around.

"He's lighting up the party though! That's for sure!" Taz laughed. As the party slowly went on winding down Jones prepared to leave. "Thanks for having me," Jones said to Taz as he walked out of the gate down towards his home. He could hear the sirens blaring close by as Jones got into his car to drive away. The party was a successful gathering that had worn him out after a long day of dancing. Although Jones had embarrassed himself in front of Taz he had continuously gained respect with his actions. An email popped up on Jones's phone. "Parties aplenty. Be there soon!" Taz's name was now written on the bottom rather than the spam emails Jones had been getting beforehand. Jones was now solidified completely with Taz as he laid back down on his bed. The bruise on his leg swelled down as he closed his eyes to rest. "No rest for you," Mira said. "Take a look at what Nepharius is doing." The whole village was gathered around in a circle chanting with Nepharius as two men lay on the ground. "What happened?" Jones said quietly to himself as he surveyed the area. "The two guys were defeated by Nepharius," Zaya said echoing through the forest into Jones's ear. "Shh, or they will catch on that you're here Zaya," Jones said in return. "Don't worry, I'm speaking only at the exact frequency that you can hear Jones. Nepharius can't hear you." Zaya reassured Jones as he looked forward. "Nepharius beat the two men completely for rights into the village's vault. You know those YouTube videos Nepharius sent you?" Zaya questioned Jones as he stared in awe and horror at the situation. "Yeah, I remember," Jones said. "This was one of the four mysterious places he kept ranting about. That he would one day show up under Khatu'un Mak' took." Jones took a step back as the temple in the background started to glow. Electricity came about the entire temple as a waterfall started going down the stones. Each stone had a light blue entrance as the shadows lurked about. Each shadow came out without a face walking through

CHAPTER TWENTY – WARRIOR RADIO

the forest as if each one was ready to stomp on the village people. "The entrance to the temple of imagination."

The leader of the village said as he got up. "Time flows nowhere here but our imaginations keep it in tune with the rest of the world." Jones rubbed his eyes to be sure he was seeing the world right. The YouTube video about the temple was real. This meant that every other place had been as real as well. Nepharius videos held the keys to the ancients. Jones ducked instinctively as the temple shot out a display of fireworks. "It's time that you two enter the temple." The leader said as he pushed Jones and Nepharius forward towards the entrance. "If you don't enter now you may not get another chance." Jones jumped as he covered his mouth. Nepharius jumped behind Jones as the two of them fell into a short portal towards the ground. Forest trees all around the two of them sprouted up showing signs of electricity. "Inside of this tree lies somewhere the relic of imagination." Jones walked forward a few steps before the blue tunnel disappeared. A giant werewolf howled in the background as Nepharius put up a shield around the two of them. "With this shield, nothing in the real world can hurt you while you focus all of your energy here." Nepharius led Jones further towards the wolf as the two of them put up their fists. Neither of them knew what to do. Jones picked up a stick and threw it. The wolf morphed into a dog chewing on the stick. "I get it, it's our imaginations in here too."

Jones willed upon himself a small knife as the two went through the forest. After a few minutes of chopping down the forest black space entered where there was a tear between the forest and the imagination. "The land will hide what you want from what it has. The leader said as he tried to communicate with Jones and Nepharius's minds. The static voice tried to get through to Jones and Nepharius. A whirlwind of sword and wind passed by the two of them as the connection streamed from their consciousness fought. The two of the streams reconnected as Jones threw electricity into it. "I can hear you loud and clear now!" Jones said. The leader commanded,

"Jump!" Jones and Nepharius both jumped as a tree rose from the ground flashing lights. The two of them rose towards the stage where a small relic lie. "Only you and Nepharius could see something this small, on the atom side." Jones's eyes widened as the relic of imagination had a tiny glow. Each bit of the diamond sparkles as orange and black appeared in the background. The shadow people outside grew closer to the village as Jones reached for it. "It's mine!" Jones said as Nepharius ran slightly behind him. Jones put up a small wall tripping Nepharius. "No! Only I can touch it." Nepharius said. "You're wrong," Jones replied. "I'm my own entity!" Jones said, grabbing the gem. Jones fell over as he passed out. The tree around the two of them shriveled as the relic now lie in Jones's hand. The shadow people disappeared as the whole village stopped dancing. The temple's light was now but a dim light radiating from the Gem in Jones's hand. "Yes, you see?" Nepharius said

Jones coughed. "Yeah, I'm still here," Jones said barely standing. "How?" Nepharius said, wondering how Jones was still alive. "You are not me, Nepharius," Jones said as he imagined away the tree. Jones fell back asleep waking up in his bed back at home. "My soul is still in grave danger." Jones said to himself as he walked about in the darkness. He could still feel the cold feeling of the warm-looking gem in Jones's hand. Nepharius took the gem and put it into his pocket while Jones fainted in his other state. "I have control now!" Nepharius said. "We still must get one more item." He said taking control of Jones using his imagination to create a cart. Nepharius hoisted Jones into the cart as he slowly dragged him back to the village.

Chapter Twenty-One – Split Soul

Jones got out of bed and got dressed in his shoes as he got ready for the first day of school. His clothes were messy as he grabbed his books ready to already fall asleep in class. As Jones could barely keep up with his body being in two places, he sat in his car turning the key. "Uh…" Jones said to himself with the feeling of a hangover as he turned on his car. Jones turned on the music and put it up to almost full to keep himself awake. "Today's the first day of class." He mumbled to himself with his books sitting in the car seat. The school was only a fifteen-minute drive where food and a mall had been built close by. Jones pulled up in the parking lot on the other side where he parked in the back. College kids alike were blasting music as well as taking a quick walk towards their classes. Jones walked in towards his first-class sitting down right next to a lady with black wavy hair and green painted nails. "Lily." She said right away not wasting any time to reach out a hand as she smiled. "Lily, nice to meet you." She said again not getting much of a response from Jones. "Hi," Jones said callously as Lily sat there staring at her phone. "I saw you in the city, I had been watching you a little bit and was too nervous to say hi. Who knew you'd be in the same class?" Lily said. Jones smiled, "Oh cool, what was I doing?" He asked in return. Lily laughed, "Dancing like an idiot out by the pier." She said, speaking her mind right from the start of the conversation. Lily had a striped black and white sweater on along with a black skirt. A small bow was tied on the back of her hair.

"I see," Jones said in return, not knowing what to say. "So why were you there?" She asked. "What were you really doing?" Jones replied right as the professor walked in to introduce himself. "I was practicing for a movie slot." He whispered to her. "A movie slot?" she asked, questioning him and now interested in the conversation. Lily put her phone down as the room felt warm to Jones. He could feel the energy in the classroom as the professor started calling out names. "Yeah. You see there's this guy called Nepharius who wants me in his…" Jones paused for a moment. "Did I say Nepharius?" He asked Lily, waiting a moment, to talk more to himself than to her. "I need water." Jones got up and went over to look for the water fountain as he excused himself from the classroom. "I'm here, it's Jones." He said to the professor as the man nodded. The professor continued to call out names as the door closed.

The sun was extremely bright to Jones's eyes as he blinked heading over to the water fountain at school. Sounds of people walking, doors closing and opening, and even the wind blowing all ramped up into Jones's ear. "Yeah, I did hear about that shooting by the pier. It was pretty sad." A student said as he walked by the water fountain. Another student walked up to Jones, "Hey man, you've been sipping water for like five minutes." Jones nodded, "Oh my bad." After adjusting to the sunlight, Jones walked over back towards his classroom where the lights were now dimmed. "Today we will be learning about a method." The teacher said as Jones already started falling asleep in class. "Sir, pay attention." The teacher said ousting Jones as he pointed towards the board speaking softly as to not come off as rash towards the class. Jones woke up, "Sorry." He said as the professor continued his lesson. Lily started taking copious amounts of notes as she tried to understand the theories behind the teachings. "Do you need notes at the end? You've already missed a fourth of the class." She asked as Jones sat there flipping in and out of his sleep.

"Yeah, that would be great." He said to her with his eyes darkened completely. Jones started to question his sanity as the room seemed less

CHAPTER TWENTY-ONE – SPLIT SOUL

like a classroom and more like a village. The seats morphed into logs and the people sitting down became village people. Almost as if each soul was interconnected with one another the visualization popped out at Jones. "Jerky?" Lily said as his view of her as a village person offering him meat extended itself. Jones grabbed the beef jerky nodding his head as Nepharius now stood at the front of the class pointing to a holographic board and showing them the entryway to their temple. "Drakhuthun gufruthus," Nepharius said as Jones now was paying attention to the board. "It means we are all gods, gods who can create. The one who controls the creation of the mind controls all" Nepharius laughed as Jones sat up in the cart viewing the campfire. The village people were sitting there with their sticks and planted skirts clapping after Nepharius. Jones could see the sadness in their eyes hidden behind their need to follow his orders. "Yes, and now all that's left is for me to use this to get to where I need to go!" Nepharius said, holding up the gem. "That's it, the article," Zaya whispered towards Jones. "I know," Jones said back to Zaya. The vibration went through the air as Jones saw each wave head towards the ground. "Know what?" Lily said as Jones mumbled to himself waking back up. "Oh, know the theory," Jones said, covering himself as the class continued forward. A series of strings and theories filled the board that Jones had no clue about as he lied to Lily. "Oh, good then you can tell me about this one."

She pointed to her piece of paper calling Jones out. Jones stuttered for a moment, "Ah… it's…" he said stopping, "Okay you caught me. I was dozing off." He whispered as the professor gave the two of them a stare to be quiet. "Five more minutes." Jones looked at the clock as class was about to be dismissed. "Yup, just five!" Lily said, offering her notebook to be copied down. Jones took it and did. So, taking pictures with his phone to keep the notes on hand. "Thanks." He said zooming in to make sure each picture was legible. "Get some rest. You look exhausted." Lily said as she walked out the door. Jones went afterward as the professor stopped him. "Jones, it's only the first day but this cannot continue." The professor said with a warning. "If this continues, you'll have to go to after hours.

I've seen it happen many times." The professor nodded, "Clear?" Jones nodded back. "Okay. I'll try to get some rest." As Jones walked out of the door back towards his car, he thought about the interactions.

The school was a great place to meet people. Jones wanted to pass, he wanted to get into a good school after this one. Jones headed towards his car where the fence lay as he thought about Nepharius about to wreak havoc on all of Humanities imagination. As he was about to turn on the car lily came up to his window. "Hey! Where are you off to so soon?" She said, knocking on the car door. "Oh uh. home." Jones said. He couldn't tell if it was the music in his car that was influencing his emotions or if it was Lily's smile. Jones was starting to feel a small attraction to Lily's demeanor. Even though he understood that the two of them could never be together Jones had decided he would treat Lily with respect from afar. "Okay, well. Hungry?" Jones said, offering Lily a small meal. "No, I can't. I have to get home to the garden for my family. I'm not really supposed to be out later than school allows me to be." Lily said, looking back over at Jones. "Ah well, maybe some other time," Jones replied. He turned the keys and moved his car out of the way as Jones sifted through the traffic created by the students leaving the school. "Well, my first day wasn't all that bad," Jones said to himself looking at the notes he held from his class in his phone. Off to the left of his phone, he saw the note he had written to his friends. The explanation of the way the world worked was drawn in a diagram only explainable to Jones as the mind map was encrypted to Jones's specific way of thinking.

"If this world is all about perception…Then…" Jones said to himself, "With that gem maybe…" he looked at his phone before the traffic light turned green. A car honked at Jones signaling him to pay attention as he focused back on the road putting his phone away. A watcher on a bike ride by at the same time saying sorry loudly as if to apologize for Jones as the rest of the crowd looked out the window weirded out by the man's comment. Jones continued towards his house as he contemplated his own thoughts.

CHAPTER TWENTY-ONE – SPLIT SOUL

His messenger went off filled with friend requests from people he didn't know. "Li' imbecile?" He wondered as he looked into the man's profile "Demi-Human hunter." Was written under his description. Jones' eyes widened as he pulled over to understand what was going on. All of the people Jones had talked to were now appearing in his profile. As he blinked his eyes the profiles would go blank. "I want to see you," Jones said to himself looking back at each profile. As Jones said that the profiles became clear again. "Heh, so that's how the watchers hide so well." Jones laughed to himself for the first time in a month. He checked the road and got back on it feeling hungry. "Guess I'll grab a bite to eat." A burger joint lay off to the right as Jones went towards it. People stood outside vaping as Jones went in. A Lamborghini among other cars sat outside as Jones felt the energy of being watched. Jones opened up the door as he went towards the counter. "Hey, I've heard of you." A man said to Jones. "Join us outside, man." The man invited Jones to the crowd. "Can I order first?" He said. "I got you, Jones. Two fries and a shake, right?" The man laughed. "You read my mind, didn't you?" Jones no longer smiling, wondering if he would be in danger again. "Enjoy the moment." The man said vaping.

Jones walked outside of the burger shop to where the fancy cars were. "So, what do you do?" Jones asked the man. The man smiled, "Pass me a follow, I sell these things." He pointed at his vape pen. "I sell them in hopes people will get off their cigarettes. Always apologizing for people's addictions, I guess." Jones nodded, "Oh I see. Why not make it vegan style?" Jones said to the man. The man laughed, "I'll throw in jerky tasting bubble gum too eh?" Jones laughed back, "Well, hey no problem man. My burgers are almost ready." Jones said, getting ready to walk back into the store. "Alright."Jones knew he would most likely never see the man who sold vape again but had a conversation worthwhile. As he picked up his shake and his burger, he watched the crowd disperse. Jones went towards his car drinking the shake as he contemplated being able to eat his packaging. "Nuisance,' I tell you. Plastic is too damn efficient at holding and destroying the world." Jones said to himself. "One day." As he put his foot on the gas pedal aiming for home. "So, what happens when you give a person too much time to think and nowhere to go?" Jones said "insanity, a world of escape into nowhere land around one's own mind."

Jones acted as if he was speaking to a crowd. Nepharius was listening to his every word as he drove home. "That's right, insanity because one's own mind can't create. We as humans are built to create and when we can't we break. When we break, survival mode kicks in. "The entertainment we turn to, to learn about stories because we have no other ways to motivate ourselves to create the ideas we're making," Jones turned towards Nepharius. "Do you understand what will happen if you disallow those a chance to use their ideas? To create and add on to your own?" Jones said seriously to Nepharius. "Our world, our home will collapse in stagnation. When we stagnate, we die. We stop wanting to network, stop wanting to reproduce. We stop wanting to move forward in our everyday lives." Jones raised his voice. "Do you plan to kill us all Nepharius! Do you!? I won't let it happen!" Jones shouted at Nepharius from the cart that he got out of interrupting his conversation with the village people. "You foolish arbiter. Sit back down!" Nepharius said, clenching the gemstone. Against Jones's own will he sat on a chair as the chains locked him in place. "I'll find a way, Nepharius. I already have." Jones said. Nepharius smirked, "You'll be going for a long swim soon. Don't worry Jones, I won't tie you up. I'll have you swim behind the waves I create with this gem as I deactivate everyone's memory." Jones wiggled in the chains as Zaya silently watched, waiting for the right time to break Jones free. Every store had its own nuance in which Jones had walked into. A flash of thought ran through his head as he memorized the ambiances that fit each setting. If a store had anything written group-wise, chances are Jones could find those people. "Mafia Central." Was written on a restaurant that Jones had accidentally walked into. He recalled the man patting him on the back as he thanked him. "Yeah. If you need any help…" Jones's mind flipped back to him chained in the chair as Nepharius continued explaining his plan. Looking around the village for a possible way out Jones searched for leverage he

CHAPTER TWENTY-ONE – SPLIT SOUL

could use to break the chains.

Zaya whispered again from afar, "Stall for as long as you can. I'll figure something out." She said as Nepharius finished writing on the hologram that floated within the village. "We will follow you to the end." The village leader said as Nepharius thanked the strange man. "Lift Jones over there and carry him on your back towards the ship," Nepharius said as Jones got lifted on their village man's back. This man was tall with white long hair, stripes ran across his face as his breath of mint flowed out through to the other side. With each breath, Jones could feel the energy extending out from the man's body. Women and men both picked up their weapons and staff as a small crew of less than twelve headed towards the ship on the beach. Zaya ran fast headed towards the other side of the ship as crew members slept by the side waiting on Nepharius's return. As Zaya snuck on the brazen ship she went back towards the cabin where Jones's only chance of escape would be from the leaving point. Jones tried to stall for time by kicking and making a ruckus as the village soldier told him to continuously stop squirming around. "Smack him out," Nepharius commanded.

The man took the back of his short-sided stick and smacked Jones, knocking him clean out. "Shit," Jones said, fully awake as he drove towards his driveway semi-dazed about what he had been doing before. Jones finished his burger and rushed inside putting his backpack on the bed along with his brown felt hat as his mind raced towards what to do next. As he sat there on the bed his mother came around to check on Jones. "Are you ill?" She said as she looked at him. Jones put his hand over his forehead. "I'm fine Mom, just thinking." Jones had been caught up so deep in trying to escape Nepharius that his real-time kept intermixing. His train of thought was spiraling out of control as the two worlds were completely connected from his viewpoint. Jones got back out of bed as his mother went back into the kitchen to avoid the possible conflicts the two of them might have. She sat there making dinner, getting ready to serve it for the family. "Why don't you come to join us tonight?" His mother said as Jones thought about it for a moment from what little thinking he could do. "I have to study. Class is going to be tough tomorrow." Jones said, giving out an excuse as he thought about his other worries.

"Okay, I'll put it in the fridge." His mother didn't expect or notice a thing as Jones thought's continued to race. He put his backpack down by the drawers as he went over to the shower to try to clear his mind. A shaver sat on the corner as Jones blinked. The shaver started to reflect green and blink green light self-cleaning itself as Jones blinked again. "What's this?" He said as he picked up the shaver. Jones had left a green laser pen that his mother put on the counter previously. The green laser hadn't been turned off. As the green light disappeared the shaver stopped as well. Jones took the green laser pen and pointed it back on the shaver getting no results. "I'm going to go out for a short drive." He said to his mother. "I thought you were going to study?" She said in return looking at Jones. "At least eat some dinner first." Jones's mother looked at him firmly annoyed that he wasn't cooperating with basic dinner plans. "Alright. What's for dinner?" He asked from the restroom trying to relax his mind."It's mashed potatoes and chicken with broccoli." She said back to him, raising her voice. Jones replied quickly, "Sounds great! I'll be right there!" He said quickly getting dressed to walk around the corner. As the plates were all aligned perfectly with folded-over napkins Jones took a seat at the dinner table. "Butter's on the corner." She said pointing to it. Jones took the bread and butter and filled his plate to the max. "So how was your first day back?" She asked. "Learn anything interesting?" She added on instigating a conversation in hopes to learn how he was feeling. "It was good, met a cool person at school and learned some math,"

Jones replied as he scarfed down his food almost as fast as he put it on his plate. "Sounds like a good start." She said, Jones replied, "Yeah I learned a lot and have notes already. Seems like it will be a hard class but still fun." Jones finished his plate getting up to rush over to the sink. "Alright, I'm going to finish getting ready and go out for a walk," Jones said. "I'll study

CHAPTER TWENTY-ONE – SPLIT SOUL

right when I get back." His mom nodded as Jones went back to his room to prepare. "Pleasant Hill is waiting for you, Jones. The big clock that you were at is ticking." Mira said, running through his head. "A guy named Brown is at the phone store. Find him." Mira trailed off catching Jones off guard giving him no time to respond. He continued to get ready for his outing.

Jones put on his black Jeans and brown felt hat as he walked forward towards the door. Putting in one of his CDs where hardcore music played. He stepped on the gas and headed out towards Pleasant Hill. Passing one of the cars Jones smiled at him as he put his hand out to move the car out of the way. The car slowly swerved towards another car as the highway cleared up. Jones continued to step on the pedal veering hard towards the left of the highway. Off the exit, the car almost turned over. Jones caught the wheel keeping it from tipping as he stepped on the breaks. Jones headed towards the parking lot next to the giant clock that was ticking forward. "I have to find Brown huh?" Jones said to himself running into the phone store as a guy with headphones over his shoulder looked at him. "How can we help you?" He said, taking them off. "Looking for a man named Brown." Jones said, "How do those sound?" He took the headphones trying them on. "Like a theater. Pretty sick right?"

The man bragged slightly. "Welcome to our watcher's extravaganza shop. Names Ware." He pointed to his two friends, "This is Naomi and Star" the two of them bowed. "Yup! We are!" Star said to Naomi as they smiled. "Well alright," Jones said, confirming he was in the right place. "Run back and forth. Take the physical." Ware said in a rough voice. Jones ran back and forth as fast as he could. "Best record you got huh?" Jones said. Naomi laughed "You need faster shoes huh?" She laughed. "Alright, I'll take those." If we could have a tissue that self-heats itself after we use it so we wouldn't be throwing these away all the time that'd be great." Naomi complained to Star as he went over and got to work on the shoes. "What are you going to do to them?" Jones asked out of curiosity. "Oh, we're going to boost them for your trip back home!" Naomi said looking over at Wares who was wearing a black rounded hat. Jones noticed it, "Where did you get that hat?" He asked Wares smiled. "Got it after I threw a person off a cliff. I mean our hats do represent us; don't you know?" A man sat on the corner of the store. "Wares shut up." He said slouching over. "Kid come here." The man was strikingly old wearing a brown hat with brown clothing. "Hey, Architect kid! Heard you were making a car and need some help. Also heard about Nepharius from Mira." Naomi and Star kept working on the boots twisting in various tools as the two of them were using items Jones had never seen before.

"I can't even imagine what— "Jones cut himself off as the shoe now showed blue. "When you're done with Nepharius. Come back here and we'll help you out." Brown said as he walked into the back of the phone store disappearing through the back. "He's kinda mysterious, that Mr. Brown." Wares said. "Took me in as a kid,

I started tinkering and here I am." Wares said laughing. "Anyway, you can't hang here too long so I'm going to have star pretend to sell you a cellphone." As a customer walked through the door Star grabbed Jones and put out a phone. "Here you go!" She said smiling as her voice squeaked happily. Naomi hid her tools as Wares put back on his headphones. "Alright," Jones said, putting on his shoes that felt lighter. "Here's $134 for the cellphone," Jones said, handing over his cash. She smiled as she went back to work. Jones went out the right door thinking about Nepharius who was keeping him in chains. Every time Jones closed his eyes all he saw was darkness. The imagery wasn't going through his mind. Jones looked at the clock watching the time go by as people aimlessly walked down the streets. "Mira!" Jones called out loud in public as people looked at him walking down the street. "Mira, you listen here!" Jones said again as more people stared now wondering what was going on. "Shh, they are looking at you, Jones," Mira warned as Jones quieted down.

"How is Zaya, why the shoes? It's already too late as I can't even get in!"

CHAPTER TWENTY-ONE – SPLIT SOUL

He said. Mira took a step back, "Jones, quickly now. I'm guiding you as fast as I can to contact our friends in the Universe. You have the right idea. For now, hide these shoes." Mira instructed Jones as he rushed back to his car ignoring any stares on the street. Jones got in and started to drive home. As Jones was driving home with the shoes hidden in his trunk he thought about the next day at school. Jones knew that his parents would be questioning where he was within the confines of the few hours he had taken to sneak out. He knew the questions such as, "Where did you get those shoes? Where have you been? Where did you go?" would be the questions asked at the door right when his mother saw him. Jones was prepared to make up a story, "Yes mom, I got distracted by talking to a friend at the store. An old buddy of mine works there." Jones said to himself practicing in the car to get it straight. "Went just down the street in Pleasant Hill." He said to himself. "What are you doing?" Mira said, questioning Jones' antics. "Talking to myself, trying to cover for these new shoes. My mom's not going to believe a word I say you know." Jones replied to Mira half paying attention to the road as a watcher came by with a wheelchair. "You can get those shoes mailed next time!" He shouted indirectly for Jones to hear as the rest of everyone around them looked at Jones as if he was crazy. As Jones got into his home, he looked around slowly noticing that the lights had already been shut off. The lights were dimly lit on the table as music had previously played in the house. With the player active Jones went towards his room hoping to not make any contact with his mother. As he carried the shoes with the tools inside of them. Jones, I ran around the corner throwing them into the closet. "Jones, what was that noise?" His mother said from the other room. She had been watching T.V. "Where have you been again?"

Jones thought quickly as Mira had told him to. "Pleasant Hill, hanging with a friend." He said, trying not to incriminate himself into more questioning. "Well, tell your friends you have school from now on. You have to focus on finishing your final courses and graduating." His mother said angrily. Jones nodded as he went towards his room. He had gotten away with her not finding out about the brand-new shoes he bought. "Okay. Now put them on." Mira's voice went through Jones's head again guiding him towards where Nepharius had cut Jones out. "Why?" Jones questioned. "These shoes will add extra energy to your other half," Mira said. Jones, self-conscious of his door and being seen lying in bed, put on his shoes slowly while lying down. His vision blurred as he hadn't slept well again. Blinking his eyes, his room and the jungle where Nepharius had been dragging his knocked-out body merged into two. Jones felt dizzy as he awoke. Nepharius looked back at him as the villager with the club noticed him grabbing his head. "Wait," Nepharius said as the villager put up his club again. "Don't knock this foolish man out yet." Jones looked up at him as his feet felt light. The tools were active on his feet as the two shoes Jones wore felt the same now. "Press the left one at the right time." Mira said, "Right in the sole, it will have an extra kick." Mira laughed. Nepharius looked around. "Someone else is close by, aren't they?" He said looking at Jones, who refused to speak. "You see this boat Jones?"

It's taking us to Criminal Island. Our final stop, where all four hundred of my comrades are. This gem will eradicate that fence at my will." Nepharius laughed. "Come." He said as the villager turned towards Nepharius. Jones reached down to the sole of his foot pressing it inward. "This is Star's automated system. Please hold onto your feet, if you don't you may lose them! Cheers!" A happy shout came out as the shoes boosted Jones forward. The chains wrapped around the Villagers Club as the chair broke. Pieces flew all over the place as the club broke further into shards jamming in the chain. Jones's shoes kept propelling Jones forward from behind more than the villager could hold on. Knocking him over and spiraling out of control the chain broke hitting a rock. Jones smacked the ground rolling over his head as the system went off again."Star's warning. You've lost function. Will defunct now." The shoes were powered down as one of them showed a small hole in it. "Okay. No warning?" Jones said to himself angrily directed at Star as he sat for a second trying to recuperate. Nepharius took the villagers after watching and told them to stay taking a few with

CHAPTER TWENTY-ONE – SPLIT SOUL

him. "You two, stall this nuisance and run!" Nepharius warned as the two villagers crackle jumping forward. Nepharius turned to run as Zaya came out from hiding coming back with help. "I found you some backup!" She shouted coming along with Bey in tow. "Heard you had some trouble, Jones!" She shouted from far away.

The two of them charged towards each villager tackling them. Zaya threw Jones some headphones, "Use these to focus!" He put them on as music played into his ear. Jones felt powerful waking up as the villager rushed him. Jones was able to focus on something moved to the right dodging. He grappled the villager as Bey swung a right fist towards the other one. "Woohoo! This is a ball. You never told me you had this side of you!" Bey shouted as she rolled around with the villager smacking him twice. Jones pushes the villager onto the ground smashing his face in as Zaya took a piece of wood. "Catch!" She said as Jones reached out grabbing the wood. He threw it down right into the villager's leg as the grey man screamed. Jones's headphones fell off into the dirt. He looked around noticing the other villager had also been knocked out by Bey's first charge. "Nepharius is on the run. I don't know how you got here, Bey…but I'm sure glad you are." Jones laughed, wiping his forehead as he stood up. One of his shoes was on and the other was off. "Jones, there's not much time left," Mira said. "Nepharius will be taking off soon." Jones nodded as the three of them started racing towards the boat. "Jones hurry up!" Zaya said as Bey followed behind. "Maybe we can make a cart in this space to move along faster. Jones, what do you think?" One of Jones's shoes was still working from his left foot, "Stars program here! One engine is still at a fourth capacity." It responded to the two of them conversing as Jones stuck it on the back of a plank.

"I'll hold it if we take that cart over there," Jones said, pointing towards the half-broken chair. "Grab anything that looks like a wheel" he instructed as the three of them looked around. "There!" Bey said, pointing to a few small round boulders that had been chipped away. "With these sticks, this shoe and these small rockets won't hold long but should get us close!" Jones said excitedly as he looked at the angle. "Bey hold this." Jones threw the stick towards Bey as she jumped surprised by the throw. "Hand it to me next time ya dope!" Bey complained. Jones laughed, "Sorry!" The three of them put together the cart with the shoe held onto the back. "Hop in," Jones shouted as Bey and Zaya ran towards the creaky sticks and stones. "Hope this works." Jones put the shoe in the back as he tapped the sole again. "Star's initiation. Go!" It said as the shoe imitated propelling the three of them forward. "Woah! Hold on to yourselves!" Jones shouted as Zaya laughed. "Cart sick!" Bey shouted out loud as she continuously felt irked. "I'm cart sick!" She said, repeating herself as she almost puked over the side. The cart wobbled back and forth barely holding on as rocks, trees, and various debris passed by. Jones could feel the wind from within his room blowing on his face. One of his shoes was dirtied and taken off as he was sitting on his bedside in the dark. He was mumbling to himself as his mother walked in hearing noises."Jones?" his mother said, with a worried expression.

Jones sat there on the bed as his mother tapped him on the shoulder. "Jones woke up." He looked at her for a second half awake. "I heard you say something, so I decided to ask if you were okay, why do you have one shoe on?" Jones thought for a moment before replying. He looked up at her, "Oh, I guess I passed out midway into sleep." Jones said, attempting to alleviate her worries. "Are you having trouble sleeping again?" She asked as she scolded him at the same time. "You have school tomorrow. You need to get some rest. If you're having trouble sleeping again, we'll get you something." She put both of Jones shoe's in the closet as he laid back down. "Okay, mom. Thanks." He replied getting back under the covers surveying what had happened. One of the shoes had a dirt stain on it from a few moments prior. "Bey and Zara need you. You need to go back Jones." Mira said, urging him to pay attention to them while the cart sped through the jungle. Jones sat back down as the cart came into view. A rock stood out in front of them. "Jones! Watch out!" Bey shouted from across the

CHAPTER TWENTY-ONE – SPLIT SOUL

way as Zaya jumped abandoning the cart. Jones and Bey hit the rock as the beachside came into view. Tumbling over themselves the two of them rolled down the hill. Jones stumbled into a tree stopping and breaking his fall as Bey hit a rock knocking her out cold. Zaya got up brushing herself off as she came out almost unscathed from the cart's breakdown. "Jones stood up. Use your creativity or something! Nepharius is about to take off! Look!" Zaya said pointing towards the ship.

Jones looked over at the crew members boarding as a rope was tied down at the edge. Nepharius had already boarded the ship standing at the front as he gripped the stone in his hand. Nepharius sat there staring out over the ocean as if he had accomplished a lifelong dream. Jones couldn't understand Nepharius hatred towards the creativity of humanity or his hatred towards people among their actions. "Psst Jones," Zaya whispered as Jones rubbed his head and got up. "How are we going to get on that ship?" She asked him concerned as Nepharius tapped his foot. "I'm not sure yet. I'll think of something." Jones replied. Nepharius stood there waiting for the two villagers expecting their return. He knew that Jones might be a match for them but couldn't place the delay on their return. "Jones must have won," Nepharius said quietly to himself as he spits off the side of the boat. "I knew I shouldn't have trusted them to do the job. My crew is much more trustworthy." Nepharius said quietly to himself ready to leave. "Let's go boys!" Nepharius called out as one of them went onto the beach reaching for the rope. "There!" Zaya pointed out a window that had been opened below deck. "We'll sneak into there!" She said, "Bey doesn't have to come along, does she?" Zaya asked Jones as he thought for a moment.

"No, it's best she doesn't. Her soul may wander but it won't be involved until I can fix this whole separation of our consciousness that Nepharius had created." Jones grabbed Zaya's hand and ran down the beach as Nepharius got off the bow of the ship. Jones was used to seeing Nepharius check his crew members. He knew from watching that Nepharius would go for the wheel. In that instance, Jones ran with Zaya headed towards the window below deck. Seashells and rocks moved out of the way sparkling from being touched as Jones ran as fast as he could. The crew members didn't notice as their focus was on preparing to leave. Jones leaped up towards the window jumping up as the boat tilted off to the left. He grabbed onto the window successfully pulling himself into it as the wooden floors felt glossy, fully washed. "Come quickly," Jones said, waving Zaya over, helping her up into the ship. The two of them shut the window as crew members started to pour in. Jones looked quickly for a place to hide with Zaya a foot away. "Look!" Jones said as a treasure chest lies with nothing in it on the right side of the room. Jones ran over to it with Zaya and got in closing the trunk behind them. "Nepharius will be pleased with us." One of the crew members spoke as a villager sat in the rowing seat of the cabin.

"Yeah, yeah! We learned the fighting techniques he taught us to a T!" The other crew member held up his hand-throwing a fake fist laughing as the first crew member started joking. "Not to mention when Nepharius uses that gem properly humanity won't remember a thing!" Jones eavesdropped from the treasure chest trying to understand what the two crew members were saying. "Yeah! He'll wipe their imagination clean! No one will be able to come up with a new idea and no one will know why!" The two of them laughed together as the villagers started rowing. Jones and Zaya rocked in the empty treasure chest as his hand fell on Zaya's foot. "Hey, watch out!" She was surprised by Jones's movement. He reached to cover her mouth as she referred to his mind. "We can communicate like this too, stupid!" She said as Jones relayed it back. "Shh, do you want them to hear us?" He questioned her as she quieted down. "We have to destroy that crystal. The golden piano broke its seal but I think it will still work." Jones said to Zaya. Mira's broken words tried to go through Jones' mind but did not affect the sound, which jumped in and out. A tape recorder playing backward over and over sounded through as he grabbed his head.

CHAPTER TWENTY-ONE – SPLIT SOUL

"Ugh." "Jones…. where…Jones." It repeated as the ship grew further from the beach. In the complete darkness of the treasure chest, Jones could only guess where the ship was headed next. "Jones woke up." A hand shook him while he was in his bed. His mother was standing right over him as he looked her in the eye, taking a few seconds to adjust to the reality around him. "What?" He said as the alarm buzzed. "You have to get to school. It's your second day already." Jones got out of bed looking at the clock as he realized it was already 12:11 PM. "Damn!" He said to himself realizing he was already twenty minutes late. "Alright thank you, leave my room please so I can get ready," Jones said to his mother urging her out of the room. She went out after nodding her head acknowledging that he was serious about his school. Jones looked at the shoe in the closet as both of them had damage on it.

"Where was I…?" He said to himself wondering where he had wandered. "One of your friends called, said you were looking through his bushes for something." His mom said. "Did you lose something?" Jones replied right away, "Yeah my wallet." He said lying again. He quickly got fully dressed leaving no time for a shower as he raced out of the door. The warm sun was shining again as Jones turned up the music and headed out to his school's parking lot. After a few minutes of driving, Jones pulled up and parked. The parking lot was empty as the few stragglers hustled towards their class. Jones ran in the door and sat down as the teacher looked at him. "Jones, you're late." He said drawing on the whiteboard. "Hey, Lily." He whispered. Lily looked over at Jones, "Got any idea of what's going on here?" He said to her expecting a response. "Can't think of any," Lily said cheerfully, writing down her notes as the professor wrote on the board. "Can the class tell me any ideas on this answer?" Jones surveyed the classroom for a moment expecting a response but got none. "No ideas?" The teacher said, "Well then, the math answer is twenty-four." The professor went on to explain it as Jones looked around the classroom worried. "Lily, tell me a new color. Any color." Jones asked with a worried voice. "Blue." She said, "Blue is not a new color." Jones said, "You know, like if you mixed purple with blue." Jones replied, raising his voice a little. "Quiet down Jones." The professor said in return as Jones grew more worried about the situation. Lily shook her head l, "I don't know what's going on Jones but I think you should stop. I can't think of anything, ok?" She said, irritated by this, "You're late again. Here are the notes I took." Lily said, handing them over as Jones thought to himself. "Damn, Nepharius has already acted. In a world without ideas…" Jones sat there feeling defeated for a moment as he copied down the notes and mathematics written on the board. "No new progression for us. It's over." Jones said. "Don't give up yet," Mira said to Jones, encouraging him again. "Nepharius may have the gem but that doesn't mean he's won his way." She said to Jones. He nodded his head paying attention to the math class as he wrote down the notes. "You're right, Mira," Jones replied.

Jones got up asking to be excused from the class as he ran towards the front door avoiding the people around him. Jones' world spun as he realized he was stuck in a nonexistent state of mind. No one understood the split of Jones' mind in between hopping in and out. One side tired and the other side dropping down. Still, Jones continued to place himself outside as he ran towards his car. Jones looked at the car door and started driving towards home as a bright white light over the city propelled them forward. Jones felt stuck between both worlds stuck between which life he wanted to live. "Harver!" Lily yelled as she saw Jones racing home. "You forgot your notes!" She said, "Your notes!" Jones waved her away as he started the engine putting his foot on the pedal. He went into multiple worlds at once feeling it in his head. With every waking moment, time passed until he came too. "I'm at home." He said to himself walking in his door headed towards his room. The howl of a wolf came from afar as Jones shook off the sound. He ran into his room forcing himself to focus on one world so he wouldn't be split in half. The treasure chest on Nepharius ship shook. Nepharius laughed belching loudly holding the gem in his hand towards the sky. Sunlight hit the gem activating the rule Nepharius had set into place. The rule to wipe out everyone's imagination started to creep into

CHAPTER TWENTY-ONE – SPLIT SOUL

everyone's mind. "Damn you Nepharius!" Mira said as she swooped in from above. "I'm coming for that!" Mira tried to grab it but Nepharius acted. The gem fell in the water on his command. This is how it should be in its silence. Mira missed hitting the ship as she rolled over her green and black dress grabbing onto a log. The idea orbs around Mira's neck that she carried around fell to the floor as Nepharius laughed. "What a waste of good food," Mira said, disappointed looking at the idea orb necklace on the ship deck. "Weakling. I was prepared for you!" As he kicked Mira to the side. Mira got back up running towards the back of the ship past the mast. "Jones!" She said running towards him as she grabbed him from one world. The voice echoed through Jones's head as he lay there on his bed. None of his ideas responded as he yelled at the world. The world slowed down to a time point as Jones jumped up for the gem. Running out of the chest with Zaya in tow. "Fuck." Jones said seeing Mira fall as Zaya jumped forward aiming towards the gem. "No!" She latched on as Nepharius struggled. Jones ran up as he moved forward to punch Nepharius. Nepharius keeled left as Jones pinched him again pushing him back to hold the gem. "My ideas and world!" Jones said as he took hold of the gem. "Play it Zaya!" Zaya ran to the golden piano to play the middle C keynote. Zaya played the golden piano notes dropping in further as the vibrations flowed out of it. The four legs pushed together as the light beamed up piercing through Nepharius. "You want things to end so soon?" "Not this way!" He said reaching for Jones as the two of them fell through the water as the water turned into clouds. "This is my world," Jones yelled, pushing Nepharius further away from them.

Jones dropped as the world went pure white. A few minutes passed as Jones woke up noticing Nepharius lifeless in white space right before him. Jones got up grabbing the gem. "I can rebuild what we've lost. I can rebuild this space." He imagined the world around him recreating it as the whiteness filled with the city of Jones' thoughts. "Jones!" The crowd cheered as he lay there in his new spot. "Jones you did it!" Mira said now more awake. Jones fell over as he looked down the space. People gathered around as the world spun. "Okay, we have to pick up this crazy." The ambulance said walking by the crowds. Against Jones' will he was picked up and moved away. Jones woke up as his blankets were half off of the bed and half on. The sun shone through the rooftops at him giving the feeling of pressure from the light of the sun. Jones got up walking over to his drawer as he took out a shirt and put it on. His head felt a bright light as he tried to get acquainted with himself. He couldn't as he wobbled back and forth falling back into the bed. "What's going on?" Jones said to himself

Mira walked up to him. "You fell over and passed out from that gem, remember?" She said, reminding Jones of who he was. "Mira, why are you here?" Jones said, trying to get a hold of the situation he was in. Plastered on the walls were a white flower papered wall. Jones didn't know the difference as he sat on the bed. "You're at your house." Mira said, "Quiet down. You're finally awake." Jones rubbed his head looking out of the house. "Yeah. I see." Jones said, realizing that he knocked over Nepharius. "Wait what happened after that?" He asked Mira. "After you knocked the gem and caught it. You used your imagination to re-create our lost world. You then freed the people's minds. Then after Nepharius wasn't coming up from the ocean you broke the gem. Thus, when you passed out, I took you home. You've been a walking zombie since. Waking up and going to school not knowing what to do other than your mind's routine." Mira scolded Jones as she stopped yelling. "You've gained your freedom, Jones," Mira said, tossing him the document that branded him as a criminal.

Jones signed it and passed it back to Mira. "Call us anytime," Mira said as she left. Jones got up and got dressed. He walked around the corner to see his mother sitting next to the T.V. with the couch and lamp on. Jones checked around to make sure that his world was oriented with himself. "Mom?" Jones called out to her wondering what the reply was. "Shh! I'm watching this, we can talk after. Don't you have school tomorrow?" she scolded. Jones smiled, "yeah, never mind." He said walking back into his

CHAPTER TWENTY-ONE – SPLIT SOUL

room. Everything seemed to normalize around Jones. He flopped back on his bed and went to sleep. The psychiatrist walked by patrolling the area. Nighttime was beginning to fall, but Jones couldn't sleep. Neither could his roommate. "So…it sounds like you were really after him, this Nepharius guy. Did you know Nepharius means evil?" Jones's roommate asked curiously. Jones laughed, "Yes, Nepharius is exactly that. A purity of what humanity would consider being "evil." Our true enemy of extinction, non-development. His roommate laughed, "You're an interesting one Jones. I'd like to keep reading if that's alright with you. You're saying that our plains are connected?" Jones nodded silently. "Keep on reading, if you truly want to see the world from this perspective the answer is in my written journal." The roommate picked up the book and started reading again, he slowly sank into his bed. His roommate's voice was heard clearly as the footsteps of the psychiatrists echoed through the hallways. Jones yawned as darkness fell over the building.

Chapter Twenty-Two – Cleaning After Nepharius

Two months later, Jones was in his last semester in school. He went through the parking lot over to where the center stood. "I hear they are renovating the garage." A man spoke to another man. The construction workers sat on the sidelines talking about the entire new mall development. Jones knew that he had influenced people around him and laughed silently to himself. "At least one good thing came out of it." Jones got into his car and drove home thinking about his next steps. "School, that's where I need to be." He said to himself. The third day at school had already come. Things seemed normal around where Jones would go. As he walked into class, he was no longer late. "Hi, Jones!" Lily smiled as she happily greeted him to sit down. "You finally aren't taking my notes!" She said laughing as he sat down in time. "You haven't been late either ever since you got back." Lily tapped Jones back lightly as the professor came in. "Everyone names yourselves for today." The whole class started naming themselves while waiting for the first real lesson. "Jones we were unable to find Nepharius." Mira's voice rang through Jones' head as he listened in the classroom. "What do you mean unable?" Jones said half complaining and half in fear of the worst. "Yes, Nepharius survived… somehow. There have been reports of him on the go for the other piece. The gem may not be in his grasp, but he still has a few tricks up his sleeve." Jones sighed as he called himself out to the professor naming his name.

CHAPTER TWENTY-TWO – CLEANING AFTER NEPHARIUS

"Jones T. Harver, musical professional!" He said loudly. The class laughed as Lily sat back to scold him. "Jones! Embarrassing." She said as Jones sat back down. He heard Mira's chuckles echo around him as his eyes focused on the board again. "Right." He said to himself going back to reading what was on the board.

Jones sat there scratching his head as he slowly copied what was on the board. It had already been three days since the news of Nepharius's escape. Like before, most of the watchers had gone back to their original jobs. Other's had sat down on the corner again making dealings on their markets of galactic conscious currency. Some watchers still had no place to go roaming the streets looking for other watchers to give them a home. "This is no healthy way to live," Jones said to himself thinking about the comrades tossed aside. "Once someone and now an entire story, washed away on the side due to something in their lives." Mira was the only one who had been in contact with Jones after the crash of the world, making sure that his mind and body had stabilized. Both realities were colliding. "Hey, Jones. Have you slept well at all lately?" Mira questioned him as he continued to drift off taking down the professor's notes. "Yeah. Actually, better than ever." Jones said, replying to Mira having a sense of peace within the words he said. "Knowing what you know Jones. Don't let anyone know." Mira said. "What people don't know can't hurt them right?" Jones replied in return. "What happened to Zaya and Bey? What about the ship?" Jones asked. "The ship has been taken in with Nepharius's remaining crew. Zaya has been returned to her music tour and Bey is back at home resting." Mira filled in the gaps of what had happened as Jones sat there in class listening to the professor.

He sat there staring at the notes smiling to himself as to not give his position away. The professor finished up the notes. "Next week we have another exam." He said as the rest of the class groaned and went out the door. "So, I'm headed home," Jones said to Lily as he walked out the door. Lily smiled nodding her head. "Sounds great!" She said walking off the other way. Jones went towards the middle of his school where the cafeteria had been developed sitting down by a star-patterned design. "This place would be great for an entryway," Jones said to himself daydreaming again. He didn't want to go home right away. Jones called Ottie, "Hey man, what's up?" He said sitting there. Ottie picked up the phone for the first time in a while. "Hey man, your laptop is all good right?" Jones sat for a moment staring at the blue sky slowly running by. "Yeah, it is. I can finally make some more songs." Jones said as he sat by the star pattern with gray over it. "When are you coming back here?" Jones questioned Ottie. "Soon?" He asked curiously. "Yeah, probably soon. California is pretty dope." Ottie said in return. "Alright, I'll be waiting." Jones walked further down the street towards the back-parking lot where he had parked. For the first time in a while with nothing happening around Jones he got used to the peacefulness.

"The watchers, I guess. They are where they are because the watchers want to be. I know you want to give them a place, Jones. I suppose no one gave them a chance to get reintegrated. Tossed out from their societies since day one. That's why the watchers are the way they are." The voice echoed through his head. Jones couldn't make out who it was as he tried calling back. "You see. People who are so depressed that they go into their own little worlds to escape reality. These people would rather be on drugs because they don't want to accept the realities they live in. Watchers, watchers are much the same as your kind." The spirit of music's voice became clearer as Jones sat where he was and listened. "Watchers have no place to go. They never left but couldn't integrate. So, the streets were their only comforting home. These people didn't want to work for someone else's dream. Well, most of them…" the spirit of music sounded disappointed and sad. "One day I won't have to watch the watchers anymore." The spirit of music sighed as he had a sad tone in the vibration of his voice. As Jones looked up at the sky it started to rain. The spirit of music had connections to the heart of the earth that if he were captured or damaged would have great consequences. Jones

CHAPTER TWENTY-TWO – CLEANING AFTER NEPHARIUS

kept his observation to himself as he got up ready to go to his car. "I have to get out of the rain my friends. I will talk to you later." He mumbled to himself as he walked further over to the back gates. As the rain fell lightly, Jones sat in his car thinking about what he had done. He had stopped Nepharius from destroying people's imaginations. Jones wondered what other possible problems were out there. As he looked around him, he could feel the watchers walking, waiting, and developing their tools in secret. Jones could feel the presence of Zaya and Bey. He knew that his life would be different than before. Jones stepped on the gas of his car and started to head home as his books sat in the back.

"You still have yet to develop your car." A voice said through Jones' mind. "Who is it?" The voice's tone lowered, "One of the three men you saw making it. Are you coming for a ride or not yet?" The man said, inviting him. "I still have more to do. I can't yet." Jones replied, "I haven't earned this hat yet." He said quietly. "You're right, you have yet to stop Nepharius completely. He is going for the map next. Although humanity is saved and may never know what you have done for them. You are still a hero because of what you have done. However, your celebration is short-lived. Other watchers still consider you an attachment to Nepharius. Mira paused for a moment contemplating her statement, "a villain across all of the galaxy."Jones stopped for a moment to think as the light turned red. "How does a thought-form? Imagery? Is it our imagination of two ideas like I said to Mira that propels us forward?" Jones sat there contemplating for a moment. "It's more than that my friend, it's people who had an idea wanting to get it out to others. The inspiration of others propels the world forward. There will always be yin and yang. Good and evil and people stopping humanity's progression because most of them are afraid. Afraid of their loss of power. You must understand that there is a whole other universe unexplored outside of ours that we see on the same plain. You are one of the free ones. Able to see the similarities of us watchers and to project that." Jones sat there taking in everything the man was saying. Although he was no longer surprised by what he was hearing, Jones smiled at the answer. "What do you want from me?" He asked the gentleman who was now standing in front of him wearing a brown felt hat as well.

"I want you to accept the world of watchers. Nepharius isn't the only problem in our universe." Jones thought to himself, "When the car is ready will you give me a test drive?" He asked. The old man laughed, "There are so many places to explore my friend." As Jones was driving his car the rain around him kept pouring. The sun came out leaving a little hole in the clouds as if the warmth of an entity was watching over him. "With Nepharius unbreakable shield that he put on you as a protective curse and us on your radar, you will be well looked after by our ever-turning wheel of fate. Do what you must do but when you are ready come to us. The man then faded, turning away as the red light turned green. Jones turned his car up to full volume and headed for his house to rest up since the incident. The next day Jones woke up and looked at the clock. It struck 9:00 AM as he meandered over to the fridge to get out the cereal that he liked. "Mom, there's none left," He said to himself, opting for yogurt instead. "Why don't you go shopping before school?" Jones' mother said as he thought about all the people supporting him upon his adventures. "Lily doesn't know yet," Jones said to himself rubbing his hand in between his eyes as he recalled all the past images that raced through his mind. Jones gave out a big sigh as he went out the door with his backpack on. "Today is going to be the first normal day in weeks." Jones thought to himself throwing his backpack in the back seat of the car as the books tilted off to the side. "Ah, shoot, nuggets, and craisin I'm late again," Jones said to himself. "Hey Lily, can I get the first pages of notes?" He texted as he stepped on the gas pedal trying to blend in with society. As Jones drove down his street, watchers waved to him to say good morning. Trashmen, gardeners, people running and talking all stopped to look at Jones as if to show that they knew who he was, why he mattered. Jones didn't know a single one of the people as he approached the red stop sign-waving but ignoring the watchers at the same time. Jones smiled and continued to drive towards his school. He parked his car by the gate as he ran towards the school door where

CHAPTER TWENTY-TWO – CLEANING AFTER NEPHARIUS

Lily was waiting. "What's going on here?" Jones said curiously as class was waiting outside. "Our professor hasn't come in yet." She smiled as her ripped jeans and blue shirt sparkled from the sunlight. "Said he had to take care of a paper run." She kept smiling, oblivious to Jones already having lost interest in the conversation. "Oh. Alright cool." Jones replied, staring down at his phone as he searched the internet. Although Nepharius had been taken care of, news across the galaxy spread of his escape. Spam in Jones's mail congratulated him while the other half ridiculed him. One email stuck out to Jones, particularly the bold letters written across the top of the screen as he stood outside next to Lily.

"Welcome to the world of the universe. We here at council five saw your attempt to stop Nepharius. We would like to cordially invite you to our hall. Watchers in the world of the universe are still in need of help from small problems to big ones. You have been chosen to help solve these problems as you journey on in life". Jones looked down at his phone to be sure the spam mail wasn't being misread. "Council of five, huh?" He said under his breath. Lily looked at Jones. "Something bothering you?" She asked him as he stood there thinking about it. "I don't have the notes," Jones said as the professor started walking towards the door. "No problem, I can help you with those notes." He said as he opened the door, "One of the teachers told me you've been busy. I understand." He said as he smiled. Jones looked back at the teacher confused as if he was in on it as his phone flashed. The text messages changed saying "hit here for hologram and other news." Jones looked down at his phone as he tapped the news button. "In other galactic news today. Jones T. Harver scoured the world in search of Nepharius stopping him from an imagination block on humanity's lifestyle. A well-known criminal seemed to have inside disputes with his friend as a family feud broke out. There have been no comments accepted or made by everyone involved. We hope to get more information and commentary soon."

Jones blinked again as the newscaster changed back to everyday news. "On today's news, a man accidentally ran his other friend out of business. In the small coastal town of Santa Cruz, four cops chased the suspect down to the gas station as the suspect held his friend hostage." The door unlocked as the class went inside. Jones put his phone away taking his usual seat next to Lily. "Hey, Lily. Did you get my text about San Francisco?" Jones asked her as she stared blankly at the board. Her mind was elsewhere as if she was dreaming. "Yeah, it was beautiful." She replied half in tune with the conversation as the professor started naming out names on the board. "We have a small task for you." Mira's voice echoed again as Jones took out his books. "What is it?" Jones asked back, staring at the board. "Come down the Iron Trail at 2:00." Jones nodded his head slightly as the professor called out Jones' name. "Okay, class. Today we'll learn about theorems." Jones zoned out as the day went by trying to wrap his head around the concepts. After a few hours, he left the class without saying a word to Lily or conversation. Instead, he rushed towards his car to drive home. "Time to head to this trail." He said to himself driving towards where the sign was. Jones had previously walked a little of it before but had always turned back a fourth of the way through as he got tired. At the start of the trail, two wooden pikes lay directly apart from one another. Each one had ridges going through them as if the poles hadn't been touched in years. He stood there for a moment looking at the cement between the two as he slowly walked through taking his first two steps. Trees and grass in various colors of green to dark green sat out on either side. Jones started to walk down the trail as he looked down to the right side where the wind was telling him to go. Trash and cones alike pointed forward down the dam that had been empty from rain for four days prior. Each one of the pinpoints pointed forward towards a bridge that lay brown and rusted into perfect condition as the fence cross-cross pattern stuck out. As Jones walked forward further an old inactive Army Base stuck out of the side with multiple army tanks ready to be deployed at any given moment. Barbed wire stuck out along with bunkers and various other vehicles stored away next to the dam that kept pointing Jones forward. "Jones take a seat." Mira's voice echoed as Jones sat down on the bridge.

CHAPTER TWENTY-TWO – CLEANING AFTER NEPHARIUS

A man ran past him at full speed going up the rusted ridges to the top of where a person would crush their bones if they fell across the side. "Is this the energy you were telling me about?" Jones said to Mira as onlookers wondered why a man was talking to himself asleep on the bridge side. "No, I called you here because I want you to meet with the council of five. Follow the wind and head straight across the bridge into the school. You've been there once before." Mira said as Jones walked further to where kids were dancing. Two of the teachers were talking calmly with one another as Jones sat there reading the stress levels as they spoke. "I heard last you swam across the entire ocean with the whales." A man spoke to a woman as her pupils went from small to slight dilations. "Yes, I heard you went to study some of the best medicine on a hike through India." She said to him in return. Both of them turned towards Jones as he sat on the corner of the stage. "You're, back aren't you? A little late but back." The man said as the both of them calmly looked towards Jones. Neither of them felt stressed as they relaxed from the intense conversations the two of them were having. "Yes. I am." Jones sat there, "Heard the council of five had a concern they wanted me to check out?" Jones questioned as he sat there on the corner of the wooden stage watching one kid slowly walk in.

"Yes, we have a request. There's a watcher that's very old, upsetting neighbors in downtown Oakland. With no place to go, we want you to bring him back in to get help. You see…he's a great fighter of his time. We figured you may be able to find him. You seem to have a knack for this, my arbiter friend." The man spoke as he held his hand up to stop the woman from further interrupting. She was about to interject. "I got this, it's okay." He calmed her down. "We have to teach now. Please go." His brown hair and green eyes gazed upon Jones as it flowed further than usual. Jones nodded quietly as he left walking out of the schoolyard. He ran excitedly down the Iron Trail back towards his house, the cones in the dam now pointed the other way as the wind flowed behind him telling Jones when to walk faster or slower. Telling Jones when to expect a person looking at him. He was able to read the wind in parallel with the earth as to blend in with society like the spirit of music had warned. As Jones got home, soup waited for him on the counter preceding another interaction with his mother to navigate. "Made some lunch!" His mother said excitedly. She was happy that Jones was taking school seriously. "I heard your grades went up lately. After this semester ends there's a possibility of you going to a better school." She smiled as bread lie next to the bowl of soup. "Yeah mom, I'm all for it". He replied as he ate the soup relaxing by the tableside. "An old fighter huh?" Jones thought to himself as he gulped down his soup ready to go forward with the task.

"It's three. I'm going to study outside for a while." Jones said to his mom after eating. She nodded, impressed by his newfound study habits as he went back outside opening the door. Jones got into his car turning on music this time playing it softly. Jones drove off to BART five minutes from home to park by the gas station that he saw every day. As Jones parked near the BART, he walked up the stairs paying the new way going through the door. "Next time is free." The lady waved and smiled as Jones gave a confused look but smiled back. He walked up the stairs towards where the sign placed itself in red scrolling by. "Still no bars on the edges," Jones said, shaking his head as he imagined the bumps in color-coding rather than its black and yellow. With soft music playing to make the wait more suitable in an empty train. Watchers around Jones were playing with their items and engineering different things building ways to protect themselves from the outside world. Jones quietly listened to music as he got in the BART. Feeling like he could no longer leave the house without his phone he made sure the music would keep him on track. Shutting out the outside world as he sat down in the back of the BART. In jeans, a black t-shirt, and his brown felt hat. The BART train took him towards the West Oakland stop. "This is Demi-human hunters' territory," Jones said to himself, understanding where he was. Getting off of the BART train, Jones walked further over towards the cracks and graffiti that wrote "Sun across the stars." He peaked at it as he walked further down the street. "Where am I going to find this old man?" Jones said to himself as he started aimlessly

CHAPTER TWENTY-TWO – CLEANING AFTER NEPHARIUS

walking down the street sides. Houses alike had cactuses and items on the side blocking the stairway up to them as he walked through various places. Seeing a couch on the front doorstep Jones sat down feeling defeated by the task. He knew he couldn't ask any ordinary neighbor or they would question why he's looking and call the cops on him. With his head in his hands, he slowly fell asleep in the sun. Three hours later Jones woke up with the time reading 7:00 PM. "Damn." He said to himself realizing it had become late. Lost in the city of Oakland, Jones started walking in search of the BART feeling that he had failed. Multiple people were out and about as some places were closing. Jones heard music playing and decided to follow it into where a restaurant lie. His phone only read only 2% battery.

"Hey sir, can I charge my phone here?" He asked the waiter showing his plug and cable. "Yeah, you can stay here until closing. You have to leave when we do." He said as people laughed in the background. The cook flipped his tongs as the smell of glazed onions wafted through the air. Jones looked at the map finding his way back towards Bart. "Hey, where do people walk around here usually?" Jones said as the waiter passed by with a plate of food. "Usually around the 5th." He said from his perception. "Thanks," Jones replied in short. As his phone charged Jones picked it up and left quietly taking a walk further towards where the man may be. Passing by the ripped-up couch he had slept on, the weather changed towards rain. An old man carrying a rug walked forward as he had a small slash in his eye. His beard went down towards his pants as the rug he was carrying provided cover from the rain. "The fighter," Jones said to himself. By a small stroke of luck, he had found him. "What do you want?" The fighter said with one eye open as he stared at Jones calmly. "I was told to find you," Jones said as the old man kept walking forward. The old man turned around waving Jones away as he kept on walking forward during the rainfall.

"Wait!" Jones said, chasing after the man carrying the rug. The man turned around, "You better get yourself home, kid! It's dangerous out here!" Warning Jones as he continuously walked forward. "Mira, I found him," Jones called out. The man turned around as he heard Jones' voice through the galactic space. "You found me?" He said looking up at the sky briefly and then back at Jones. "You're the fighter, right?" Jones said, questioning the old man. He stood there. "Yes, I used to fight karate back in the day. How did you know? I also know Kenpo." The man said, keeping a stern face. Jones looked at him noticing the time. "I'll be back soon," Jones said. He had completed his mission of finding the fighter. Noticing that he was getting onlookers outside of the building Jones cut the conversation short. The old man walked forward with his grey hair as the rain and wind blew his way. His sandals hit the ground as he continued to carry the rug forward not knowing where he was headed. "To walk is just to walk, Jones. As long as I keep walking forward it doesn't matter where I fall." The man laughed as he wandered off. Jones walked along with the cement towards the other side. "Hey, old man! Where's the BART station?" The old man pointed to the left. "Back that way, kid." He smiled for the first time trying not to show Jones his emotions. Jones started to wander back as the smell of old dust and the sound of people echoed through the neighborhood. He walked back towards the BART feeling accomplished as he happily jumped through the streets excited about his find. Jones followed the man's direction as it led him around the corner directly back to the BART.

"Chemicals." A man said as Jones passed a building where a lady with blonde hair in a lab coat was walking. She smiled as Jones waved her down in the night. "Is this the way to the BART?" Jones asked. "My phone died." The lady smiled at him, "Sure it's right up those stairs around that corner." The lady pointed to them as she continued to quickly walk away. Jones walked towards BART wondering why the council of five and Mira was hunting the fighter. By now it didn't matter to him what they wanted as long as he decided they were the "good guys." After all, the CIA and gangsters could be considered good guys in a world of hidden

CHAPTER TWENTY-TWO – CLEANING AFTER NEPHARIUS

corruption between the watchers. Jones himself was already branded as a criminal who was illegally trying to smuggle artifacts across the ocean due to Nepharius' crafty wording and actions. Jones sighed as he walked up the stairs of the BART talking to himself. A man sat there by the side on the bench as he watched Jones. "Yeah, yeah, I got him. Don't worry, he's dead for sure." The man spoke as Jones overheard avoiding that man's world. "Not a place I want to be," Jones said to himself as he got on the BART riding his way home.

As the BART was going through the tunnel three men in purple shirts showed up. One of them put down their boombox and started dancing after saying the announcement. A brown box with a slit in it saying "donate five dollars here." was held as the three of them started doing flips and dislocating their joints to impress the crowd. Jones woke right up as he looked them in the eye. Instead, the man didn't ask Jones for money but rather gave him a fist bump telling him to rock on. As the three of them seemingly appeared while the BART was moving, they disappeared just as fast. The crowd clapped giving them well over seventy dollars in that short amount of time. One old lady scolded them saying for them to be careful of their joints as she also paid the man. Jones sat there contemplating the motions that had happened throughout the night as he rode home. "Sometimes it's not that I'm not interested in your world within our own. This world is similar, isn't it? That's why all superhero movies, Uncle Walt and the rest of the ideas always come back to us. Us here on earth." Jones didn't speak a word as the thoughts flowed through his head about how old items could be improved upon with a simple tweak. "Mira, why do you want the fighter?" Jones asked, sending out a signal through his mind trying to call out to her.

"The fighter may be a lead to the map relic. Nepharius isn't dead, remember? He's after the map for power to move anywhere he desires at the cost of another's life. He can't stop humanity anymore with the Idea Gem, he's graduated to murder." Jones sat there contemplating the matter as the BART slowed to its first stop. "Getting off, young man?" A gentleman said sitting next to Jones. "In a couple of stops." He said blandly as the world faded back onto normalcy after the men's performance. Jones smiled as he went back attempting to contact Mira again. This time he only heard the echoes of his voice. After a few minutes, Jones decided to take his headphones and place them in his ears to attempt to block out the noise. How music in an instance changed his entire world from a silent train ride to a situation. "Do I feel happy? Do I want to see the world as sad? What do I pick?" Jones said to himself as the second stop hit. "All of the songs with their titles. I can hear all of them needing me." Jones said to himself as he stared around the train. He could feel the watcher's eyes piercing on him unsure what would happen after his name was plastered all over the galactic news. Jones put on a heroic song as he sat back waiting for the journey of that night to end. "I think I get it now. Every time I go out with this intent I will be pulled into these mini-worlds if I accept someone's request. All I have to do is listen to their viewpoints." Jones' mind started to connect the dots. "Now arriving in Lafayette." The BART train conductors said over the microphone. "This is my stop," Jones said to the man sitting across from him as he got up and started walking towards home.

Jones stopped to see the old war veteran. He looked across the stairwell as the taxicab was written on the side. Feeling tired he walked to where the green painted car with yellow words stood. A man with long hair sat in the car smoking a cigarette. This time, Jones got in asking about the previous man who had driven him home before. There were no pretzels or water as the leather seats felt used up. "Hop in. I'll take you," The man said. "Where is the old war veteran I met," Jones said, asking the man as he paid. "I have an IOU for a little bit of money with him." The man looked back at Jones. "Oh yeah, yeah, he left recently. It's alright." He stuck his hand out the window while talking to Jones waving his hand with the wind. "It's a calm night tonight." The man replied, signaling his desire to be ignored. "Yeah," Jones said in the back looking out of the window.

CHAPTER TWENTY-TWO – CLEANING AFTER NEPHARIUS

He felt down that he was unable to pay back the man his ten dollars. "I guess I'll have to settle paying him back when I see him," Jones said, trying to cheer up as the two of them got close to where he lived. "That'll be fifteen dollars." The man said. Jones held out his hand and gave the money. "Thanks." He replied, feeling the awkward tension in the car. Jones who struggled reading situations before could see them so clearly. Each face he saw was as if he had lived in their shoes before he even fully got to hear their stories. All of the telltale signs stared him in the eyes as he moved towards the front door of his household.

"Here is my stronghold." Jones thought to himself considering it the home base that he hadn't worked for. "Falling right into my lap to do something worthwhile." He said to himself opening the door as he felt watched by Mira. "I'm home!" Jones said, seeing if anyone else had replied. There was no answer as he grabbed food from the fridge as usual. Jones wandered over to his room as he pulled out the math books, putting them on the table. Lily's notes in pictures had been pulled up on his phone as he started to copy each one down. "You know, you can go to school to study." Mira's voice ran through Jones' head. Everyone wanted to help, egging him on to succeed. "As you should." Mira continued. Jones laughed to himself in his room. "Don't should yourself." He said in broken sentences as his thoughts only went through the various scenarios. Jones finished copying down the notes as the DAW sat there staring at him. "Your creativity is what matters. Why not put some emotion into the galactic universe?" Mira encouraged. Jones started to write as he closed his eyes listening note by note. Imagining the feelings, he was putting out there in that moment. He pictured the fighter walking through the rain as he wrote in A-Minor hoping to capture the same feelings. The night fell as Jones finished up his song. He got on his bed for a peaceful night's rest. Tired of uncovering various operations for the council Jones prepared for the next day.

The clock struck 2:00 PM as he had overslept from the night before. He yawned, rubbing his head as he got up towards the computer. The song was still staring back at him as he hit export. "With this, it's done," Jones said to himself, happily feeling accomplished. There had been no reach out by the council as he went into the kitchen to grab breakfast. "How's school going?" his mother said first thing in the morning as Jones poured himself a bowl of cereal. "Well, it's going." He replied, reaching for the milk. "I'm going to stay a little extra to study," Jones said, considering the concepts that he had to learn. "That sounds great." She said happily, surprised that Jones was staying later for the course. He got fully dressed hopping in his car as people on his street noticed him. This time Jones accepted the watcher's invitation allowing himself to briefly hop into their viewpoints. To hop into their worlds as he saw them waving. With a slight wave back and no hands on the wheel, Jones kept on driving subconsciously making his turns towards school. "Slow down." One of them yelled as Jones zoned out while driving. He slowed down accordingly trying to respect the wishes and will of people as he read into them. Jones' control was increasing every time he used his power. His thoughts narrating as he thought back to the day, he trespassed on the hospital property. Jones recalled himself picking up his sweater that he had left near the generator. "Don't forget Jones. When your body is weary, these electrical lines exist to propel you forward." Mira said. "You know if people were able to walk in busy streets like San Francisco or New York and generate energy for things by simply walking over them, we could have a lot of input," Jones said Mira. "I'll consult the council of five someday." She said, smiling at the idea. Jones could feel the warmth of her energy as he walked up the stairway towards his class. "Well humanity needs it, I think..." he trailed off as he got distracted by people walking by as they happily conversed. Jones got to the door and opened it, taking his seat next to Lily. "Hey," he said. She looked at him and waved, "Heya stranger. Prepared for the exam?" She asked. "What exam?!" Jones said in return, worried for a moment. "It's in a couple of days. Haven't you studied at all?" She said, questioning him with concern in her voice. Jones recalled himself being distracted by making a song. "Uh not much, that's why I'm going to after-hours," Jones replied, trying to sway away Lily's suspicions. "After hours..." he trailed

CHAPTER TWENTY-TWO – CLEANING AFTER NEPHARIUS

off.

She looked at him. "Jones? You alright there, buddy?" She said, continuing to question him. "Yeah, yeah, I'm fine." He said thinking about the various responsibilities that he had to accomplish. She shrugged her shoulders and turned back to the board to copy down notes. This time Jones was also paying attention as the professor started his course. "Today's class, I want you to think of a project. A project you can use to write about math used in today's society." Jones raised his hand. "Can I write about multiple universes?" Jones said out loud holding no regard for the man at the front of the room. "Well… uh, it's an odd request, Jones. But I will approve it." The professor said as he tried to calm down the class from laughing. Jones smiled as Lily turned to him, "I hope you understand quantum theory." She said to him, rolling her eyes. Jones looked back at her and shrugged, "It's a school project. I mean it's not a big deal, right?" Jones said in return. "What are you going to do Lily?" He asked her as he sat down reading the board. "I'm going to the study lab to stay after class." She said, grabbing her bag. After an hour class finished. The entire class got up and ran out of the door headed to the study lab as Jones walked up the stairs towards the door. A few computers sat in front of them as he and Lily started discussing their notes. "Hey, can I join you?" A man said from behind them with black hair. "Tom." He blurted out not waiting for a reply from either of them.

Jones and Lily looked at one another dumbfounded. "Sure man. Take a seat. So, what do you do?" Jones said, hitting it off right away. Tom sat down. "Professional cyclist but I don't do it anymore," he said. "Oh, why?" Jones replied as the cyclist looked at the table."Didn't feel like it anymore. When you've done it over thousands of times it loses its luster." He said as he put his notes on the paper. "Teach me this." Tom pointed to the paper as formulas were written across the top of the page. Jones and Lily started teaching him the equations as he sat there listening. Jones wanted to ask the expert of cycling all about it for Nebulous magazine but wasn't sure the timing was right. Two engineers sat across from a different class writing their theories on the board as Jones put his head onto his hand twirling his pencil. "What are these for?" He asked them both. The woman turned towards him. "For uh… chemistry." She said precariously. "Oh, I don't understand this at all," Jones said, rubbing his head. "Jones…psst." He heard Mira's voice. "Jones, the council of five want to see you. It's important. The men got into contact with that fighter or so. He's said to be a lead into Bohemian grove. Know the place?" She questioned him as Jones looked at the board. "Bohemian grove?" Jones said back as Mira was now standing there writing the location on the board. "Yes. It's said to be where the fighter wants to go. He wants to confront an old group of arch…" she stopped for a moment, afraid to finish the word. "Archenemies? Archers? Arch builders? What is it, Mira?" Jones asked her curiously. "Archons." She said, Jones laughed, "I used to play video games with those things in them. Archons can't exist here" Jones said. "Where do you think these ideas come from, Jones?" Mira rebuttals. "Do you think humans pull them out of their ass? No, humans get them from scriptures. Real places, including yourself." She said angrily Jones sat there for a moment. "So, you want me to meet up with Mr. Fighter carrying a damn rug and checking out someplace called Bohemian grove where archons meet?" Jones said, questioning her. He was overheard by Tom. "Bohemian Grove is a place where billionaires discuss matters, right?" Tom asked Jones as he grabbed his attention. Mira had disappeared from writing on the board as Jones focused on the conversation at hand. "You know, it's kind of weird when you talk to yourself," Tom said to Jones as he sat there realizing he wasn't blending in.

"The spirit of music would be mad," Jones said thinking about the warnings he had continuously received. "Thinking out loud Tom," Jones said as Lily and Tom both looked over at him accepting his poor excuse. "I've got to go," Jones said as Mira reappeared at the door. This time she was no longer dressed in green and black as her red blouse hit the floor. "Figured I'd blend in!" She smiled, Jones smiled back. "No one can see you." He

CHAPTER TWENTY-TWO – CLEANING AFTER NEPHARIUS

said, scolding her. She laughed, "Not yet but one day these students will!" shouting as Jones moves forward towards his car. He stopped to take a drink of water thinking for a moment. "Why does the council of five need me to go with the fighter? I already found him for you." He asked her curiously and she smiled back. "Cause your key spark in the world might be there. A key to manifesting the future that doesn't exist. Nepharius said, remember? We are our own gods." She said smiling as Jones continuously walked towards the car. He didn't want to argue as he sighed "I better not fail my assignment because of this. I have an exam coming up, you know." Jones mentioned she laughed again. "As much as I like you, Jones. You have quite a sour side." She pouted as Jones opened the door to his car.

"Don't you have some work to do or Nepharius to catch?" Jones said, questioning Mira. "I'm supposed to be watching over you as well. The galactic government rules, you know?" She laughed again. "Aside from that, what would I do if one of the last arbiters disappeared again?" Jones blinked his eyes and Mira was gone. As he drove down the road towards his house he thought of where to find the fighter. Surely the council of five had the tools to find this watcher. Jones knew he would have to consult with them to understand how to find the man in Oakland. "I'm home," Jones said, announcing himself as he arrived. No answer was received as he walked through the house. Jones sat down at the table where food was already ready. "We've been waiting for you." One of the members said ominously as they sat down in Jones's house. "I'm from the council of five. The two of us. You can call me Hestia and my friend here is Yule." The man sat oddly with long hair almost down to his waist side as a belt with a little C written off to the side stuck out. Jones stood still for a moment, motionless as the man pulled out a map. "Your fighter is here. When you're done wondering how we got in and if anyone can see us you can take the map from me." He said pointing to a spot in the road. "Lucky for you we have contacted the fighter. Unlucky for him, he's still talking to himself on the streets. Some of these damn watchers refuse or just don't know how to blend in" Yule sat there silently nodding as Hestia kept talking. "I tell you,

Yule. Some people have a real nerve going on about them. These damn archons hiding out in Bohemian Grove" Jones sat there for a moment, "I have no idea where I come in, in all of this but I'll go." Hestia smiled, "Good, 'cause you're still a criminal anyway until you finish this mission." Jones tried to shrug it off as he went over to his refrigerator to grab a bite of food. "Yeah well, Nepharius fooled a lot of us," Jones said quietly as he seemed unthreatened by the council's presence. "Look, I want this done by this week Jones. These guys are meeting in their monthly place and we need intel to know what they are planning.

Make sure the fighter keeps himself in line. That old guy doesn't listen well, it's why he's always swearing at people on the streets. You know, the mind thing and all…" Hestia trailed off as Yule finished. "Jones, be careful. Don't let them see you and don't let the fighter light anything. It's a damn forest you see? We don't want to have to call the rain runners." Jones questioned, "Rain runners?" He wondered. Jones had heard of these people before. The people who had prayed to the clouds and ran with them to make the rain pour. "Yeah, these people exist. You've seen one once." Yule said. "Be quiet Hestia. He already knows we've been watching him for a long time, say nothing else." "Hey". His mother said from behind him. "Looking at maps to travel?" Jones replied quickly, "Yeah, got an invite to a friend's place. Wanted to see how far it was because my app is down. I'm done with it though." He said rolling up the map and putting it away under the drawer. "Anyway, my day was good. I already ate." Jones said trying to stop any suspicion of his mother. "Okay. If you need anything let me know." She said walking to the other side of the room to complete more office work. Jones sighed as he went into his room waiting for the time to pass by. As night fell it would be his task to go and find the fighter and take him to the bohemian grove. "How do I get a man who talks to himself to cooperate with anything?" Jones ridiculed the man without realizing he was ridiculing himself. "Mira, what do you think?" Jones said quietly, trying to call upon her.

CHAPTER TWENTY-TWO – CLEANING AFTER NEPHARIUS

"I don't. I do." Mira said in a few short words as Jones looked at a picture of Einstein hanging over his head next to the black and gray Jeep. "I do huh," Jones repeated back to himself as he sat there. "I think I have an idea." He said smiling to himself before falling asleep from the exhaustion of schoolwork. A few hours later Jones woke up as the clock struck 7:00 PM. Mira was sitting in Jones' computer chair listening on his headphones to the music he had created. "This is pretty good Jones." She encouraged as she continued to move her head to the music. "What are you doing in my room?" Jones questioned her as she sat there listening in. "Protecting you. What are you doing in your room? Why aren't you finding the fighter again? The council pointed to where he was." She said as Jones shook his head. "This is as bad as Nepharius isn't it? If I go, I'm going to get roped into something I don't even want to be a part of. I'm going to end up the same way Nepharius does, won't I?" Jones complained as he put on his shoes. "You already agreed to track the fighter and take this mission with the watcher," Mira said sternly for the first time since Jones and her spoke. Jones was taken back by Mira's voice. "Yes, I did. By some council who has apparently been watching me all this time. Some council that I don't even know about! You want me to go out of the blue and take down some archon grouping?" Jones sighed. "I just dealt with Nepharius roping me into this whole damn world of everyone and now this?" He threw his hands up walking towards the computer chair. "Give me those headphones back. I need it." Jones said, taking it from Mira as she sat back quietly watching. Mira patted Jones on the back. "This is to clear your name, Jones. I requested that the council reach out to you. They offered me this mission but since you stopped the pirate king, I figured it's a good way to clear your name." Mira sighed. "You know you're really ungrateful." She said, annoyed by Jones. "If I wasn't at work, I wouldn't even talk to you!" Mira lashed out as she disappeared from Jones's view. Jones put away the headphones properly as he put on the rest of his clothing and the brown felt hat reaching for the doorknob.

"If it weren't for me. You wouldn't even have your own imagination, Mira."

Jones said, unmoved by Mira's complaints towards Jones' treatment of her. Mira remained silent, still upset as Jones walked out the door. His car sat shining in the night as the moonstruck near the center of the car. The night sky was clear as the stars could be seen from afar. "Have to remember that we're all stardust. Keep remembering it, Jones. We're all the damn same". He said to himself as he started to drive the car into Oakland. This time rather than using BART to pick up the man, a car would be much easier. Jones was in no mood to chase a man who doesn't cooperate. The car turned down the same street where the red couch lies on the sidewalk. The old man was nowhere to be found although there were traces of him having been there by the Chinese rug laid out on the sidewalk. "Hey! Fighter!" Jones called out to the man as few people were around. "Fighter, are you out here?" Jones called again as he started to walk down the street. "All of these people are feeling unloved and not having a path. That's why they are out here." Jones said to himself as a man with a tent stared at him while sleeping away the day. "Fighter!" Jones called out again as he walked further towards graffiti painted across a wall showing sun, moon stars, and the earth. "World peace as one." Had been written against the wall as a presentation of togetherness was painted. "Fighter!" Jones yelled out loudly this time attracting attention to himself. People watched Jones as a man walked towards him. "There you are." The fighter opened his eyes, staring at Jones with his best up one.

"Hey, what do you want from me, kid?" The fighter said as he rang out his long white beard. "The Bohemian grove or something like that," Jones said to the fighter as his eyes seemed surprised for a moment. "Bohemian grove huh? Yeah, I can show you where that is. I don't know what you'll find there other than a bunch of cracked-out people in a forest." The fighter said in a warning tone. "Heard archons were meeting around there?" Jones said to the fighter. The fighter laughed, "Whatever drugs you're on I want them. Okay, I'll humor you and take you to that damn park. Got a car? Cause I sure as hell don't." The fighter laughed as he now stood in striking distance of Jones. Jones, feeling no threat from the man's energy nodded

CHAPTER TWENTY-TWO – CLEANING AFTER NEPHARIUS

as he started walking back to where he parked the car. "My rug better be dry by the time we get back." The old fighter spoke his mind looking at Jones as he got in the car. "Do you smoke?" He said, reaching for a lighter in his pocket. "No, I don't," Jones replied as the man pulled out a lighter. "Not in my car anyway." Jones finished his statement, hoping the fighter would catch on. The fighter laughed, putting the cigarette in his ear. "Alright Jones, not until we get there." The fighter started as the night went on. "So, what got you into this position anyway? Without money and living this way?" Jones asked the fighter. The fighter laughed, "What does it matter to you?" He said curiously, trying to understand Jones' motive. "Nothing really old guy, trying to simply understand how experts go broke or get to where they are really," Jones said, speaking his mind. "Well, it ain't nothing." The fighter replied. "My wife and I didn't get along and when I couldn't walk well anymore, I was kicked to the curb from my job. When you have no friends left and can't fend for yourself, that's it around here, that's when I hit rock bottom." The fighter explained. Jones listened closely. "How far is the drive to this place anyway?" Jones asked the fighter. "Bohemian Grove's pretty far from here. I reckon it'll be a while". He said, seemingly happy he was getting a ride.

"Listen, why that rug?" Jones asked. "Meditation to speak to the galaxy, also my last keepsake." The fighter said. "You know they are my only friends around here. At least the guys at bar A2 talk to me." He sighed. "Guess when you have a cut in your eye people view you differently. I'd rather look like I'm talking to society than blend in with damn humanity. Wish I could just escape here, build my house in the forest on some land or some shit". The fighter tensed up reaching for his cigarette. Jones put on some light music to try to soothe the fighter's soul. As Jones turned on the car radio it started to play country music. The old fighter sang along to the words as the two continued their drive. The fighter put away his cigarette remembering Jones' words. After a few hours of driving straight, the fighter pointed to a corner and first wedge.

"There. Supposedly the meetings are supposed to be tonight." The fighter said. "What meeting?" Jones replied curiously. "I don't know, some people meet up and discuss weird things. Heard some pretty cool and also messed up shit coming from around here." Jones drove the car further down the road seeing a small trail. "That's it?" Jones asked the fighter. He smiled back. "Yeah, that's it." Jones parked the car off to the side as the two of them got out of the car and started walking. The forest was flourishing, deep with the green trees as the fighter took a cigarette out from his ear. "Give me a light, why don't you." The fighter said. Jones reached over and helped the man cover up the cigarette as it lit up his hand. "Think we'll need to fight?" Jones asked, questioning the fighter. "Unless you believe archons are real or some shit, I don't think so." The fighter replied. Jones prepared himself as the two got closer, noises started to travel in the background. Jones blinked his eyes. Yule reached out echoing through his mind "Archons." Jones and the fighter got beside the trail hiding in the bushes as one of the Archons discussed their plan. "No, you don't understand. These humans will never expect it." One of them discussed as the other scratched his head holding a piece of paper. The candles were lit brightly as bouquets of food were served to them in the middle of the circle. One of the Archons reached for a duck pâté as he munched down on the cracker. "Don't you see it? If we put gold here in the business and crash the market, the market will crumble. All it will take is something to keep people's attention away from our task at hand." The Archon turned to the other as the party went forward. "Yeah, that sounds good. Let's sway them with books, gold, and newer technology." The two of them laughed, snacking as Jones looked into the circle unable to believe what he was seeing.

"So, the Archons really exist?" Jones said to himself as the fighter took the cigarette out of his ear, lighting it with the lighter. "Yeah, these damn sons of bitches been planning things like this from the beginning. Even Mon-san has been showing up around here." Jones turned to the fighter questioning him as he whispered, "Mon-san? Who's that gonna be?" He

CHAPTER TWENTY-TWO – CLEANING AFTER NEPHARIUS

looked at the fighter's cigarette as the two of them stayed crouched within the bushes. "Sh, they'll hear you." The fighter said as Jones blinked again. A group meeting of private corporations had met there to discuss matters of the world. Jones was standing right in the middle of it not realizing the two people were joking about humanity. "Hey, fighter, I think that's all we needed. The place you know?" He said feeling an ominous force shivering as the wind blew forward through the forest telling Jones to leave the space. "Yeah, yeah. Let's stay a bit longer." The fighter complained of feeling comfortable about the whole situation. Jones walked backward as the orange light illuminated through the forest. Dirt kicked up towards Jones as he coughed a couple of times. "What was that?" One of the archons said from afar."Shit, I thought you said you didn't believe in archons!". Jones said as he grabbed the fighter's arm. The fighter turned to run with Jones "They heard you dammit Jones." He scolded as the two of them started running away.

The fighter dropped his cigarette in the dry grass as the two of them ran as fast as they could through the trail back towards Jones' car. "Get in before the whole group comes!" Jones said as the two of them reached the car. In the distance, a group of people starts looking around as the cigarette slowly burns in the ground. "Shit you didn't put out your cigarette, did you?" Jones said, questioning the fighter. "Who gives a fuck?" The fighter said in rebuttal. "Take me home, this ain't fun anymore." Jones looked out in the distance, "I'm sure the group will catch it." He said to himself as the two of them leaned over. "I'm going to clear our footsteps," Jones said, going over to where the two of them had run. He started kicking up dust and stepping left to right with the shoes. Jones then got in the car in a rush and started driving away. "Yule! Yule!" Jones cried out, "Okay, you win. The archons really exist. What's our next plan?" Jones said, trying to contact him. No one answered as Jones started to take the complaining man back towards where he found him. "Kid, drop me off and never contact me again." The fighter was irritated at the whole scenario. Jones nodded his head as the two had driven through the night, almost arriving back home in the morning. Jones quickly dropped off the fighter and headed straight home. As he walked through the door his mother slept on the couch watching T.V. Jones snuck into his room to sleep until next midafternoon as he had to get to school. "What a weird night." He said to himself in an attempt to calm down.

Chapter Twenty-Three – Archonic Disaster

The next morning, Jones woke up staring at the ceiling. His eyes were heavy and his clothes smelled like pine from the forest he had visited last night. "Good morning." He said, trying to see if anyone was awake yet. His mother had gone to bed. Suddenly, a T.V. the report began. "A weird stakeout ends in disaster." The reporter said, "A group of mysterious people met at "Bohemian Grove" where many of the people could not get outside of the house as the fire burned. Traces of the fire started by a possible cigarette that had been dropped potentially by one of the gatherers. The people burned in the fire have been unidentified. However, one of the people was an unfortunate billionaire who owned three corporations." Jones stood there taking a moment to note the irony of the phrase unfortunate opportunity. Jones watched the T.V. as he blinked again changing the program, "In galactic news today, archons were found to be plotting to take over in the forest. A police investigation found that many archons had been gathering there for years. Some remains were found as others seem to have gotten away thanks to two brave soldiers who accidentally attacked the archons base and damage had been dealt to their organization." Jones couldn't believe what he was hearing on the news as he stood there in shock. "This is all my fault…" he said to himself with his hands in his head. "No, no. I am not a killer." He repeated picking himself up. Jones quickly shut off the T.V. Before any of his family woke up.

"That damn fighter almost got us in trouble". Jones projected up through the galaxy as Mira picked up the signal. "Jones, it's okay." She said, trying to comfort him. "You did a good thing Jones." Mira floated over to him, grabbing his face. "Back away Mira. I don't need your counseling. Why do you try?" Jones questioned her as she stood there. "It's time you tell me, you've been helping me all of this time without telling me anything." He said angrily as she sat down on a seat silently mustering up the courage. "I'm the other side of you Jones." She said, "The council of five. We are all part of you. Manifestations of the now that are missing. No one can see or hear us but you. You have a special capability; you can bring us into your reality." Mira stopped as Yule stood beside her. "Yes Jones, we're here for you." He said as the clock struck 9:00 AM. "Stop it! Get out of here!" Jones said back wanting to escape from them. He grabbed his backpack and went out to the car to drive back off to school. "Don't try to run from us, yourself, and what you were brought here to do," Yule said. "If those damned cigarettes had a clipper or small filter on the end of them to properly put them out this wouldn't have happened!" Jones replied.

Yule replied quickly, "We'll think of something to prevent this in the future for the careless. We didn't think such an old fighter would not pay attention. He's a grade-A well-known black belt and should know better." Yule scolded as Jones parked, sitting looking down at his hands. "This is going to be branded as a murderer in my world and a hero in the next." He said as he put his hands in his head. "All I can do now is wait and pretend this never happened. I never went there." He said to himself as he got out of the car walking towards class. One of the students looked at him as he talked to himself. "What?" He said, trying to alleviate all suspicions. "Are you practicing for drama or something?" The person said as he walked by. "Yeah, I have a few classes." Jones lied as he walked further towards his classroom where Lily stood. "Hey, Jones!" She waved to him completely clueless about what had happened previously. "Hey, Lily…" Jones said, trying to hide his emotions and mood. "How's the project going?" She said smiling. "Not so great. I couldn't think of anything last night. I had

CHAPTER TWENTY-THREE – ARCHONIC DISASTER

trouble writing about the theories of traveling through different plains of the universe." he said. She laughed, "You picked a really hard topic. Tried Wikipedia or YouTube?" She continued not letting Jones finish, "You know we have this thing called the Internet." She joked around as the professor came up.

"Morning class." He said as he opened the door, cutting off their conversation. Jones waved back, "Good morning sir." The professor looked at Jones curiously, "You're early today." He said it as if Jones was hardly ever on time. "Yeah. I know." He said quietly, taking his seat next to Lily. Jones kept running the situation through his mind over and over. "I thought these were insanely smart people. They didn't even fireproof their damn place in the forest. With all of that money, you'd damn well think…" Jones trailed off in his mind trying to calm himself. "It wasn't me directly, it wasn't even me at all, so it doesn't matter. That fighter has nothing to lose." Jones thought to himself as the professor started to write the formulas on the board. He sat there for a moment as Jones relaxed his shoulders. "No one knows. It's fine." Lily could see the worry in Jones' eyes as he contemplated the news that was spread. After all, Nepharius is still out there ready to attack humanity in other ways. Jones focused on the board and copied the notes. This time they were becoming clearer as he started to recognize the patterns in things again. "I can see it. Multiple connections that make sense. Jones took them and started jotting them down as math came easily to him. Jones took notes to prepare for his essay on travel through the universe."Jones are you there?" Yule reached out to Jones as he continued to try to pay attention to class. "Go away, Yule. I have to pass this." Jones said, trying to focus on the board. "You can write about interstellar space travel later. I have something important to tell you at this moment." Jones tried waving away Yules' echoing voice in his head. Unable to get Yule's voice out of his head Jones gave in.

"What is it?" Jones said with an irritated response. "Well, you know how watchers have no place to go. Why are we helping them right?" Yule said.

"No idea, though they simply needed a place because they had nowhere to go in the society," Jones replied, not caring about Yule's reasoning. "Well, Nepharius is after that map because he wants to stunt society's growth. He has always believed that power over the people and their ideas will keep society in check," Yule said. "We need the watcher's strength against Nepharius's crew. See, by governing the watchers who have nothing and helping them out we can put them to work in our society. Ours here at— "

Jones cut him off. "Yours there at what? The CIA who wants to lock us all away because we're dirty criminals right?" Jones rebuttal angrily. Yule took a breath. "Well, no… that's kind of how it fell into place. It wasn't our intention." Yule quieted down not knowing how to continue. "Yeah, well you did, intentions or not. It's messed up Yule. You should dismantle it after you're done with Nepharius. Give these people a real chance at life rather than be slaves to your sickened society. Born just to die with the illusion of choice. Born just to copy the same ideas already out there rather than looking at how to improve. All for what? Your control over society? You're no better than the very man you're trying to stop." Jones stopped before he continued sensing Yule's distaste for the backlash he was getting. "Fine, Jones. Next time there's an issue, talk to Mira. Clearly, your reserves with me are strong." Yule said, disappearing. "That's not what I…" Jones said, trying to reassess what he had said. "I'll focus on class…" Jones said quietly to himself as he copied down more of the theories on the board. "In times of humanities in need we tend to overlook parallelisms." Jones started to write. "Sometimes when walking down the street we take improper glances at objects or movements. This in turn sparks another idea. Where do ideas come from? Well, as explained previously these ideas come from mixing two versions of something. In theory, we get these ideas from different worlds. Worlds we are temporarily seeing through traveling of the mind. These travels however do not create physicality's in our actual world. Unless… we can touch those in what we see imaging and recreate it in the world of our own. By two separate plains aligning to the same…" Jones stopped writing as Lily looked over at his essay.

CHAPTER TWENTY-THREE – ARCHONIC DISASTER

"Woah dude, did you smoke some hardcore weed or something? I don't even follow." She laughed looking at Jones. "Well, those who are crazy enough to think big and want to change the world all at once usually do…" Jones said in return trying to save himself from getting laughed at. He knew based on what the other watchers had said that Jones was better off not trying to explain to Lily where these ideas came from. "Watchers, huh?" Jones said as he started to think about it. Lily poked him on the shoulder bringing him back to the classroom. "Hey, want to study again before our next exam? You left in a rush last time without a word. Like, kind of weird." Lily threw in her words to try to cheer up the situation. Jones's facial expressions were clear that he was still troubled in his head from incidents that she had no clue about. To Lily this didn't matter, she liked Jones as a person and supported his demeanor. "You know, you're a little weird Jones. A good friend but a little weird. Let's study." She encouraged Jones to continue forward with his essay and mathematics course. The clock at the top hit 3:00 PM as the class got up. "Don't forget our exam. First, one might be taken home due to circumstances but don't hold your breath." The professor said as the class smiled and then sighed in disappointment. "Aww, sir! Come on!" A few students said as the whole class went out of the door. "So, Lily. What's new?" Jones said, asking her as the two walked together.

"Well…I've been working around the mall selling clothing and such. It hasn't been much but…" she trailed off looking at the sky. "Hey, do you daydream Jones?" She asked him as the two of them walked. "Yeah, all the time," Jones said, surprised by her question. "Sometimes when I'm listening to music I feel as if I'm transported to that moment in time." Jones smiled, "If it's good." Lily turned to Jones and looked at him wondering what was on his mind. "What's your peace?" She asked him. "Where's this coming from all of a sudden?" Jones asked back, not understanding Lily's point of view. "I guess… have you ever seen that computer default background that comes with it?" Jones said. "The flowers in the background, the little blue sky, and hills you can run across? Or the beach and water with so little going on?" Jones continued to talk about his place as Lily chimed in, "Yeah! It has a red brick house in the background, a windmill, and maybe some feed outside. There's no animals or pets." Lily added, "Like a connected mind portal?" Jones laughed, "Now you're getting it. With the right music, I feel I can always put my mind there. Maybe the watchers who are on one of the world's biggest commodities, drugs, go there sometimes when they feel lost. So, lost they don't feel like coming back." Jones said with misfortune and sadness in his voice. "One life can change so many; one life can change none." You know most of these statements are said by big people, but some of them are said by the people with nothing. I believe, perhaps with guidance, that most people who are there can wake up." Jones continued, "Maybe their brilliance reflects what these people wanted to become. What these people ramble about are things they wish to have or become." Lily replied deep in thought based on Jones' words. "That's why none of them recognize where or why they are there huh?"

Jones said in return. "Yes, those poor souls only have an escape to turn to because these souls envisioned something more. Or fell out of love with something that drove them. So, they get stuck in their past." Lily continued, "Jones, stay in your own place here. Don't get stuck in that world. You may never return." She sighed, "Stay here. Stay with yourself and know you're able to inspire many. Even if you don't know it yet!" Lily said worked up by the conversation the two of them had. "Hey, you hardly even know me and you're on about treating myself better?" Jones shook his head, "Well, thanks for caring. I suppose…" he trailed off looking at the sky as the two of them continued to walk towards the steps next to the study hall. This time the place was virtually empty except for a few people. "Oh yeah! The arbiter books!" Jones said to himself, snapping his finger in his ear. "What are you doing?" Lily asked Jones in confusion. "Well, there was this musician who taught me how he remembers stuff.

He does it by snapping his fingers Every time he says something." Lily looked at Jones and laughed, "Alright. This is kind of ridiculous, but I'm

CHAPTER TWENTY-THREE – ARCHONIC DISASTER

starting to understand." The two of them sat down at the table and started going over the notes as Lily taught Jones the concepts he had missed. "It makes sense now," Jones said as he happily folded up his paper and put it in his bag. Lily smiled as her phone hit 6:00 PM. "Hey, I have to head out." Lily smiled as she ran towards the door with her books in her bag. Jones went outside after her, but Lily had already left. Jones sat there wondering for a moment if she would be okay driving home. He put on his backpack and walked towards his silver Jetta. Jones put on relaxing music and thought about the arbiters as he drove towards home. "I need to read up more on myself to understand what an arbiter is," Jones said as he went home. As Jones got into his car he prepared to go straight to his room. Jones floored his car as he got close to his room. There was the book of arbiters sitting in blue and black. Jones opened up to read it further.

"Arbiters exist to blend in the world as you already know between time continuums. Sometimes seen as best friends they will latch onto purpose... found a baby one kinda close. Been monitoring it for weeks. Will see what else arbiters can do - Nepharius - " Jones continued to read as he highlighted different words with his fingers. Patterns upon patterns appearing in front of the text. Slow, feeling fast like the tree's in the wind. "Somewhere arbiters are continuously moving even if they are already dead. With the inability to truly die they need to write themselves out of existence as they wrote themselves into existence. Arbiters are meant to complete the tasks given to them. During these times an Arbiter's speed is immeasurable at getting the task done. An arbiter may become blurry to one's view while traveling from one conscious stream to another." Jones kept on reading trying to decipher the words as he sat thinking about himself. "All this time...Nepharius took care of me but misused me for my power." Jones couldn't help the realization. He closed the book of arbiters as the world spun. "Now I understand. Now I get why travel is so possible between..." Jones stopped in mid-sentence as he felt himself rewriting the world in his mind. "I have to get control over myself," Jones said as he fought with the mind state of reality. Fast seemed slow, skipping seemed easy and the mind that called upon what it wanted for what it wanted. "Get back to the natural state, where everything's in balance," Mira said to Jones as she appeared in front of him in red. "Come on." She said, pulling on him, waking him up. Jones realized that he was on his bed as one of his legs was tugging on the chair. "So dizzy," Jones said as he got up for a drink. As Jones recovered, he looked around him. "The arbiter I was meant to be?" He said to himself as he got down on his bed. "Guess I'll need to go into that place," Jones said to himself. He closed the book and headed down to the library to return it.

"I'll rewrite my own history. My own experience as an arbiter." Jones said to himself as he put a pen down to finish the words he started. "A universe on a parallel plain can be accessed through slowing down motion to speeding uptime. Therefore, when an atom splits, time splits along with it. The atom opens up three more holes to allow one to jump into many plains at once. "This will be sure to get me an A," Jones said to himself as he smiled, shutting down the computer. "Every time something bad happens. I always try to think in a positive light. Even if my own mind is creating the disaster in the world." Jones said to himself trying to reason with himself. He wanted to make sure that his mind didn't affect the world as much as he thought it was. Jones got on the internet and started to look at pictures of cute cats and dogs as he understood why humanity looked for these escapes. "This is life for one's mind, one's mind is one's temple," Jones said to himself keeping a distance from those he loved. "Yet, this is no way to live. Facing the hard realities and tackling them rather than sugar-coating myself with dogs and cats isn't going to overcome the problems we face today. These are hard problems that stagnate society." Jones continued, "If we are slowly compounding this information over time in the same arenas, eventually someone will hit the right pathway. Like if all these plains split evenly there must be a pathway created through my mind for my happiness." Jones sighed as his mind raced. Mira and Yule along with Bey among others raced through Jones' mind. "All of these people helped

CHAPTER TWENTY-THREE – ARCHONIC DISASTER

me get to where I am today. Even Nepharius who is still on the run helped me shape this society around me." Jones thought to himself as he loaded up the DAW and started to make a song. "These are the feelings I'm going to put into my song. This is how I will reach people timelessly." Jones laughed to himself as he started to click place by place. "Fear is the only problem in society that will stop many from progressing. Blind fear, not cautious fear." Jones thought to himself as he played the first keys to the song. Eventually, after a few hours of writing it into his computer, the song was ready to go. The sound had reached out with timeless feelings as the galactic conglomerate of people heard it. The music radiated through the space of the galaxy as each face that passed Jones smiled. "A song that will make people smile." Jones thought to himself as it played. The spirit of music sent Jones a text message. "Hope you're well. Busy watching over the earth but that tone wave is so relaxing! With love, the Spirit Of Music."

Jones smiled at the text message, "So unconditional love is to love without any attachments. This must be why parents end up loving their children in such a way." Jones started connecting sayings with feelings as the song echoed throughout the room. Jones laid on his bed thinking about the Bohemian Grove fire as he kept swimming forward in blackness as if he was trying to keep his head above water. The beach stuck out to Jones as he swam towards it, not seeming to get any closer to land than where Jones first started swimming. "I have to get to land," Jones said to himself in his sleep as he twisted and turned in his sheets. Putting on some soft music. Jones hoped to drown out the sound and change the scenery of his world. The one place where he felt most comfortable, he had hoped to dream up again. Jones felt as if he had finally been able to sleep for the first time in weeks. The next day Jones woke up hitting the alarm clock. This time he got up on time ready to take the first exam of the class day. A text from Lily had already called out to Jones asking him where he had been as he sat there rubbing his eyes. "Oh, I slept in. On my way." Jones texted Lily quickly realizing he was late for his exam. "Shit. I even got up early today! Damn!" Jones said as he scolded himself for not being at school on time.

Jones proceeded to throw on his black T-shirt with jeans and head for the door. "Are you hungry?" His mom shouted as she tried to get Jone's attempt in his rush to leave. Jones replied, "No Mom, thanks!" He said as he headed for the door. "Oh, Doctor K. called to thank you for being a good patient. He's retired now so if you need someone to talk to it will be Orin!" Jones' mom shouted, Jones retorted "Okay!", slamming the door behind him. He got into his car and turned the volume all the way up as he sped off towards his school. Trying to focus on the road he paid no attention to the watchers who were moving to try to slow Jones down to normal speeds. "C'mon garbage man I don't have time!" Jones said to himself as the truck slowly went forward from being out in front of him. He moved around the garbage truck as it made its turn to try to turn onto the freeway as an older gentleman with a mustache slowly pushed his cart across the walkway. Jones was losing his patience as he got onto the freeway. "Stop forcing me to obey the speeding laws. I'm late!" Jones said towards the galactic universe as he sped towards the school. He was already warned not to move people against their will as he sat there worried about the exam. Although Jones was tempted, he did not move people out of his way as he had done previously. Jones went into the gate with his Jetta and parked in the fenced-up parking lot as cement piled high next to the spots. Jones got out of his car and ran as fast as he could towards the door where the professor started handing out the exams. "I'm here, sir! Sorry, I'm late." Jones said as the professor handed out the tests to the classroom. "This is our only in-class essay. The rest will be "take-home" essays. You're very lucky I'm patient with you." The professor said Jones sighed in relief. "Thanks." He replied, taking a seat next to Lily. Lily jokingly covered up her test, "Hey, no cheating!" she said. Jones smiled back, "Well sorry!" He replied, rolling his eyes. "Kidding, glad you made it on time!" She said smiling. "Here's a sharpened pencil, we can't have our own." Lily handed him the pencil. Jones blinked as if he caught a glimpse of it with a sensor on the pencil. "This is how you know they are official for the class," Lily

CHAPTER TWENTY-THREE – ARCHONIC DISASTER

said. Jones shook his head as he noticed the pencil with green tape on it. His mind drifted again as he prepared for the exam.

"Alright!" Jones said as he started doing the test. "While the world is out here in turmoil. I'll keep pushing forward. All of these people are pushing forward so I should too." Jones kept telling himself as he continued to do his best towards the test. "Like a cog in a machine of ever turning events. I'm here to document. My arbiter description does say so." Jones thought further as he recalled the math formulas that Lily had taught him. Jones continuously marked down most of the right bubbles as he turned in his test. "Sweet all done," Jones said, handing over the paper to the professor as the professor smiled back. "Good job, now I'm sure you have other things to do." The professor said to Jones. "Yeah. I suppose so." Jones said back as he left the classroom and headed towards his car. He pulled up the essay on his phone and started writing more. "Once you have embodied multiple plains and exhausted your body's outer elements the inner mind will take over. As your senses become strengthened so does your ability to sense the energy around you. Your gut feeling for survival will also increase allowing you to communicate with animals, run faster than you ever have before, and increase movements. Be wary. If you go in too deep, you will crash and it will be hard to come out of this state of mind." Jones looked up from his phone as multiple students walked outside to their cars. He decided it would be better if he left before the crowd came. Jones put his music up all the way and headed out towards fast food. "I'll have one bucket of chicken," Jones said to the man in the window. As soon as he saw Jones, he went into hyper motion moving about the place to make the chicken in an above-average time. Jones sat there and watched as this became normalized for him. "Thanks," Jones said as the man nodded watching Jones move his car into the parking lot. "Well, alright," Jones said to himself as he received a text. "Hey, it was hard in there but I'm just out. It's good to be out." Ike had sent him a text message as Jones sat there happy to hear that his friend wasn't continuously held captive by the CIA.

"I'm stuck on these pills for a while though." Ike texted continuing the conversation. "My mom has me basically on a no see- anyone policy though. Let's make music soon." Jones replied to the text. "Yeah man, glad you're out. No more crazy talk. If ever again, keep it secret." Jones wanted to keep his friends away from the watcher's world as he sent the text to Ike hoping it would reset the damage he had already done. "Yeah, it's been good for me. I'm no longer eating and smoking a lot." Ike texted again, "My mom's been pretty happy about it and we're getting along too." He continued. "Man, they must've really done some correctional stuff wherever you went," Jones replied. Sending a laughing face as Ike texted back, "Oops." With a monkey face. "Let's finish the album soon," Ike said, ending the conversation as Jones looked out at the road. "Yeah. We will." Jones texted back putting away his phone as he started driving back towards his home eating the last few pieces of chicken. "Hey, this is your dad," Jones's dad called. "I did a little research on the guy you were talking about, Nepharius you called him right? He'd been dishonorably discharged from the military. The man is wanted and has a whole bunch of stuff going around him. I advise you to stay away, you won't be able to come back here for a while until you're settled. See you soon, love dad."

Jones' voicemail rang through his phone as he shivered at the idea of Nepharius coming after him physically. Jones knew that he had spied out where he lived so it didn't matter if he was in Hawaii or California. Although he didn't feel particularly threatened by Nepharius's crew or idealisms, he did fear for his family at the thought of what Nepharius might be able to do if the two of them met face to face again. After all, he was almost able to best Jones in the battle of wits between him, the CIA, and all of the mythical towns Nepharius had already robbed. "Okay dad, I understand." Jones said to himself, "Not until this is completely over will I go back there." Jones started driving home, Mira echoed through his head. "Okay listen, I know the last mission didn't go over as we thought, the archons did burn up but are now on our tracks. On top of this, there are other watchers in need. You must talk to Yule soon Jones. We need you."

CHAPTER TWENTY-THREE – ARCHONIC DISASTER

Mira said, trying to coax Jones into talking to headquarters again. "I'm not so sure I'd like to talk to Yule again after what he said," Jones said in rebuttal. "I'll buy you food!" Mira offered. "How are you going to do that? I haven't brought you into this world yet." Jones said back as he drove his car down the highway. "I'll get one of your friends to do it. All I have to do is reach out to them, right?" Mira laughed as she sent a text through Jones' phone to one of his friends. As if Mira already knew which friend of Jones was hungry, he replied right away.

"Yo! Massi here, what's up Jones?" Jones replied to the text. "Oh, hey Massi, I heard you had food," Jones said Massi replied quickly, "Food and Booze! I'm ready to come over whenever" Mira smiled, "Have fun, Jones." She said as Jones put his phone in the side of the car upset that Mira had essentially been abusing his privacy. However, Jones ended up smiling. He texted Massi. "Yeah man, that sounds great. Come on over." Jones said as he got home. Massi appeared in his car a few minutes later blasting grime music out of his car. "Hey! Good to see you, man. You kind of, like, disappeared on me for a bit there. How have you been?" Massi said as Jones went up to give him a pat on the back. "I've been good, been good. I've been recovering really well. You said you wanted to make a song, right?" Jones said in return as Massi stood there for a moment. "Hell yeah, I do! it's the only thing keeping me sane in these hard times. Load up the DAW and I'll get out a drink or two." Massi said as he pulled out a bottle of Vodka. "Man don't bring up all the weird old places and stuff again. Saying look at these buildings with triangles on top of them and all of that. You were kind of freaking me out, man." Massi said. "Yeah well, good to keep an open mind, right? I won't though." Jones replied laughing it out not wanting Massi to know about the world of the watchers. "Well anyway, pizza and booze always hit the stomach," Jones said as the two of them hopped on the computer and started to make a grime track. "I've been out on the streets lately. Some of these cats say they've really been listening." Massi said. Jones looked at him awkwardly. "Listening to what though?" He replied wondering what Massi was up to.

"Yeah, listening to songs. You know, the words and all. Taking these singers to heart. It's weird but I guess it's not weird having an idol and all that. You know we should fly to China and be famous. Jones, that's what we should do. The world is so vast, what are we doing here just sitting around and stuff?" Massi laughed as Jones sat there listening to him ramble. There was a comforting part about Massi beyond his rough edges. As Jones recalled Toby and the others who had been locked away, he had grown used to rambling. The crazy and random no longer felt crazy and random. Jones felt as if he was outside fate itself, not letting it catch up to his every move. "Yeah, well let's get into it!" Jones said as the two of them started to make the song based on how they were feeling. Jones sat there wondering how his exam would be as the day went on with the two of them sharing a drink. "You know it's not all about us. I mean in music it is when we're making it. Being famous and all of that isn't all it's cut out to be." Jones said. Massi looked at Jones, "Well maybe just having our stuff heard would be nice." Massi said as he downed more vodka than what seemed socially acceptable."That's a red label. Really shouldn't be drinking too much of that." Jones chimed in, noticing that it didn't have gold or blue on it. "Well, it's for the fancies of the bottle," Massi said laughing. Jones looked at Massi and then down at the label. "Nah, you're right it's because they want to be fancy," Jones said in return as he laughed. After a few minutes, Jones finished the song with Massi as the two of them kept playing the tune over and over. "This makes me feel like I'm in Saudi Arabia. These violins are in such a cool scale, like fuck man." Massi said joking around as Jones sat there attempting to listen in for possible mistakes.

"Yeah, it kind of does huh?" Jones said back to Massi as the clock struck 7:00 PM. "Hey, I have to go. My girl is texting me." Massi said as Jones looked at the computer feeling empty. Ottie and Jones' trip to Los Angeles came flowing through his memories as the sting of failure stuck. "Hey, if a killer killed a man, who was a killer would it be right or wrong?" Jones asked, wondering for a moment if his actions at Bohemian Grove were acceptable. "I don't know. A life for a life is always the fairway, I guess. No

CHAPTER TWENTY-THREE – ARCHONIC DISASTER

one deserves to die do they?" Massi said as he put on his shoes reaching for his skateboard. "I'm going to get away from here one day, Jones. I'm going to go to China or someplace far away from this place. Or let's get big, go to London." Massi rambled on with the beer in his hand as he hopped on his skateboard. "I'll see you soon. Don't do anything stupid." Massi said Jones smiled back. "Yeah, yeah. Thanks for coming over," Jones said, waving to him as he left out the door. Jones looked up at the sky as the entire world felt still.

"It feels like I'm in a painting that hardly moves," Jones said to himself watching the night sky clouds slowly move by. "All of this feels so surreal. If the world stopped altogether it would be awesome and peaceful at first. Then it might suck." He thought to himself standing there. "Who are you talking to?" Yule echoed through Jones' mind. "I heard Mira finally got to you. Are you ready to speak with me further?" Yule said, expecting Jones to lash out as he had done before. Jones simply shook his head up and down. "Yeah, I'm back in. The world will know my name Jones T. Harver. Or even if it doesn't. The world will know without knowing change ever happened. Until I'm long over with." Jones said, trying to seek pride in the work being offered to him. "I can't offer you currency or a livable wage for this Jones. I can however offer you stars new equipment and our next watcher I want you to connect with. The problem is that you would have to attend Sonoma State University to find him. I heard long ago one of our agents followed this watcher. He went AWOL and has been out of touch since. Heard he was studying the damn books to build some great equipment. Amazingly, the man understands these. I've tried to read the book myself, sensical? None of it." As Yule kept on rambling Jones nodded, taking his words seriously. After viewing the archons talking to one another Jones believed that there could be bad watchers out in the galactic consciousness stream. "I'll go but I want you to be in constant contact. Tell me next time some crazy guy is going to be in your sights." Jones said with a hint of anger not losing his composure as he laid back down on his bed. Yule looked at Jones as his blue coat with golden detailed patches went all the way down to his feet. "Jones, remember when Mira said she's rooting for you to pass the class so you can get into a better school?" Yule paused for a moment expecting Jones to respond as he brought up the question in fear of Jones's rejection. "Yeah, what about?" Jones said not finishing as he listened intently to Yule.

"It was all for this mission. We need this or there will be another potential collapse." Yule told Jones as he lay there looking up at his rooftop."What am I to you? Some pandemic team? Some damn guard you can call on anytime you wish? I know you guys have issues but ever consider my life as well?" Jones said in a harsh tone. "I'm doing this for me. Not to play into your hands." Jones said as Yule nodded. "We're on your side, Mr. Harver." It was the first time Yule had addressed Jones with the utmost respect. "Slip of the tongue." Yule corrected himself as Jones said nothing, waving Yule to leave him alone. "Listen, I know you're the head guy of this operation and all…have my best interests in mind," Yule said to Jones. "After all, I am a watcher as well. I need to live somehow." He said disappearing slowly into the distance. Jones put his arm over his head as he thought about the book of arbiters. As he rolled around uncomfortably unable to sleep in the current situation Jones got up and headed to his desk. The brown cherrywood that curved around his room stuck out as the book of arbiters lay where he last left it.

"Arbiters, Anger - Arbiters, when angry, can pull from moments in time due to their supersonic sound and memory. Arbiters can pull all centillion pieces from their minds as this species conducts inner rituals of anger practice and protection. By memorizing exact points in time or forcing their will forward through pulsating energy in front of them, arbiters can bring forth exact moments into reality." Jones read it further as he practiced what the book was stating. He felt a ball of energy go through his mind as his whole body shook. "Protection shield." He thought to himself as he felt the ball of energy go forward. Mira sent him a text of a YouTube lady trying the same thing. She ended up getting tackled completely on

CHAPTER TWENTY-THREE – ARCHONIC DISASTER

the beach.

"Make sure this isn't you," Mira said laughing as she felt Jones' ball of energy. Jones rolled his eyes as he continued reading about his species. "Arbiters, Actionables." Jones thought to himself for a moment as he read the book further, "Actionables? The hell does that mean?" He almost raised his voice in the middle of the night. "Actionables are when an arbiter is in trouble. One may call on a moment in time while others will study their opponent. Once an arbiter understands its goal this species will not stop until its opponent is no longer in its life, they become dangerous. With the basic help of friends and energy taken from within each person who has linked hands; an arbiter may use this energy to protect those whom they desire to protect. Arbiters may also sap from their "winnings" as necessary to replenish their energy that was lost during the battle. Actionables are only used in situations where there is no way out as recovery of an arbiter can take an entire army. Including but not limited to their friends, parents, situations, and timeliness." Jones laughed at the word timeliness as he sat there considering everything he had read. "Does this work?" Jones said to himself wondering when Yule and Mira would make their next crazy request. As the clock hit 2:00 AM Jones went to sleep with arbiter notes spinning in his head. "Guess It's time for school tomorrow," Jones said to himself as he rolled, overthrowing the covers back over his head. The next day Jones awoke to see the alarm clock not going off. As he reached over for his phone, he noticed the arbiter book on the floor. "Someone else had read this." He said to himself He put it back on the desk. Jones went over to the restroom cautiously thinking through every scenario as the pressure from the outside opened his window. The white tiled floors in the restroom were cleaned and empty as the shower curtain swayed in the wind.

"Someone else has been here." He said to himself thinking about all the crazy people he had met. "The army deer or that squirrel I bet," Jones said to himself, picking up his toothbrush and getting into the shower.

Jones relaxed in the hot water as he thought about shampoo that tastes like fruit you could eat. "Have I gone mad?" He continued the conversation to himself. "The world doesn't need something like this." Jones quietly spoke to himself, placing it down as he cleaned up and got out of the shower. Wearing his towel, he looked at it for a moment. "Now if this had nanotechnology to dry faster or heat dry itself. Now we're talking." Jones thought to himself. He went over to his clothing putting on his black shirt with animal beats on it. "Today I'll wear my brown felt hat off to school," Jones said looking in the mirror. "Even though I don't deserve to wear this now. I'll deserve to wear it one day soon! Jones smiled happily as he picked up his backpack headed again towards school. After a few short minutes of driving, Jones arrived at the parking lot where a construction worker was plowing away. "This'll be done real soon." The worker said out loud as the other worker signaled with his hands. "Yeah, it will be a nice pathway to the back." The sounds of their voices bounced off the parking lot and disappeared into the distance. Jones got out of his car and started walking forward as he tripped over one of the cement rocks that blended in with the dirt. "If these were colored while they were building and repainted later, we wouldn't have this problem," Jones said, annoyed by the rocks in the corner. "Yeah well, the weed killer is a worse thing kid." One of the construction workers overheard him as Jones punted the rock.

"What do you mean?" Jones said curiously. "It's given to so many people, cancer. Not as a label or warning. It's the number one cause. I can't say much more than that." The man said. Jones thought to himself as the guy spoke. Another watcher dressed as a construction worker told him information from the World War II days. "Industrialism huh?" Jones said as he put on a song with that in the title. The construction worker smiled, "Gotta be bat-shit crazy to live in this world sometimes." He said as he went back to work. Jones took his statement without regard as he went further into the school towards where his usual classroom was. "Hey stranger!" Lily said, inviting him to sit down next to her. "Haven't talked in a while. It's good to see you!" She said loudly as Jones sat down. "It's been literally

CHAPTER TWENTY-THREE – ARCHONIC DISASTER

two days. If that?" Jones said in return. "Well yeah. I needed an excuse to say that it's good to see you." Lily said, rocking in her chair. Her long black hair was braided up in colorful beads as her nails were painted lime green. "What are you doing over the weekend?" Lily asked again as Jones contemplated his thoughts. "I don't know, maybe go out to a party with my friends," Jones said, feeling distant from Lily's cluelessness about the entire galactic universe. "That sounds fun! Can I come?" Lily said as Jones wondered more about the world that still seemed unbelievable to him. "If you can get out. Don't you garden for your parents or something?" Jones asked out of curiosity as Lily sat there frowning briefly. "Yeah, I have to garden. You're right, I probably should stay in." She said as she realized that Jones' lifestyle was completely different than hers.

"Alright, well text me if you get bored," Jones said to Lily as he smiled. "Yeah, I will." She replied as class started. Jones thought about the words that Massi had said previously about the watchers being out there listening to everything he had said. "So, if I take my phone..." he thought to himself. "I have a plan of how to gather their attention. Jones smiled as the professor started writing on the board. "Good to see you, Jones. You look happy to be here." The professor joked as Jones was clearly stuck in his own thoughts thinking about his next steps. "Yeah, I'm almost done with writing my thesis," Jones said to the professor as he laughed in return. "Well, that sounds like you've been engaged lately. I'm happy one of my students has started to care." The professor started drawing down all of the scores on the board. "See these ninety-three percentiles on the board? This is where most of the class should be. Only three people made it here on yesterday's exam." The professor stopped not saying any names hinting at Jones' success. "Those at the top please continue to study. Our next exams will be taken home. I expect the grades to go up. You will have more time and access to notes and other resources." The professor hinted at his disappointment as the students quietly said yes to themselves. "Okay, now who can tell me why we have quantum theorems?" The professor asked as Jones looked back at him. "Quantum theorems exist because we can see multiple matters at different periods down to their very atoms. To see how these atoms interact at points in time not easily visible or trackable. These theories can tell us what would happen if the atoms did split at the subatomic level, creating a rift in time. This rift in time wouldn't necessarily be an exact copy from the split atom but rather a connected reality." Jones said to the professor as the class sat silently for a moment.

"I'm not sure what you said but it sounds good Jones. That wasn't the answer I was looking for." The professor continued as no one's hands raised. "Think quantum computing." He hinted as the class grew weary by his theories course. One other student raised his hand. Jones looked over to his left, noticing the biker man sitting in the corner. "Quantum Theories. These are theories that came from the word quanta revolving around energy and matter." The professor smiled, "Very good Tom. Did you Google that?" He joked. Tom held up his phone pointing it towards the professor as he followed up with his joke. The class laughed as Tom put away his phone. "Yeah, maybe." He said in reply to the professor. "Besides the representation of money. Quanta is the term we use to represent energy in our daily lives. When this energy gets disrupted then that's supposedly one way the world will shift around us." The professor continued his course as everyone started taking notes down. Lily looked towards Jones as she gave him a troubled look. "I got another low letter grade." Lily frowned while whispering to Jones. "I saw your grade. Help me out please?" She asked Jones as he sat there thinking about all the notes Lily let him copy.

"Okay. I'll help. That Tom guy really seems to know a lot." Jones said acknowledging the man in his class. "Yeah." After an hour in class, the professor let the classroom go home. "Jones, I expect great potential from you." The professor said as Jones raced towards his car trying not to get caught up in staying later than he had to. "Hey Trexor, let's go out." Jones texted Trexor as he went towards his car. "Yeah man, I'm getting out of class now. Meet you by your car?" He texted back. It had been

CHAPTER TWENTY-THREE – ARCHONIC DISASTER

a while since the two of them spoke and Jones wanted to keep up with his friend. "Sounds good. Where are we going?" Trexor said questioning Jones. "Exploring in the city," Jones said in return as he thought of the people wandering the streets. Jones would be able to get some answers on Nepharius if he explored the lost watchers. He knew Nepharius had already talked to most of them. "Trexor, I'm going to need you in your right mind, tonight," Jones said as Trexor nodded his head. "I won't babysit you like last time but yeah, it's the city. Come on man, of course, I'll pay attention."

Jones laughed, "Nothing super weird ok?" he said. Trexor struck one back. "I'll be sure to pick up the weirdest, craziest person and have them talk to you." Jones smiled, "Yeah, yeah right." he said, turning on the radio of his car. "In today's news an idol is coming to town. There are gatherings of protest over the Bohemian Grove accident. People are demanding that security go up around cities and towns." Jones turned off the radio after a short time. "Reggae music instead?" He looked over at Trexor as he shrugged his shoulders. "Okay, why not?" Trexor responded sitting back listening to reggae play in Jones' car. The two of them drove Jones's car towards the city as the light was going down in the sky. "Do you ever think of how much time we waste?" Jones asked Trexor curiously as his buddy was singing to the song. "I don't really think about it. I kind of go with the flow and do what needs to get done. Are we going to that bar street on the mission?" Trexor asked as Jones thought about it. "Yeah, we are," Jones said as the two of them got to San Francisco. "There's a corner here." A man stood on the side of the building next to red bricks. The sign said "business owned by." The sign was crossed out further as Jones and Trexor looked into the corner. "What do you think of Jones?" Trexor asked to see if Jones was okay with leaving his car there. "As good as any. My car has nothing in it besides party days of puke, piss, and crap cleaned out over the years, Jones said jokingly making light of the situation. "Yeah, doubt some crazy old guy offering parking for five bucks wants anything from you. You have nothing anyway." Jones laughed as he gave the man five bucks. The old man thanked Jones for wanting to converse further as Jones cut him off. "Sorry sir, I have to be somewhere tonight," Jones said to the man, realizing he might be a watcher. "Yeah, somewhere such as drinking at a bar."

Trexor chimed in. "Jones T Harver. Oh, Jones. Ridiculous." Trexor continued as Jones walked further down the road listening to the music in one ear as the other was listening to people outside. As Jones walked further ahead towards the people in the city one man sat down dressed in red and a blue cap. He tossed a quarter in his box squatting down as Jones approached the man. "Don't touch me." The man shouted at Jones in a low but threatening voice. "No plans to. Need directions?" Jones tossed a quarter into the box as the man who was tempered grew less. Three other men stood by him dressed in black hats and a pinstripe suit. "Black hats. Killers, crime watchers." Jones thought to himself as he used caution. The two men approached him, "Need directions huh?" Jones nodded, "Yeah, we're musicians headed to the bar. Well, he's a teacher." Jones said. The two men looked at one another, "Oh alright. What bar?" The two asked as they started to open up. "Roxi's bar," Jones said. The men laughed, "Oh Roxi's is up the street that way. Want some crack?" One of them offered. Jones shook his head, "I'm cool thanks."

The men laughed again, "Man this guy is always about the women and their snozzes doing snozz things." The other man laughed, "Want some crack?" He repeated himself as Jones continuously rejected the Watchers' request. "Do you know about space pirates?" Jones asked the man. The man laughed, "What now?" He replied, "No, haven't heard of him. I recognize that song you're playing though." Jones laughed as Trexor approached them both. "Come on Jones, who are you talking to?" Trexor pulled him away. The man shouted again, "Stay safe out there! I'm sure you'll find him. When we listen, I recognize that song." The man said as he pulled out his crack pipe offering it to his friend. Both of the men were older, missing all of their teeth as they laughed despite their situation. Jones continued down

CHAPTER TWENTY-THREE – ARCHONIC DISASTER

the street towards Roxi's bar. As Trexor caught up to Jones he waved him down. "Yo, what was that about?" Trexor asked Jones, questioning his stop. "Sometimes it's good to help people. People who are scared easily become not so scared once they see our actions at the moment. It's not knowing what will happen or the speculation of what could happen that keeps people in their cage. This added fear in the mind itself, where the mind is already trying to conquer one's own issues." Jones rambled on about fear to throw Trexor off about what he was doing, looking for the trail on Nepharius in the streets of San Francisco. "That's it! That's Roxi's!" Jones said excitedly Trexor followed behind him. The two of them opened the door.

"What'll it be, fellows?" A man with a felt hat greeted the two of them with a hearty laugh. "Whiskey on the rocks for me." Trexor said, "What about you Jones?" He turned to him signaling Jones for cash in his wallet. "One Moscow mule sounds about right," Jones said in return. "Coming right up." The bartender said as he went to grab the two drinks. "So, Jones, you've been kind of on and off lately," Trexor said as he waited for a whiskey pour. "What do you mean?" Jones said in return. "You sound like some crazy conspiracy theorist who doesn't even research or have critical thinking skills," Trexor said. Jones turned to Trexor uncomfortably looking at him. Trexor has been keeping tabs on Jones without him realizing it. "Yeah well, most of the world lacks critical thinking skills. How am I any different here? What's freaky is normalized. What's normalized is becoming freaky." Jones stopped for a moment as the bartender handed both of them their drinks. "That'll be two Croxi," the bartender said.

"What?" Jones said in return. "Twelve dollars and a two-dollar tip," Trexor chimed one as he paid for the drinks. Jones didn't ask the bartender again thinking he might have misheard him. "I'm going out for a cigarette in a moment here. Want to join me?" Jones took the chance to briefly separate from Trexor. "I'm okay man, I'll chill here," Jones said in return as he looked at the bartender. "Okay. Whatever you want." Trexor said as he went outside of Roxi's bar to go talk to the people outside. "Did you say a different currency?" Jones signaled the bartender over. "What? Oh, earlier? That was a joke I do to be sure people aren't too drunk to order." He said, trying to alleviate Jones's suspicions. "No, I'm pretty sure you mentioned the galactic currency," Jones said in return. "What do you know about Nepharius?" Jones instigated as the bartender's eyebrow twitched. "Hate that man." The bartender revealed his position to Jones. "Look, if you want more information that'll be another Croxi." The bartender said as Jones sat there annoyed by the request. "Alright, fine. Fine! Here's your damn money." Jones said as he gave him five dollars. "Nepharius is a man who used to frequent these streets." The bartender started talking as Jones listened intently. "He used to come down parading with people and beer. Dressed up in crazy and wacky costumes. Kept saying how one day he'd move to Brazil. If he didn't make it, he said he'd go back to his place. Steal some big thing from Kha'tgon or some shit." The bartender got a request for another order. "Look man that's all I know. I've got other requests here." He said as he wandered off to the other side of the bar. Trexor came back waving after his cigarette. "Jones buddy! How are you holding up?" Trexor said curiously. Jones looked back at him as he finished his Moscow mule. "Fine yeah. Think I'll explore a bit." Jones said to Trexor. "You know, no one really cares what we do out here. It's kind of weird to consider, don't you think?" Jones said as Trexor raised his eyebrow jokingly in curiosity.

"How so?" He said quickly replying to Jones as he finished his whiskey. "Let's go outside for a moment," Jones took his cell phone out as Trexor talked to him loading up SoundCloud. "Here," Jones said as he played his phone on max volume with the music blaring, holding it up in the sky. Jones started walking forward through the streets as Trexor followed, "What are you doing?" He asked Jones played the song. "See? No one cares." Jones said recalling the time he practiced aerobics on the BART in the middle of a crowd. "Woo! We listenin'!" A shout came from the corner Jones smiled. "Alright, maybe a few people care." Jones put away

CHAPTER TWENTY-THREE – ARCHONIC DISASTER

his phone as Trexor stood there for a moment. "Are you good to drive? You are kind of freaking me out I guess." Trexor said, "Let's go back to Roxi's and head home." Jones nodded as he got the information he needed. By a stroke of luck and one point of interest, he would be able to find Nepharius next move towards the artifact. Jones didn't understand why the bartender hates Nepharius. He went back and sat back down at the bar as people danced on the floor. "Hey, tender'" Jones said, shortening his words. "Why do you hate him so much anyway?" Jones asked as the bartender looked up at Jones. "Cause' that old fool ran me down into debt with his magazine. I used to work for him before I went down to work for a bigger company. Now I run this bar. He ran off with the money and I never saw a damn Croxi." The bartender said. "Know why I call this Roxi's bar?" Jones silently listened as the bartender leaned in close. He could smell the whiskey on his breath. "Cause' it's a reminder of the currency that damn man ripped me off from." The bartender turned around and went back to serving before Jones had a chance to say a word.

"Alright," Jones said to himself as Trexor went back over to the bar calling Jones outside. "Cab's here man. We have to get back. School day' is coming up and we can't be out too late." Trexor said, signaling Jones to the car. "Alright let's go," Jones said as the two of them left Roxi's. "So… how's your studies going?" Jones asked him as he sat on the other side of the car. "Studies are going alright. Doing history class and all of that." Trexor sat there for a moment as the windows rolled down in the cab. "As the teacher says, history tends to repeat itself over and over until someone changes it." Jones nodded his head. "I guess people don't really like change so they believe what worked on a small scale works on a large scale as well." Yule echoed through Jones' head as Jones' world spun. "That's exactly right Jones." He chimed in. "which is why you should be recreating the world as you go on looking around. You've done it before." Jones waved his hand in the wind. "We're past that. These ideas will surface on their own once written. That's the funny and ironic part about it. Once it's written it can be written over a thousand times but the truth will always be there.

Unless some crazy evolution of balance changes it again." Yule took Jones' sarcasm. He laughed. "True story. Pay attention, you and your friend are almost home." Jones looked back at Trexor. "Thanks for going along to the bars with me. It was a good time." Jones laid back in the cab seat and relaxed as Trexor waved his hand back. "Yee bruddah." He said in return. Yule took Jones' sarcasm. He laughed. "True story. Pay attention, you and your friend are almost home."

Jones looked back at Trexor. "Thanks for going along to the bars with me. It was a good time." Jones laid back in the cab seat and relaxed as Trexor waved his hand back. "Yee bruddah." He said in return. As the lit-up night grew darker Jones knew he was getting further away from the city. "Almost there." The cab driver said as a watcher on the street holding up a sign. "Free us soon." Jones blinked again as the cab continuously went towards home. "Free us soon." Jones thought about the sign to himself. Without understanding what it meant his head kept spinning. "Was it Nepharius who had a handle on all of the watchers on the street? Was Yule not telling him? Jones' thoughts kept running as the cab arrived at his house. "See ya later, Jones," Trexor said as he took a cab towards his car which he left at the school. Jones waved his friend off as he went in towards his house. "How can I build an empire when the weight is against me?" Jones said to himself as newspapers lie on the table. "I can't keep up with the daily lives of everyone. This is too much for me to remember." Jones said as he started reading the newspapers dating back to two weeks ago. Yule has told Jones to keep on formulating new ideas but Jones was unable to due to the buildup of falling behind. Jones started to freak out as he went into his room feeling exhausted. "I give up. I can't keep up with everything going on." Yule echoed again to Jones."Remember Jones, you have the council of five on your side. Each one of us can keep up with each idea if you'll tell us what to focus on." Jones sighed, "That's your job, you came to me with a bigger issue." Yule snickered, "True, it is my job to organize everything." Jones turned over as he still felt the feelings of being drunk taking over. "We'll deal with it in the morning," Jones said

CHAPTER TWENTY-THREE – ARCHONIC DISASTER

before falling asleep. Jones got up the next morning and got ready for school. "Where are you?" A text went to his phone as Lily sent a worried face through to him.

"The professor is starting class in five minutes." Jones sighed again, "Been late to it so many times I don't think it matters at this point." He texted back laying there for a moment contemplating how he would tackle the problems. "Look at your chart, Jones," Yule said echoing in his head. "Good morning Yule." Yule sticking around in the house no longer bothered Jones in his day-to-day life. By now every statement that was said to him had become normal. "I've got to get ready," Jones replied as he cut out Yule from his mind. "Yeah, we know," Mira said. "You too?" Jones said back to Mira. "Yeah, me too: today I'm going with you to meet someone." Jones looked at Mira curiously. "Who?" He brushed his teeth slowly. "I'm going to meet one of our inventors. You met them at the phone store. We have a new piece of equipment coming in and you'll need it." Mira said as she wandered to his right. "Can't you picture me in person already? I feel like we're so far away." Mira teased.

"Not yet," Jones said as she slowly egged him on to come into existence. "Well okay," Mira said, dropping her joking manner. "I'll catch up with you later at school." Jones looked at Mira for a moment, noticing the ideas around her necklace. "Once an idea is made, we tend to simply build and expand on that combination of ideas huh?" Jones said. Mira smiled back. "You've got it! Haven't felt like eating one in a while. You must be doing a poor job." Mira said in a scolding manner trying to hold in her laughter. "Okay, I have to go seriously." She said, finishing her statement. Jones got into his car after getting dressed and headed off to school. He parked where he normally had been parking as a toll booth had been installed. "What's this for?" Jones said to himself analyzing the toll booth. "Collection fee's coming soon." Jones looked at it as the toll booth said "place your phone here to be charged by the application." Jones saw the QR scanner on the side of the booth as he parked. "New changes are coming in," Jones said to himself as he walked back up the stairs to his usual classroom antics. Lily was sitting there smiling. Jones looked at her for a moment. He smiled, "You know, you're pretty cool sometimes." Lily looked back at Jones, "Uh… thanks?" She said, "When you're done living in your own world, we have another exam to study for and you have another essay to write." She said, bringing out the paper in front of him. "So, look here. The professor said that when an atom splits, even though the two never touch there's still a reaction in the middle of them. This reaction possibly creates an opening." Jones shook his head. "This isn't like a creativity project into an upside-down world. This is different."

Jones started writing. "To understand how another plain opens up is first to try to understand why writing makes us feel better," Jones said. "Let me explain. When a person's thought goes through their head. Not being able to write it out builds up the pressure of wanting to write it out in the mind. As this pressure builds up, we drown in our own thoughts because we're creatures who need interaction. So, through these thoughts and the need for interaction, we subconsciously open up portals or new ideas as we currently call them in today's society. Our existing matter doesn't ever touch but what does touch us is the energy created by these "portals" from our very own ideas. Rather created from two atoms after being split up trying to reconnect. This creates massive amounts of energy. This energy is then generated from our thoughts which are considered to be what I call "moving energy" and not the physical kind! Music, writing, vibration, serenity, and energy moved around by different methods release us into different mindsets. All of these mindsets are a world in itself carried by each person who has their own story." Jones sat there explaining to Lily. He continuously wrote as he spoke. She sat there and watched him growing more interested in what he had been researching. "Okay Jones, I get your point to some extent. Still, keep an open mind to the other possibilities." Lily said in return. "Oh, get ready. The professor is coming." She said as the professor went through the door.

CHAPTER TWENTY-THREE – ARCHONIC DISASTER

"It wouldn't be so bad," Jones said. "These other worlds. It'd at least be interesting." He mumbled to himself thinking about the watchers. The images went through his mind so quickly that Jones remembered the keyboard on his phone by mere image projection from his mind. "Photographic memory or photographic projection? Is this a thing? If not, it should be." Jones thought to himself as the professor started writing on the board. "Wait, equipment. Mira." Jones thought. "I wonder how she is doing." Jones raised his hand to excuse himself. "I need a restroom break." He said to the professor. "Go ahead." The professor said back to Jones as he left the room. Jones went out of the door and walked down the hallway as he took his short break. A vending machine sat outside as he sat staring at the food. Jones swiped his card waiting for the chocolate to drop as he stood there. A fellow student walked up to him. "Hey, I know you. You were in my…" the student stopped to think. "Art class, right?" He said as Jones looked over at him. "Yeah, hey. You're that guy who makes apps right?" Jones said, replying to him as he took his break. "You know what a cool app idea would be?" Jones started to talk to his classmate. "Oh, not this again," Kali said in return, showing no interest in Jones's idea. "Kali, hear me out," Jones said as he waved his hand. "Fine, what is it?" Kali said, seemingly annoyed.

"Well, you know how when you walk into a restaurant right? There're ingredients to make different types of foods. What if we had an application that could show you the probability of what something would taste and look like by simply substituting ingredients once the original dish is made." Jones was about to continue as Kali cut him off. "How would that work though?" Jones continued, "App scanning technology. Scan each ingredient and what the dish looks like. As the dish changes matchmaking learning will read it and change with it. This can then compare it to the taste of other foods. The raw data of each ingredient simply has to be inputted." Jones said excitedly. Kali looked at him. "Well, tell me how you want the layout of the app and I'll consider it," Kali said as he walked away. Jones took his chocolate and opened up the wrapper as the smell went across his nose. "Now if we could only get rid of this plastic in food." He repeated to himself as he went back to the classroom. "Jones, where did you go?" Lily asked as he sat down next to her. "To the restroom. You heard me, right?" He said to her, feeling annoyed by her lack of attention.

"Oh." She said before resuming watching the professor write on the board. "You know, some woman came looking for you. I thought I heard someone anyway. Outside of our door, they were shouting your name." Lily said. "None of the class seemed to notice as music played from the room across ours. Still, they were shouting that they were Mira and had something important for you." Lily went back to looking at the board as Jones sat there contemplating what she had said. "No way, this isn't possible". Jones said quietly. "That woman, Mira. Was she wearing green and black? Did she have a weird necklace on?" Jones asked Lily. "What?" Lily said. "I don't know. I only heard a voice." Jones relaxed. "Oh. Probably your imagination." Right then Mira's voice echoed into Jones' head. "I'm right here, stupid! And I'm wearing a yellow frilled dress today," she said. Jones smiled. Mira's voice was warm and calming to Jones. Although the two of them could never touch Jones couldn't help but still support her. "I got you the equipment Yule asked me for," Mira said. Jones shut his eyes for a moment. "An all-purpose green and black compass with a tracking device built in from Nepharius. When you grabbed the gem a small piece of his shirt fell off. We were able to put it into the equipment. As long as we have this energy tracker, we can find Nepharius from the buildings around town. He might even be at to your own backyard!" Mira said proudly as she showed it to Jones.

"I'm supposed to be paying attention to class right now. We can't act until I get into that next school, right?" Jones said, asking Mira about it. "You're right, at least with this we can beat him ahead of his own curve." She smirked as she handed over the compass. Jones took it as it disappeared into his pocket. Lily tapped Jones on the shoulder. "Jones, were you sleeping?" Lily said curiously. "Uh, no, no. Simply focused, sorry." Jones

CHAPTER TWENTY-THREE – ARCHONIC DISASTER

said, trying to keep her suspicions as low as possible. "Oh, alright then. You've been kind of weird lately. Want to study after this class?" Lily asked him as he sat there for a moment thinking about the compass. "Yeah, I have to finish this essay huh?" He said as the professor stopped writing on the board. "I'm here. If you two keep talking I will have to separate you." He said hunting at the both of them to be quiet as he taught. "Sorry, sir." Jones apologized as the two of them quieted down to take notes. "Good. Now, today we will watch videos on more theories." Jones zones out as he imagines the videos popping out in 3D. Instead of tablets, there were screens on the desk. "Jones, pay attention." The professor said again as Jones sat there trying to stay awake. "Alright." He said as he watched the video. As the man spoke about different mathematical theories off of the projector Jones watched the reel. He started to think of ideas that hadn't changed for the last fifty years. "Maybe this is why the world is still so boring for so many people," Jones said to himself drifting off. Even though there were no windows to look out of, the lights were bright. "After this video class time is up." The professor said Jones sighed with relief. "What a day." As the classroom clock hit "time to leave o-clock." In Jones's mind, he got up and headed towards the study hall. Lily followed him over to where the stairwell stuck out. "Jones, can you help me understand this theory?" Lily asked as Jones attempted to learn it himself. "This is pretty complicated," Jones said, scratching his head. Lily took her seat. "Uh… yeah, that's why it's the last required course before we graduate from this school dummy." She said, mocking him.

"Yeah true," Jones replied feeling detached from the humor she was trying to portray towards him. Jones started to write down the base formula on the piece of paper deconstructing every piece as if it was a building block. Moving around the theory until there had been some sense of a match. "I think I understand but it's a little shaky," Jones said. "This theory about energy transfer still makes little sense to me." He sighed, "Guess I wasn't meant to be a scientist." Jones continued trying to crack a joke to lighten up the mood from his rude attitude earlier. "No. I guess you weren't meant to be a scientist." Lily laughed as Jones continued to work through the problem. "Found it," Jones said to himself more than to Lily. His work ethic went so far that he was determined to get the answer. "What is the answer, professor-in-training?" Lily joked again that Jones sat there. "38," Jones said. She smiled. "Nice one. Hey look, I found something." Lily said as she flipped pages in the book. "All the answers are right here." Jones laughed as Lily spoke. "Yeah? True, that's not the point of this at all." Jones said in return. He got up and put his seat back to the table. "If these chairs are locked in place and spun out from below, that would be easier. Or folded into this desk." He thought as Tober crossed his mind. "That carpenter could have built it. I'm sure of it." Jones smiled to himself. "Aren't you going to invite me for food?" Lily asked as Jones sat silently, processing the world around him. "Cafeteria is right around the corner," Jones said. "Alright, let's go there," Lily responded as she picked up her backpack and headed over to the cafeteria.

Jones sat down at the plain tables as hardly anyone was eating. Most of the students had gone to their classes or were studying their books quietly. Jones picked up an empty cup and slid it across the metal towards Lily. The cup stopped right before her hands as she reached for it. "Hey Jones, when this class is done, what school are you going to go to?" She asked him curiously. "Sonoma." He said right away. "Somewhere up there sounds like the place I want to be. There are parties, wine for days, and green yards of roses wherever you look. The people seem so friendly." He turned to Lily hoping she would attend the same school. "Kind of would be silent without you," he said. She smiled back. "Yeah…going to Davis," she said. "Or somewhere in Humboldt. I guess it will be pretty silent then," Lily added. Jones stood there staring at the empty cup in her hand. "Such is life?" He said as he shrugged. "Let's grab dinner and get out of school. We've been here way too long" Jones jokes, lightening up the moment. He knew that after the two of them graduated, they would not be speaking again. Lily went up to the counter and ordered as Jones stood behind her. "Pssst. Hey idiot." Mira said from a distance standing in the corner.

CHAPTER TWENTY-THREE – ARCHONIC DISASTER

Jones looked over towards the direction of her words. "When you're done playing normal life, we have work to do," Mira said. Jones smiled. "Yeah, we have a criminal to catch who's a space pirate." Mira laughed, "Being on a boat was kind of fun, admittedly."

Lily looked over at Jones oddly, "Who are you talking to?" She questioned as she turned around after receiving her food. "Talking to myself about what I would say imaging myself as an agent during graduation." Jones lied. "Okay, weirdo." Lily said, "You still have yet to order your food." Jones walked over to the food, "I'll have the fried noodles." He said as the server took them out of a big pot. "Here you go. That will be five bucks and thirty cents." The cook had been zoning out as Mira silently watched Jones from the corner. "The yellow looks good on you," Jones said quietly in the direction of Mira. She laughed as Lily waited on the table for Jones to sit down. "Hey, can I get this to go?" Jones asked the cook. The cook nodded and put it in a to-go box as Jones went over to where Lily was sitting. "Hey, I've got to go. It's too late to eat for me now and my mom's waiting at home. She's been worried lately." Jones lied again as he left. "See you tomorrow! Sucks you can't stay, thanks for the help," said Lily. Jones waved as Mira followed behind him on the way out. Her yellow frills moved in the wind as rain droplets started to fall. With each drop that hit Mira's dress the color changed showing multiple colors until it turned into stars and galaxies reflecting back and forth. "I really like that dress," Jones said to her.

She smiled, "Had Star make it for me back at the shop. It's the same material used on cars. Figured I'd ask." She laughed as she skipped along in the rain. Jones walked putting his coat over his head as multiple people took out their various umbrellas. "You forgot your umbrella again, didn't you?" She said as Jones walked faster. "When you're done patronizing me, get me a shirt like that too," Jones said in return as he got to his car. He took another look and Mira had disappeared again. "I'll see her again." He said as Jones looked down at his phone. He had multiple texts from Ike. "Can you come on over?" Ike said, asking Jones. "Yea, I'll come down," Jones said as he drove home.

Chapter Twenty-Four – Celebration Collision

"Jones! Where have you been?" his mom said, suspecting something going on with him again. "Studying at school." He said in reply heading straight towards his room. "I'm going to go over to Ike's," he said. Jones's mom was surprised. "Ike's? Heard he had some trouble." Jones replied in one-word answers wanting to leave. "Yeah." He said putting on his shoes. His mom looked at the food on the table. "Hungry at least?" She offered as he continued putting on his shoes. "Thanks, but got some take out. I'm alright for now." Jones said as the raindrops continued to pour. He walked out the door looking back at the house imagining the same material as Mira's dress imprinted in the roof and wood. "This whole neighborhood would be so cool looking during rainfall if houses did that." Jones started getting lost in his thoughts as his fear fell over his head. He wondered if Ike would ever be stabilized again after this. After an hour of driving, he showed up at Ike's door knocking on it. "Is Ike home?" Jones said as his mom answered the door. "Oh, Jones! Good to see you, hope you're well and come in." She said, flustered as the T.V. was on. The black couch sat on the corner with a chair as the house had been rearranged. Ike's walls were filled with posters attached to the wall that looked like water. "Woah. What did you do?" Jones asked Ike to sit there playing music. "Felt like being in a jungle. Since there's no jungle here I created my own." Ike said laughing. Jones took a moment as he set down his phone, keys, and wallet. "How have you been?" Jones said, trying not to pry too much. "Happy to be free. I swear they do weird things in those places. To top it off, those people are crazy. One girl wanted to sleep with me the whole time and I kept saying no." He said as he played music. "Can I ask you something, bro?" Ike said, turning to him. "Were you actually crazy when you went in there or did they put you in there because you knew too much?" Jones sat there for a moment. "Listen, Ike, maybe I knew too much. Maybe I went crazy. All that matters is that we're out now." Jones said, trying to counsel Ike. "Yeah true." He replied. "Want to go for a walk?" Ike said as Jones sat there in the small room. "Yeah, that sounds nice," Jones said as the two of them got up and headed for the door. "We're going out for a walk."

His mother shouted back, "That's good. Go for a walk and get some fresh air. Ike! Take out the garbage and clean the dishes." She shouted, annoyed by his irresponsibility. "Okay. I will momma. First, give me a hug," He said as Jones waited by the door. Ike and his mom hugged and the two of them left. Jones started walking down the stairs with Ike in Mill Valley where a trail filled with plants stuck out. "It's nice to finally get out," Ike said, turning to Jones. "Yeah man, fresh air from being cooped up can really help." The two of them walked the trail while the sunlight brimmed down. "If we keep walking this trail turns into a forest. It's super light." Ike said. The two of them walked as a bicycle passed by them. "Like walking into a journey of a different world and never turning back?" Jones jokes Ike laughed. "Exactly. Let's put all these different ideas we've been talking about in our music. We'll make it timeless." Jones sighed feeling relieved that Ike seemed to be okay. "The other guys haven't contacted you since, right?" Jones asked Ike directly. "No, they haven't bothered me since I've been out. We took the podcasts down." Ike said as they walked further. "Yeah, that's good. We can be musical warriors of our own accord." Jones said to Ike in return. Ike smiled at the idea, "Nah man, let's just make music for us. Like we always do. Stay out of everything because the world is crazy enough as it is." Ike said dismissing the time the both of them had

CHAPTER TWENTY-FOUR – CELEBRATION COLLISION

spent as a fluke in life.

"Okay." Jones agreed. He would have to take down Nepharius himself and Jones knew it. "Come on, Jones. Let me show you something," Ike said. Jones followed him. The two of them turned around walking back towards his house as a dirt pathway leading up into the forest. Jones and Ike walked up to it together as trees enclosed the surroundings. Jones noticed a jacket perched up on the rocks. "Watchers must have been here too." He thought to himself calmly as Ike looked around. "Place is pretty sick huh?" He said, clearly proud of his find. Jones smiled back. "Bro this place is pretty sick." As he grabbed onto a branch that had encircled the spot. The trees were clear from all rain acting as a giant umbrella as the two of them sat on a rock. "Guess a lot of kids used to come around here at night," Jones said as Ike put up his shoulders. "I have no idea. I guess. It's a good smoking spot after all." Ike said "You don't smoke anymore I heard," Jones said to Ike. "Yeah, I can't," Ike said in return as Jones and Ike laughed. "Let's get back to your spot and work on some music," Jones said as Ike nodded. "Let's grab some food too. I have a lot at home." He said as the two of them walked back down the hill towards the walkway. As the two of them, Jones wondered if it was right for him to continue tracking down the watchers. He wondered if meddling in the battle was the right thing to do. "Hey, Ike. What are we going to do with all of this music when we're done?" Jones asked him. Ike didn't seem worried. "I don't know. We're making it for us. What does it matter?" Ike said curiously. "True," Jones said. He thought to himself, "I guess it's not right or wrong to take on this battle. It's if I want to do it for me huh?" Jones continued walking as the two of them saw Ike's house.

The stone pathway leads up the stairs back towards his apartment. The two of them opened the door as the wind lightly blew. The rain now subsided as the two of them went into his room. "Put in these headphones and get to work." Ike laughed, "Jones! You cannot leave this room until I have my song damn it." He said in a mocking tone as he acted as a lead producer.

Both Jones and Ike laughed as Ike loaded up his program. "Sunny day." Ike said, "Music captures emotion so we'll call it after today." Jones was no stranger to how the watchers communicated directly. If he could make his original songs, it would be a direct way to further join together against Nepharius. After the night out with Trexor, he realized he could gather them together through music. Ike and Jones loaded up the program as the two of them shared various ideas between one another making the song slowly between chords and observations the two of them had made. "A mixture of video game-style music with orchestra, people riding on bikes and panning. Mix everything we can think of together. I want to build a story with sound effects in the middle as well." Ike and Jones kept on sharing ideas as the song was finally made. "This is how we can communicate our story," Jones said excitedly as the two of them talked. Ike went into his kitchen and made a smoothie bringing back chia seeds to Jones as he sat there watching from the side.

"It's amazing to see how much we've grown in music," Ike said as he turned to Jones. "Here it is." Jones looked at the raw chia seeds and ate them all. "It's like trying to chew on mini flakes of wood," Jones said. Ike laughed, "Oops." He chuckled as the two of them continued to joke around. Jones was able to rest properly again, clearing his head for the essay that he was going to be finishing up for his class. As Ike snored, Jones lay next to him with his pillow over his head. The water and jungle helped Jones go to sleep as his friend snored even louder. Jones kicked Ike's foot. "Hey man come on. I can't sleep like this," he said. Ike looked up, "Sorry bro." he said. Ike fell asleep again snoring. Jones got out of the bed and went towards the black couch where he was able to drift off to sleep after being cramped. "Finally," Jones said to himself thinking of the accomplishment that the two of them had made. "Jones." a voice he recognized went through his head. "I'm coming to change the world again." Jones froze momentarily, not knowing how to respond.

"Nepharius," Jones said one word as it went throughout the galactic

CHAPTER TWENTY-FOUR – CELEBRATION COLLISION

universe turning voices towards him as Nepharius spoke. "I can track you now. I'll find you." Jones said Nepharius didn't respond. Silence followed throughout the night as no one dared try to intervene. The feeling of energy and fear was the only thing left as morning came. Jones woke up rubbing his eyes as his leg was half off the couch with the other one on. The red blanket covered Jones in his pajamas as Ike stood in the kitchen already making a smoothie. "Yo, are you hungry bro?" he asked curiously. Jones rubbed his eyes. "I have to head home. Be sure to mix that track." Jones said as he collected his stuff. "Alright bro, good music session. I'll send it to you through messenger when you get home." Ike said excitedly. Jones got in his car and started to drive home contemplating Nepharius voice. He felt that Nepharius wanted to say more but knew that the man the whole universe wanted was trapped. Conjured up by his faults and plans where isolation and war would be Nepharius's only way out. Jones turned up the music of Ike's past music that the two of them had made as Jones studied their faults. "This should be improved here," Jones said to himself

He yawned, turning onto the road. After an hour of driving, Jones arrived back at home. By now his mother had grown used to Jones coming and going randomly. She no longer seemed to worry as long as Jones mentioned where he was going and had dressed properly. Jones has learned how to be normal and blend in with society as the spirit of music had instructed him to. The brown felt hat sat on Jones's baseball caps as he picked up his backpack. Quickly getting out of his sleep clothes he changed for school. "I'm off to school," Jones said. His mother turned towards him. "Jones, wait!" she said unable to reach him in time as he left.

Jones went off to school as fast as he had got home driving to the parking lot. He wondered why there were no people there as he drove around to the front side. Walking up the stairs only geese flew above the steps squawking in the distance as he looked around. "No one's here..." Jones said to himself. He looked down at his calendar to check the date. "Oh. It's a holiday." Jones said to himself patting his head. "I'm so dumb." He continued giving out a short laugh as he got back into his car. Jones decided that he should check out Walnut Creek where multiple new buildings were being built. After a few short minutes of driving, he arrived at the shopping centers around town. "Those headphones that sounded like a movie theater in my ears. I want to try them." Jones said to himself as he looked at each building walking by. Distracted by a globe on the building that said, "World book group. All of your informational needs." He walked into the shop. The bookkeeper seemed happy to greet him as lots of people roamed the store. "What can I do for you?" She asked as Jones looked around the shop. "The comic book section. Where is it?" He asked curiously as she pointed him to the direction of the books. "There." Jones made his way over as he picked up the book. "People say these people are based on heroes or drug-induced ideas." Mira came out from the shadows of the book store looking down at one of the books. "I wish I could have met some of these people in my time," Mira said. "So, do these people actually exist? They aren't made from our imaginations?" Jones asked. "Well, some came out of disasters. Others came out of situations like yours." Mira smiled. "One day maybe a watcher will write about you too! Your unknown battles with Nepharius and our ways around everyone." Mira chuckled. "Or It will be swept under the rug," Jones said, feeling cynical about the situation. He picked up one of the comic books with a yellow cover in giant red names. "Like that pilot agent guy said who always sits in that coffee shop. What's the point if most people can't even finish a comic book." Jones said

He wanted to purchase it. "Read up on some of us Mr. Arbiter.' Mira suggested. "You won't be disappointed" she continued as her dress was back to black and green. Jones sat in a corner thinking about the book on arbiters he picked up previously as he started to read into the comic book. He opened the first page and started to read it. "Found something you like?" The librarian said as Jones gripped the comic book in his hand. He got up and walked towards the register. "That's all for you today?" The bookkeeper said. Jones nodded. "That's all." After giving the librarian twenty bucks he took it outside and started to go for a walk towards the

CHAPTER TWENTY-FOUR – CELEBRATION COLLISION

post that he once sat on. A woman sat across from the bench near the water fountain where Jones hopped on it previously. She kept staring at the clouds as Jones sat on the other side to relax. Eyeing Jones as she wondered about what he was doing, she wondered about the book he was holding. As Jones blinked people started to slowly be dressed in red, blue, and white. Fewer people looked normal around him as the man sat on the yellow post that he had previously met. "Why aren't you out partying?" The old man wrote it down. He exclaimed it was mute. Jones looked over, "No one to go with." The old man smiled, "Use the trolley to Bart again. There isn't a reason you shouldn't go." He encouraged as he pointed to the trolley across the street. Jones took his book and got off the bench to join the man near the trolley. The yellow post pointed in an exact angle towards where Jones leveraged it to stand by the trolley. "Free AC," Jones said, thanking the man as the day grew hot. "Who would have thought," Jones said to himself. The trolley bell churned moving towards the BART station. The old man smiled, his red white and blue showed towards Jones. As the BART station appeared in front of Jones, he followed the old man up the stairs who smiled pointing to get on. He stayed behind waving; the BART showed up. "Alright. Guess I'm going on a short adventure." Jones said to himself, people slowly got on the BART dressed in costumes. A man to Jones left held up a flag as the other people in the BART had sparkly glasses, gold, and capes beyond recognition. Jones sat there awkwardly as a flag slid right in front of him. He picked it up heading out towards the city. The BART stopped at each stop as a person got on. She started rapping to herself about how she was a superwoman as the smell moved through the BART. Jones looked at her as she threw a blanket over her head, rapping in anger. He held his shirt up to his nose as the stench filled the place. "Had she pissed herself?" Jones thought to himself as the BART continued to move into the city. "Sit very still… don't talk to it." Mira echoed. Her voice was almost whimpering as she whispered.

"It's a true green archon. An ogre of sorts derived from the old ages." Jones sat there as the lady continued her show trying to make sense of the mediocrity of what she was saying. "Come after me, come after me and you'll see I'm super. Superwoman. It doesn't matter if you're going to beat me. I'll always come back." She sent a message as if she was trying to communicate into the galactic space everywhere and nowhere at the same time. The archon went for the door. "I'll find you, Jones," the archon said as the BART stopped. Jones held his breath as he didn't move in the seat. She walked out the door as the smell still stayed after. Jones moved through the BART doors into each next section to escape the smell as he sat back down on the chair in the next cart. The entire BART smelled of cologne and strawberries as two women sat in the back. The BART stopped, "Embarcadero is our stop. Please get off here." Jones heard over the speakers as it vibrated through the train. Jones got up as the rush of people laughed getting off the BART. Flags, hats, and costumes were around the street as he went over to pier 31 where he had been practicing on the bottles before. A man stood on roller skates with lit-up pants as lights went up and down his leg. He had a spinner with wings and a beard that extended past Jones' leg. Mira was now standing next to Jones in a red and purple dress. "It's a holiday today. You forgot, didn't you?" Jones looked over at Mira. "I don't try to remember unimportant days," he said. Mira laughed, "Try to take a load off your shoulders today. A lot is going on as you can see. Even the elite watchers are out." Jones looked over at Mira curiously. "Elite watchers?" This was the first time Jones was hearing about a difference in class of people. "Yeah Jones, that guy with wings on is an elite watcher. It looks like he's in his own little world but he's really surveying the area." Mira said with a statement that confused Jones.

"I guess watchers have a class of their own. There's always leaders of something wherever you go, right?" Jones turned towards Mira as she pointed down the street. "It's about to start," Mira replied. Jones walked by lots of people singing, running, and enjoying one another's company. Jones went over to the docks where he had previously gone before. The grass spread out across the way as a building named "Piers best." Stood a few feet away from the view. Jones took a seat in the grass next to Mira as

CHAPTER TWENTY-FOUR – CELEBRATION COLLISION

the first firework went off up into the air. Faces and shapes exploded as a mushroom cloud that dropped over the city in all white trickled over the people. "You know, I've been thinking a lot and… this whole world of the watchers. Their ways and all. I should bring it to light. What do you think?" Jones wondered as he sat there watching the firework explode as it dropped down over the town. "How would you give all of these people the perception to see into this world?" She asked Jones as her dress reflected the fireworks now back into the crowd. "I'll write about it. Change the perceptions of people all at once." Jones said back to Mira as the next firework went off. She smiled, "After you catch Nepharius, Jones. You can do what you want. If you catch him, the world of watchers will be behind you every step of the way. Most of these watchers already are." Mira smiled. She looked at Jones, determined to keep in touch with him as she slowly brought herself into a connected reality with his. People were looking at Jones leaning over if he were talking to himself wondering if he would notice them. Mira tapped his shoulder telling him to look off to the left. "I heard that a park is a good place to view the city. Head up the stairway back across the train tracks." Mira said encouraging Jones to feel for the places he was in.

Jones stood up to walk across the train tracks in the other direction. As one of the trains went by, he blinked. The train slowed down as if Jones should hop on it while moving. He was about to step forward as a man pulled him back. "Wait, man!" The man said, bringing Jones to a halt. "Thanks," Jones said quietly as the train finished moving by. Jones continued to walk across the way as a herd of people gathered to watch the end of the fireworks. Jones walked opposite towards the stairway pausing halfway in between. As he turned around the entire city glistened with lights and laughter. Jones took a picture and sent it to Lily. "Happy day off!!" He said, trying to gain her attention. Lily replied quickly, "How beautiful!" Texting back as he looked over the water. Right then neighbors lit off fireworks that tilted over. One-shot through the streets hitting a black car as Jones turned around watching it bounce off the car disappearing into thin air. "I better head home Mira," Jones whispered as he got up from his seat walking back down towards the BART. Jones walked through the streets of the city towards the BART a man yelled at him from his car next to his girlfriend. "You're nothing! You're just a brown felt hat!" he said. Jones walked through the street. "Charles! Stop it! The girl said from the other side of the window as the cars were stuck in traffic. Jones didn't pay attention as he kept on walking towards the BART train to get home. As Jones got towards the BART a man in black clothing and a green beanie approached him. "I can help you." He offered as he collected receipts from the BART train. "Oh, alright it's like this?" Jones said as he swiped his card into the BART machine. Another man sat on the end of the corner and put his thumb up as he swiped Jones' card. "So how are you living lately brother?" He said realizing the two were trying to rob him. Jones saw one of the watchers put his hand as a thumbs up."Well… not well, not well but I'm trying." Jones looked across the way.

"Your colleague?" The man instantly frowned, "I'm sorry here, take one of the receipt cards. It's got twenty bucks on it". The man said as his colleague held the card scanner on the other side. "This will get you home fine". Jones thanked the man and headed towards the BART as he looked around him. "Still no colors on the Bart platform." He said disappointedly as the sign gave the times. People sat on the circular curbsides as Jones looked at them. "If these had a triangular point people could at least lean back on them during wait times." Jones thought to himself as the BART showed up. He got in, wasting no time wanting to get back to hunting Nepharius who had set him off into the watchers. Jones wanted to free the souls left in tatters, trapped in disguise who had more qualifications than the average person. "All aboard the BART that will take you home. Fasten your seatbelts that don't exist if you're older and hold onto your liquor cause we're taking you home." The BART conducted as Jones put in his headphones taking a ride home. "Thanks." He said quietly as he laid back on the seat thinking about the day that had happened. The watchers celebrated with Jones giving him the benefit of the doubt. The people of the watchers were secretly

CHAPTER TWENTY-FOUR – CELEBRATION COLLISION

rooting for him as each one fended for themselves and he felt it. As the BART got into the station Jones hopped off walking down the steps as he looked at the one-way escalator going to the top. "This is the fastest way to the top right now? Does it work? Man, we would have replaced this escalator with something more efficient years ago." Jones laughed to himself as he walked through the BART isolating himself. He felt what the watchers felt at that moment. The watchers who used their quirky tools hidden from society to hide from people. Each one of them was secretly laughing at society as the people isolated themselves trading as if they had lower forms of communication. Yet the watchers had some of the most sophisticated communication Jones had seen. "Watchers don't just disguise themselves as broke, you know Jones. These watchers are also famous people too. This is what we call the watcher's way." Jones looked around him seeing no one as he walked home. "Remember they act and sing. It's their disguise for what they are actually doing. Those videos are real." Mira said from behind, appearing as Jones walked alone in the night towards his house. "We've been over this. It's not…not possible." He said to himself as the fireworks from the city sounded throughout all of San Francisco. "The made-up world isn't real. It's up to us to show that. Even if we act outside, off-set. No one's capturing that. Don't you get it?" Jones shouted as no one looked. The streets were empty as everyone else was out.

"I'm going home to sleep. We're left behind in this world to prove to no one while striking some balance of proving it all to ourselves. Nepharius is still out there and what have we done? Gotten arrested, thrown friends in danger, and lost our credibility that's what!" Jones walked angrily. "Hey, come on, it was a celebration today." Mira tried to counsel him as he got closer to his house. "No. This has to end. I'm going to finish school on my own accord. This pressure is getting to me. I can't keep this up for much longer." Jones continued as the road grew slim. The pathway he was used to walking through now seemed dark rather than lit. A happy sign with "be your best!" was written with a flag sticking out from it. "Is this the world? All we have to offer? All we have to offer ourselves?" Jones' thoughts carried on as lights kept off through the fading fireworks into the night. "Okay. Okay, I'll leave you alone for now… you can't catch Nepharius alone. Get your priorities in order." Jones ran faster until his house appeared. He went inside heading straight to bed as he stared at his ceiling. Jones shut down his mind completely as darkness enveloped his thoughts. No galactic space, emptiness, and space ensued.

Chapter Twenty-Five - Mira's Reality

The next day Jones woke up looking blankly at his clock. He pulled the head over his covers not feeling like getting out of bed. "Not today." He sighed knowing that he had to attend school. Lily texted him four times as the alarm kept going off. Jones looked at them leaving her to read. Shortly after three more texts came in from Lily. "Will you answer me and stop being emo?" She said as he looked at it again. Jones put the phone back down as the picture of the Jeep stared at him again. "Alright. Guess I have to get up." Jones woke up out of bed as he answered Lily while brushing his teeth. "Yeah, I'm on my way." Jones texted as he got ready for his day putting on his clothing. He put on his black beanie walking out of the door this time as the car shined from the rain that had poured during his sleep. "Is life always about getting up the next day after some sad shit?" Jones said to himself as he got in the car.

"No. It's about…well no one knows what life's about. Just live." Mira said from behind. "Thought you'd leave me alone?" Jones said in retaliation. "Yeah well, I couldn't leave an idiot to do a professional's job," Mira said, trying to take a jab at Jones. "You aren't the nicest lately but we have to get this done and if you're going to get it done might as well make sure it's right." She nodded in the back as Jones drove towards school. "Yeah, I have to graduate first right?" Jones said He drove with her towards the school. Mira nodded, "You've got less than a month left and a simple essay to finish. One or two more exams. You've got this in the bag." Jones looked towards her, "What bag?" She laughed, "Poor jokes Jones." Jones mentioned it again trying to cheer up the situation as he slowly felt better. "Yeah, poor jokes." He snickered as the street cleared up. In a few short minutes, he arrived at his school again. Jones ran up the stairs to where the class had been in session. He opened the door as the professor had already written the math on the whiteboard. Jones blinked his eyes, feeling drained from the night before as he stood there trying to process what was going on. The formula read the words "late." To him the professor said nothing. Jones walked over to his door as he sat down next to Lily. "Hey." He whispered as the professor continued the class ignoring that he was there. "You're way too late," Lily said in return. "Yeah, I was out late." Lily nodded showing Jones the text message he sent of the picture he took of the city. "Yeah, I know doofus. So, are you going to finish your essay today or not?" She said, questioning him. "Last time we talked about quantum worlds you ran off in the middle of our discussion. Even that guy Tom in the corner who we hardly know asked me about you." Lily sat there for a moment thinking, "On top of that you hardly ate lunch and have been dodging me consistently. What's going on? Do I bother you?" Lily looked back over at Jones concerned about him as she put the nail in the coffin with her last statement.

"Sorry, you wouldn't believe me even if I told you," Jones said in return to her apologizing. "It's not you or me, it's my situation Lily. You've been a great friend so far." Lily rolled her eyes, "Only if your idiot self will listen to me. Then okay. Let's study after school." She said in return Jones sat there for a moment. "Okay," he said as the professor continued the lesson. "Jones, we have another exam coming up," Lily mentioned. The professor stopped writing. "Yes, we do Lily. Very good for keeping up with the class unlike your talking buddy over there." He pointed towards Jones who sat there acting as if the professor hadn't pointed him out. "Me?" Jones said ready to retaliate. "Jones, if you pay attention in class you might be able to finish your essay. I thought you liked this stuff?" The professor questioned him as the class looked around. "I do. Sorry." Jones said defusing the

CHAPTER TWENTY-FIVE - MIRA'S REALITY

situation as fast as he could.

The professor smiled, "Great, I know you understand some of this but help others understand it too. Be quiet or go home." The professor scolded as Jones sat reading the board. Lily offered up her notes again as he copied them down onto his notebook. The classroom's four plain walls and dim lighting made a sense of plainness in the air. After the small altercation between Jones and the professor the class silently paid attention as the day went by. After it ended Lily headed for the door waving Jones to follow her. The professor called Jones up to his desk as she stood there wondering what he was going to tell him. "You've been late far too many times. You know that five percent of your grade relies on this," he said. Jones sat there in front of him. "Even if you have very decent grades you have to set a good example for the rest of the class." He continued as Jones sat there wondering when he could go. "Is something going on?" There it was, the question that Jones got annoyed by. "No, nothing is going on professor. Don't worry about me!" he said. Jones was not able to tell his professor that he had already found multiple ways and people who were light years ahead of them disguised as crazy people on the street. "Now I have to study. May I go, sir?" Jones asked as the professor stood there for a moment thinking about the answer he received. "Yes, you can go. Seems your buddy here wants you to study." Lily and Jones walked out of the classroom together and headed towards the computer room in the study hall. "Wow." Lily said, "You really let the professor put one over you." She laughed as Jones laughed back. "Well, he is giving us exams that we can take home. Makes the course way easier when you can study and have references. Some of us don't have magical memories like Mira…" Jones stopped himself. "Like who?" Lily said curiously. "Friend of mine. Has an outstanding memory." Jones said, covering his tracks. "Oh cool," Lily said as the two of them opened the door walking into the hall to sit down. "So, tell me more about this quantum world," Lily said in curiosity. "Well, legend has it." Jones jokes, "Legend has it that if we were to use our minds at peak capacity mixed with the inner imaginations of what's in front of us, we can create what we imagine." Lily looks at Jones. "Wizards don't exist, Jones." She laughed. Jones corrected her, "No, wizards don't but people who can build it in their minds first given all of the proper tools ahead of time could break it down to its very molecule. Picture an engineer trying to build a rocket.

Every little piece that went into designing can be pulled apart in their minds and built. Hell, this idea is even in a comic book." Jones said thinking about the one he had previously read. "So, what does this have to do with quantum worlds?" Lily questioned him. "Well, by pulling apart and rebuilding every piece at near the speed of light. The only thing that can travel that fast is our thoughts generated by the energy of our brainstorming, this is how we can build things. In theory of course." Jones continued. "This is what my essay is about so far and where I'm at. Except there's one problem…" Jones dropped off thinking about it. "What's the problem?" Lily said, listening in. "The problem is if people who can do this do too much. The people break, getting stuck in between their thoughts, unable to come back to the surface." Jones said. "Like a biological machine breaking down. That is, after all, what we are." Jones said, finishing off his statement. Lily day there amused by Jones ideals. "Sounds like you have understood this. "Yeah. Not everything but with this in my writing I think I can pass the course." Jones said excitedly. "Here I am still trying to understand the basics," Lily said in return pointing to the middle problem. "Even though this is in the book I hardly understand this." She said, staring at it. "That one's hard because it's an off problem with no proper solution," Jones replied, having already solved it ahead of time. "No solution?" Lily asked. Jones continued, "no more than a trick question to send you in loops. Much like when people get stuck in their own thoughts. Trying to find a solution going on loops where a solution doesn't exist. This then leads them to make up their own." Jones said. "It's kind of scary how it pans out." He said lost in his own thoughts. Lily sat there watching Jones. He packed up his book and put it away in his backpack. "I'm beat so I will head home now," Jones said as he got up. Lily waved at him, "Thanks for

CHAPTER TWENTY-FIVE - MIRA'S REALITY

helping me." She happily said. Jones waved back as he went out of the door towards the parking lot.

"I've been waiting for you Harver," Nepharius said. "My crew and I have released the movie. Pretty soon people will understand our world. We will be feared." Jones kept walking, ignoring the voice. "Until you come after us nothing will change Jones. Nothing changes unless you do something." Nepharius laughed as he faded away. Jones didn't know how to respond as he thought of the last time the two of them met on the ship. Jones went over to his car as it started to drizzle. He got into it and headed towards home thinking about Nepharius who taunted him. Jones pulled out the compass that he carried in his car. An old watch was left by Massi in the glove compartment as he stared at it. "This will find you," Jones said to himself as he continued to drive home. After a few minutes, he arrived at the house where his mom was cooking. The rain started to pour down even harder. "I have to train." Jones thought to himself as his mother called out. "Hey, Jones, welcome home!" She said happy to see him. "Thanks, Mom. Hey, do we have any weights?" He asked.

She smiled, "Weights?" Confused by his question. "No, I don't think so." Jones nodded as he put his backpack down in his room. "I'll get a raincoat." He said as he went over to the closet taking a yellow sailing coat. As the rain poured Jones walked out into the backyard by the poolside where weights happened to be. He put them around his shoulders and started to make runs around the pool. His mother stared out the window worried if he had truly healed. As Jones took each step around the pool through the rain. Nepharius whispered, "It's too late to train to catch me now Harver! I've already found where the map is! An old ally told me." He laughed

Jones continued. "It's not too late to start now. I will catch you!" Jones had come from the training outside. He went back inside hanging the coat after he had walked in circles around the outside pool. "Jones honey, do you need help?" His mom said. "Help? Why would I need that?" Jones said as he walked back inside. "You're acting kind of odd. Like a crazy person."

Ms. P voiced in a concerned way. Jones got upset, "I'm not crazy, you're crazy!" He was annoyed at her comment as he went into his room and closed the door. "Help, why do all these people tell me I need to get help? I feel I'm not being listened to. If someone would tell me they understand and listen to me I wouldn't have to repeat myself. Instead, all they do is tell me I ramble and try to force things on me. Then deny they try to!" Jones said, annoyed. Mira appeared sitting on the computer chair. "I understand you. The world may be in turmoil but the focus is you at this moment. You don't need help. You want someone to listen. That's all huh?" Jones nodded, wiping the rain off of his face leftover from his hair as it dripped down onto his T-shirt. "They will never understand. Not until you're all free." Jones lies on his bed thinking of the end of the semester coming up. He could picture everyone standing on the podium as he would get a chance to speak. "Keep on track. Don't let anyone take away the mission from you. You know what you have to do." Mira said, counseling him as she continued to sit in the computer chair.

"Your mom's here. I better go." Mira said as she walked out of the back door that had been left open. Jones lay on his bed listening to the raindrops as each droplet sounded like a different key of the music. Calming himself down from the previous interaction he picked up the mathematics book and started studying. "Jones? May I come in?" His mom said knocking. "Yeah. Go ahead." He said, trying to reconcile. "Sorry about my comment earlier." His mom said. "It's okay." Jones said, "I'm stressed and there were no weights. So, I made my own. That's all…" Jones paused as he trailed off trying not to let his thoughts consume himself. "I see. It makes sense. I brought you some food." His mom said as she tried to relate to his point of view keeping the doctor on speed dial in case. Jones took the food and ate it. "Thanks, Mom, just studying." He said as she lowered her guard. "Okay. Is it good?" She asked. Jones smiled, "really tasty!" He said in return.

His mom smiled as she left the room. Jones got onto his computer and loaded up his DAW. It had been a while since he last made a song. As the

CHAPTER TWENTY-FIVE - MIRA'S REALITY

rain fell, he titled it "Under the rain." appealing to the simplicity of the sound of the raindrops. After a few hours of toying with the program, he was able to start piecing it together bit by bit. As Ike said to Jones, creating a story with panning and sound effects in his music would appeal to many. Jones posted it on SoundCloud as messages started to flow in from all over. "The watchers." Jones thought to himself as each one posted their personality trying to reach out. "Yo, here's our song in return. Spread the word." Messages flowed from all over as Jones read them unexpectedly. As soon as he had uploaded the song and replied he stopped. Jones looked over at the rain continuing to fall as he went back down to lay down. "I suppose the watchers still understand," Jones said to himself trying to rationalize the situation he had put himself in. Between attempting to study and the music his mind started to wander. Jones thought about all of his friends he hadn't seen as he distanced himself from each one of them to protect each person from Nepharius crew, the CIA, and the hospital corporations.

"Yule," Jones said as he lay in bed. "Yule are you around?" He pushed his thoughts through the galactic space to attempt to contact him. "I hear you." Yule came out wearing his council suit in black and green as his red top flashed. "This red top goes off if it senses an energy of danger. Had Star make it for me. Pretty cool right?" He said to Jones. "These hospitals. What's your plan?" Jones sat there questioning him. "Well if you take down Nepharius. These go with it. I've heard some doctors purposely extending the drugs people have to take for more money." Yule said, annoyed. "It's not on purpose but who knows. Nepharius connections go wide. Wide and far across our galactic universe. Although you've put a dent in his plan to obtain the watchers' trust." Yule clapped his hands as he looked at his new suit, proud of the design. "Listen. I'm one of the council of five. The rest of us are busy dealing with the watchers. There is so much more you have yet to see. Free them and us for we will improve the world around us. All of these ideas floating will be made." Jones listened to Yule explain as the droplets slowed to a halt. Nothing but puddles upon one another gathered together as the droplets became invisible. Each puddle still moved to the rain and wind as if doing the bidding of physics. "It's still a mysterious world. Uncle Walt thought so. You can too. You have a similar mind." Jones looked out the window waiting for the droplets to finish. "I don't know who Uncle Walt is. I have much to learn." He replied as he slowly drifted. "Three A.M. is the loneliest hour. Why don't you get some rest?" Yule asked worriedly. "I'll try," Jones mumbled as he fell asleep.

The next day Jones woke up bright and early. His sleep deprivation felt completely gone as he got ready for school. This time Jones swore to you himself that he would be on time as he picked up his backpack headed for the door. His car was completely clean from the rain as it had built up dirt from the night before. "We caught Nepharius on the East store near the sports aisle. The golf clubs with rocket power boosters attached to them." Yule said. "Go, catch him. He's walking on land towards his goal." Jones got in his car and pulled out his compass. "I'm going to be late for school for this." He replied to Yule as he stepped on the gas of his car not paying attention to the traffic on the road. The compass started to move as music played in the background showing Jones the way towards a sporting goods store. The blue veranda stuck out under the sun where many people walked around. Jones parked his car as the sporting goods store said, "Times Hitters." on the front. Jones went inside the store as he was greeted by the owner. "Going golfing?" The man asked as Jones looked around the store. Although his state was no longer sleep deprived as he blinked the store's demeanor changed. Nepharius sat towards the back as his crew was picking up crystals. The purple golf balls shined in front of Jones as the golf club package had a rocket power design on the front. Sports pants and hats littered the aisles as Jones walked further through the store. A "try this." button stuck out into the aisle as Jones went further around the aisle towards the golf club. As he slowly crept up trying not to alert Nepharius crew members Jones froze in place. The aisle turned into caves as crew members picked up the crystals loading them into a

CHAPTER TWENTY-FIVE - MIRA'S REALITY

minecart. Jones blinked again as some people filled their carts with golf balls and clubs. "Jones. Don't take one step closer." A voice came up from behind him as he hid in between the shorts and the pants. As Jones slowly looked behind him it was the Demihuman hunter. "You!" He almost said loudly as he was surprised. "Yeah, it's me. I tracked him down and figured you might be close by." The demi- human hunter said. "Don't engage with them. If you do it will be all over. Each of those crystals has the power to blow up this entire place." Jones frowned, "He's loaded so many."

The two of them whispered to one another as one of Nepharius's crew members walked by them, not noticing as he pushed his cart. "Yes. This isn't where we will fight Nepharius. We cannot light up this place." The demi-human hunter tipped his hat forward as he watched Jones look at one of the golf clubs. "What are these for them?" Jones asked in return. "Oh, you'd love those. These are so powerful they'll hit a crystal through the wall before it even explodes." The demi-human hunter had to stop himself from laughing out loud as another member of the Nepharius crew walked by. "Come around the corner." He urged Jones to inch forward. Jones walked slowly crouched on the aisle as one of the workers came up to him. "If you're going to buy something please do so. Otherwise please leave." The man said as Jones sat there ready to retaliate. Instead, he heeded the demi-human hunters' words and headed for the door. As Jones snuck out towards the door the store manager looked at him. "What are you doing?" Jones stood up. "Be quiet. I'm trying to escape."

The store manager looked back at Jones curiously. "Escape from what?" He said looking around as a short line formed by the front desk. Jones got upset and ran out of the store as fast as he could. "You've blown my cover," Jones shouted as he raced towards the street. The store manager shrugged his shoulders as the demi-human hunter ran behind Jones. The two of them looked behind them as two of Nepharius's crew members were behind them. "You found us eh Jones?" Nepharius said as the two of them dodged through the streets. Watchers started to gather as the two crew members chased them. "Here take this!" The demi-human hunter passed Jones a purple golf ball. "One of the crystals," Jones said. He blinked as he could see the crew members clearly now. Both of them pointed towards telling people to stop Jones and the demihuman hunter. Jones threw the crystal as hard as he could as it bounced on the cement continuously. The golf ball rolled towards the two crew members as watchers scattered."Oh shit." The crystal exploded as the two of the crew members flew back into the building. Jones looked back as Dirt rose from where the golf ball landed disappearing into the distance. "Those two people were weird huh?" The store workers said to one another. "Mentally ill thieves I suppose." The two of them went back into the store as Jones ran back with the demi-human hunter.

"We got away." He said laughing at Jones as he smiled. "Yeah, we did!" Jones said back. "That will put a dent in his forces." He laughed looking at his phone as Jones realized the time. "Oh no! I'm way late for school!" He said as Lily texted him over five times asking where he was. "I have an exam today." The demi-human hunter nodded as the two of them split up. Jones walked towards his car as Mira stood by the side. "Are you okay? I heard what happened from headquarters! I raced over here as fast as I could. The wreckage looks pretty bad." Jones and Mira looked into the distance of the direction he ran from. Smoke filled the air from a burning building further away. "Damn. Zero casualties?" Jones said. Mira nodded. "The watchers scattered in time. Many of them were pleased with what happened and were already spreading the word. You must get back to school to finish your second exam." Jones got into his car speeding off towards school. "I forgot I had an exam today." He said to himself dodging traffic. In a few minutes, he arrived at school running up the steps as fast as he could towards the top. Jones opened the door as the professor looked at Jones wondering why he was sweating."Take this and you'll have to take the exam in ESL 29 instead. Although it is an open book, I decided not to take it home." Jones took the exam from the professor as he looked over at the compass. Nepharius presence disappeared. The chain clanked as

CHAPTER TWENTY-FIVE - MIRA'S REALITY

Jones put it back in his pocket and headed to sit down to take his exam. He knocked on the door reading ESL 29 as the teacher answered. "Can I help you?" The teacher asked.

Jones went in. "This is ESL 29, right? My professor told me to come here to take my test."The teacher looked at Jones as sweat dropped from his body onto the floor. "Seems you made an effort to get here on time. I'll let you take the test here." The teacher opened the door as other students sat there studying. Jones looked at the table as the rest of the students drowned out in the background. He put the test on the table, noticing the clock on the other end ticking away. "This feels like the other room. I wonder if the school was built the same way long ago." Jones thought to himself as everyone else penciled away on their exam. Jones' heart sped up as he focused on the first question. "What is the importance of quantum physics and parallelism?" The first question popped out at Jones as he stressed. "If I don't pass this we've failed." He said to himself. "Take a deep breath Jones and focus on the main goal," Mira said as she echoed in his mind. "Can you help me get through this exam? Look at the other students' papers?" Jones asked as he sat there scratching his head. "I cannot interfere with the physicalities of time. You know what would happen if I do anything before, I'm considered real on the same plane. Even if you were to grab my hand it's much harder to go into your own." Mira explained as she sat there chewing on a chopstick. Her legs were crossed as she sat on the table in front of one of the other students looking from a distance. "Focus and remember the notes Lily has given you." She reminded Jones as he finished taking his few deep breaths. Jones reached down into his backpack pulling out the notes. "Ah, I've got this." He said, reminded of the notes Lily took. As Jones pulled out the notes, he started sifting through them finding the answers to the test. After a couple of hours, he signed the paper at the bottom and walked towards the door. The feeling of relief went over Jones like a burden lifted off of his shoulder. He made his way back over to the classroom as the door said "Leave your test here. I'm out right now." Jones did so in the folder he was given. He started walking towards his car as the sunset slowly went down towards nighttime.

Chapter Twenty-Six – Flash Back

Jones recalled the first time Nepharius had welcomed him on the airlines. "I heard you had landed in Hawaii. Let's meet up and discuss our plans for the magazine!" Jones looked at Nepharius curiously. "What magazine? I thought this was a trip to get better at music?" Jones said as he texted Nepharius. Jones looked out the window with the wooden glass table next to a red couch. Fancy cups and golden displays were laid out on the kitchen counter. Jones walked out of the deck staring over Hawaii's hills as the sun filled the day. "I heard Animal Beats wanted you to do some prospecting for new clients. It's pretty crazy out here. A few labels came into town." Nepharius texted Jones as he got off the couch standing on the front porch where white lounge chairs with a small umbrella popped out. The wooden floor smoothed out and polished to give a finished feeling. "Yeah, I was going to go exploring," Jones said as he looked at his phone waiting for a response. "Well, meet me down by the shoreline and we'll talk." Jones texted back "okay." As he walked towards the door. "Going out Jones?" His dad asked out of curiosity. "Call it a company meeting," Jones replied to his dad as he went out calling the cab. Shortly after the cab arrived in front of the house. "What brings you to Hawaii?" The cab driver asked as Jones got in, wearing a typical tourist shirt. "Oh, you know. I'm here to meet a few club people on a show business trip." He said pointing to the shirt. "Oh cool. I hope you will enjoy your stay around this time." The man said happily as music played in the background.

"Yeah, it will be a good time," Jones said in return as the cab driver headed towards the beach. A bronze-painted car parked by the side with Nepharius standing by the side of it. His friend sat there as well. "We're practicing filming," Nepharius said welcoming Jones with open arms. "Latty over here has been practicing camera work while I've been practicing martial arts." He said as Jones looked around. "Hey, that's pretty cool." He said as the two of them walked down the beachside. "Yeah, man. I've got a few things to show you. Let's go over to where I'm staying after a movie." Jones walked along the roadside with Nepharius as the two of them looked at the trees. "Jones, do you know about watchers and the energy of the earth?" He asked as Jones walked across the roadside next to the beach. "A little. I've learned to sort of watch the wind as it moves through the trees." Jones said in return. "So, you're one of the wind people," Nepharius said in return. "That's sort of your element. If you're a believer in chakras anyway." Nepharius said casually as the two of them walked. "You need to watch this movie we're about to see. How they did the CGI effects and a breakdown. One day, I'm going to make one and get started up again. I need your help starting too with this magazine." He said piecing it together. "You want to be known too right?" Jones thought about it for a moment. "I don't know. I'm not sure I have much of a story to tell yet." Jones said thinking about the conversation.

"Well, if you give me some time we'll dip into other people's stories," Nepharius said again nonchalantly. Jones likes the idea of reviewing others in what they were doing. It interested him in how these people got to be at the peak of their game. Jones looked back over at the theater as no one was around. He stood by the theater looking inside. "Guess it's been rented out huh?" Jones said out of curiosity. "Yeah. Well, not many people go here." The two of them sat down watching the movie together as they got ideas. As the movie played on for two hours Jones sat there absorbing the details. Wondering what made a movie a good movie. As the show ended Nepharius got up walking out of the movie theater. Jones followed him as he called a cab. "Come, let me show you something else." The two of

CHAPTER TWENTY-SIX – FLASH BACK

them hopped into the cab. "I can't leave this island yet but I will one day." He said as the cab took them down towards a mountainside. He waved at a man who opened up a barbed wire fence as he walked into where people were moaning in pain. One man had his eye covered while others had their legs or arms bandaged. "This is the recovery station. I've been staying here a while." He said as he waved to everyone. "Some of these guys will be helping us with the movie. They know a lot more than they seem." Jones walked around briefly with Nepharius as beds were layered out with a tiled floor.

"I see," Jones said, having nothing to say. He absorbed the looks of the place, one sink in the back with multiple toilets and white. Green on the beds as people lied down making sounds from pain to PTSD anxiety. "It's time to go," Nepharius said to Jones as he took him out of the place. "Hungry at all?" He said to Jones curiously. "I'm all good, man. Thanks." Jones said as Nepharius called a cab. "I'm showing you these things because you asked to see a different world. Perceived differently than what most people see," he said. "I know you have never been on this side of the fence but you'll see. These are decent guys. Tossed aside by society's wake to be forgotten about." A man with a skull cross and bones walked by in a blue hat. "Take the bus home. Go right to the mall and we'll talk later." Jones took the bus thinking about what had happened as he sat there contemplating what had happened. Nepharius had a plan and he knew it from the start. Jones went to the mall shortly after taking the bus as he sat there in the animal beats shirt. He went into the phone store where a lady stood. "I'd like a charger for my phone," Jones said to the lady as she looked at him. "Hey, I know you. You work with animal beats. My boyfriend loves one of your musicians." It was Jones' first year and he didn't know how to respond.

"Yeah?" He said as he reached for the charger. "Can I get an autograph?" She asked Jones. "Wouldn't you want an autograph or phone call from him instead? I mean…" Jones thought to himself. Instead, he reached out and wrote it on a sticky note. "Um… sure no problem." He said, giving her the sticky note back. "What's going on?" The man asked in the back. "That guy's famous," she said. Jones looked around as the guy got up. "You're famous?" he said. Jones waved it down. "No, I'm not at all." He said as he tried to leave. "I've got to go." He made an excuse to leave the store. "Why don't you go have fun tonight. One of the label owners is playing at a club." Jones got a text from Nepharius. "Just head there. They know who you are already." He continued as Jones went away from the mall standing upstairs. "Alright." He said curiously not understanding anything going on. A man with a bandana stared at his phone with a tablet as he was pulling file folders out of his tablet as two hippies sat on the couch near him. "Hey, man can you get us directions?" Jones nodded looking up directions for them as the other man kept cutting film bits and pieces.

Jones grew curious as the two hippies offered weed. "Make someone else's day. I'm alright thank you." Jones said, rejecting the offer. "What are you doing?" Jones asked the man. "Cutting film pieces on my tablet for this band's next showing. I used to work on band videos professionally." He said "I wanted out because the whole lot of it is too crazy. You'll find out if you work in that industry. I'd love to chat more but I have to go." He said turning Jones away. "Peculiar," Jones said to himself standing around looking at the poster. "Well alright." He said again as he went over to the showing time. "If you come get a drink free!" It said at the bottom as Jones walked over towards the entryway of the mall. He had already called three cabs throughout his day to get around. Nightfall was hitting over the city as the poster sat there as if to welcome him into the party. After a few hours of exploring Jones got in the cab heading for the bar and nightclub in Hawaii. He stood in line next to a man with blonde hair and a black shirt. "That will be twenty bucks." The bouncer said as Jones dishes for it in his pocket. "I don't have twenty on me. Only my card." The man with blonde hair and a black shirt came up to Jones. "You're a ridiculous one, aren't you?" he said. "Here, I'll pay your twenty bucks on your way in." He said giving the bouncer twenty. "Looks like a fun show right?" He said as he held out his hand. "Yeah.

CHAPTER TWENTY-SIX – FLASH BACK

Yeah, it does." Jones said in return. "Names Spun." He said smiling. "Nice to meet you, Spun." Jones looked at his phone as Nepharius texted him. "The radio show knows you're there. Enjoy man." Jones looked at his text scratching his head as he went into the party. People were beautifully dressed as the entire night went by. The energy of the bar and the lights shined down in the night as Jones could see what Nepharius had said. "It doesn't matter how you dress. It's what you're doing during that time. You'll see soon." All of the innuendos passed over Jones's head as he stood around after drinks were ordered. He went up to the front to try to get the manager's attention. "Here on business for Animal beats," Jones said to himself. The bouncer came up to Jones, "Hey man, fuck you and fuck off." He said as Jones stood in the corner. The manager walked up to Jones talking to him over the turntables as the crowd danced. "It's okay. Talk to me after the show." Jones looked at him as people danced on the speakers. "Let people dance. They're trying to have fun." A shorter man said to Jones. "Yeah, sorry I didn't know," Jones said as the sound went in and out of the equipment. One of the radio hosts spotted Jones.

"Hey!" She waved pointing to him. A circle formed where Jones got inside and danced in it. "I see you over there!" She thanked him for dancing and kissed him on the cheek. Everything happened fast inside the club. Jones wasn't sure if he made a bad or good impression. "These idols are so pretty huh?" The man said. "Yeah, I suppose," Jones said, feeling indifferent and having trouble loosening up. "Let loose a little." The man said as Jones turned to him. "I threw this show. Let them dance up front and relax." He said with an inviting voice. Jones sat outside until 3:09 AM as a meeting was being held. Jones let it finish and explained a little about Animal Beats. "We'll keep that in mind." The manager said and left. As the party slowly quieted down. Jones went home thanking Spun who let him in. His flashback ended as Jones paid attention to where he was walking. "I guess for my first time it wasn't so bad," Jones said to himself. Jones looked back recalling his mistakes as he walked to his silver car in the parking lot at school. "Crazy times. I get it now." He agreed with Nepharius despite his bad intentions. Jones drove his car home to prepare for the next day. As Jones went into his house his mother greeted him at the door. "Welcome home Jones. How was school?" Jones looked at his mom and paused for a moment. "School was good. Well, it was okay. I took a test and I was late but I think I passed it." His mom looked at him. "Sounds like you studied hard and passed." She said with a smile as she hugged him. "Yeah. I think I passed anyway. Well, I tried." Jones said, trying to make short talk. "Hey, mom. Do you think ideas come from others to build off of or is society too greedy that we don't give them out because we're afraid of people stealing our work?" Jones asked curiously as the tea kettle boiled. "I'm not sure what you're asking." His mom said in return. "Why do you ask that?"

Jones looked at his mother curiously as the kettle steam stopped automatically. The water dinged with Jones standing there as if he had something to say. "Curiosity," Jones said in return. "Well, I think people are a mixture of both. Ideas can also be a mixture of both. Some people are greedy and others want to see the world thrive. Is this a psychological question?" Jones thought for a moment. "No, I guess it's more of my own curiosity and philosophical question." Jones shrugged his shoulders as she took a tea bag from the cupboard. "If you want some tea, I did make some for you." She said counseling Jones. "I can tell you need it because you're looking at the tea." Jones walked over and took some from the pot. "Mother's intuition?" Jones said curiously. His mom laughed, "Mother's intuition." she said. "I saw you've been out a lot. A package came in the mail from someone. It's directly addressed to you." Jones took the package as it read on the outside open carefully. Jones headed towards his room. "Okay! Thanks, mom." He said as he opened up the package cautiously after staring at it. The package read "From the party man. We're going on tour soon. You're a pretty crazy kid - Nepharius pirate crew. J. Cougie & the Boogie boys' ' Jones sat down thinking about it. "Signed Taz." Jones eye's drifted towards the bottom. Nepharius would learn about Jones's whereabouts soon if he wasn't careful. Although the two of them were connected Nepharius was unable to track Jones without a compass of his own. Inside the package

CHAPTER TWENTY-SIX – FLASH BACK

held a small piece of paper and a USB stick. "Use this when you feel you need to call us." Jones took it in his hands and felt it as the USB lit up in green. "Call us huh…" he said to himself, putting the USB stick away. "One day soon I'll use this." Jones put it away quickly as he turned on his computer to start writing more of his essay. "Jones, are you okay?" A text came up from Lily as he sat on the computer to start typing away. "Yeah, I'm fine. I made it in time." Jones texted Lily back as the color of his text messages turned different colors. The whole background of the phone changed as we. He blinked again looking down at his phone. "Huh, I thought it was there." He said to himself as he started to type on the computer. "Myths about quantum loops and quarks can be seen as something nonexistent. Twenty-four had given a study to mindset travel used by freemasons in the nineteen twenties. This eventually led to the development of the electric car as well as mysterious happenings during this time. It is noted that Mr. Sla knew the transfer of energy more than anyone. Although he died a lonely man. He left the world with magical inventions." Jones kept typing as the night fell.

"If Sla and uncle Walt met, I bet there would have been a beautiful riot," Jones said to himself thinking of the time. "Or any of the musicians back then in today's society." The thought continued as a squirrel popped up on the windowsill again. "You're thinking too much Jones. Why don't you take a break? Slow down." Jones looked at the squirrel as its black beady eyes peered into his. "Mach three like that doctor said, right?" Jones said in return. "I don't care. This needs to get done and things aren't finished." The squirrel moved along slowly to the other side of the tree as Jones shut his window. "You'll lose it, Jones. Heed my warning, we have been guarding you." Jones looked out the window as the squirrel disappeared. "Guardians come in all shapes and sizes I suppose." He said, sighing as he continued his essay. "Squirrel and deer. Thought my protection would be more than that." As he continued to write. Jones wrote throughout the night until early morning. His eyes turned dark from the lack of sleep from the night before. "Graduation is within the next week or so!" Lily texted Jones excited about the standing ovations. "Are you going to speak in front of everyone? I heard you were nominated." Lily texted. Jones tried texting back as he sat there blank-minded. "Nominated? Me?" He asked her about the school's choice. "Are you sure this isn't a mistake? Jones asked Lily in curiosity. "Mistake? No. You're being nominated to speak. Our professor sent out an email today!" She texted back.

Jones scratched his head out of confusion as he opened up his email. It had been a while since he checked as the spam email no longer had club invites in it. Jones had spent the time to clean it out and unsubscribe so that he would be able to easily see the real invites from Nepharius crew members. "Guess I'll get ready for school," Jones said to himself walking over to his backpack imagining the dress that Mira had on. "This could be used on backpacks too, couldn't it?" He thought to himself as he picked it up heading straight for the door. Jones hadn't bothered to shower as he was determined to be on time. After a few minutes of driving, he parked his car in the usual spot by the back parking lot and headed towards his class. This time arriving early at school Jones walked through the back-lake side where water shot out from a mini lake surrounded by grass and flowers. Ducks walked on the other side looking up at the sky as if something was there. Jones looked over at the ducks as each one of them stopped looking at him. "Right. I thought I was low energy lately." Jones said as the ducks continued to stare. Jones walked forward heading towards his class as he ignored the ducks. Cooks from each of their class poured out onto the concrete out of their room as Jones dodged them fighting his way towards the math class through the crowds. Lily stood near the classroom door waiting for the professor as she smiled. She waved her bag back and forth seemingly lackadaisical as Jones approached her. "Jones! There you are!" she said. Her smile faded. "You look like you've been hit by a train. What happened?" She asked him curiously. "I stayed up all night attempting to finish this essay. I chose a topic that has given me more trouble than its worth." He stood there leaning on the door as she chuckled. "Try not to fall asleep in class this time. Our professor will have you marked down."

CHAPTER TWENTY-SIX – FLASH BACK

Jones stared at the sky for a moment collecting his thoughts as he silently feared the loss of his grade. "Got any caffeine? I will grab a coffee then." He said to Lily.

"Wait, do you want a coffee or are you asking if I have any caffeine to offer?" She said digging into her backpack. "Here's a caffeine pill. As long as you aren't asking me for Adderall." She joked as he took it out of her hand. Jones chewed the caffeine pill. "You're supposed to swallow it, not chew it. It's not a gummy caffeine pill." Lily said laughing again. "You're too much Jones. Also, you're early for once." Jones looked at Lily swallowing what's left of the pill as the taste filled his mouth. Feeling disgusted by the caffeine that sat there he went to grab a drink of water. "I'll be right back. This tastes like a mixture of sawdust and powdered soup" Jones said, walking off to the water fountain. He sat by it taking a drink of water as the professor walked up to the door greeting Lily. "Right on time as usual." The professor said, "Where is Jones? Is he late again?" Lily stood there for a moment trying to calm down from laughing at the incident. "He's on time for the second time this semester sir," she said. "He's having a quick drink of water." She continued as the professor stood there unlocking the door. "Good. He's been nominated. I have to make sure his essay is stellar before we send him out on the podium in the next coming weeks. He had aced the last test." The professor mistakenly said blurting out the end piece. Lily responded quickly as the rest of the students and Jones started pouring in. "Good for him. Expected from that dude." She smiled as Jones looked back at Lily curiously. "What?" Jones said. "You aced your test," Lily whispered as Jones did a short yes with his arm. "About time I got something right." Jones's day brightened up as the class started. The professor stood up and made his announcement. He hinted that he was going to announce Jones had been nominated.

"As you know, class. One of our classmates has been nominated for his outstanding research and essay work. He will be speaking at the graduation ceremony. Please be sure to have your documents and ID ready to be scanned into your diploma…" Jones zoned out. "Wai, what? Scanned into my diploma?" He pinched himself as students nodded in affirmation. "Have your driver's license and your major penned down properly" Jones nodded. "This feels like the DMV." He joked, whispering to Lily who had already been holding on to her laughter from before."Yeah, at least our professor isn't zombified like most of the DMV people behind the desk." She said in return. "Okay class, please take out your notes as there will be one more exam. This exam will be taken home." He said as the entire class cheered quietly. "Thanks to one of your classmates, I'm giving this class the privilege." Some of the students looked towards Jones noticing that it could be him while others talked to one another quietly. "Right, now who can tell me…" the professor started speaking as Jones drifted off to sleep. "Looks like the mission will be complete, Jones," Mira said smiling as she came dressed in her original clothing. "You've done a great service this time." She said proudly Jones smiled back. "Although you'll be able to catch Nepharius and this is simply a stepping stone of what's to come." She warned Jones telling him not to get too comfortable with her tone of voice. Putting her hand on the desk right next to him she snapped her fingers. Jones woke up feeling the caffeine slowly enter his body. "Glad to see you're paying attention this morning." The professor said as Jones already started to zone out again. "Lily, I missed most of what he said. I'll trade you a meal for the rest of your notes this week." Jones said. "A meal and a cookie on top," Lily said in return. "You also have to help me study." Jones waved his hand. "Alright I will, that's fine," Jones said, trying to dismiss the demands quickly. Lily smiled, "After class, you can take pictures and copy what you need." Jones zoned out again.

"Great, I'll be able to get this done." After an hour of class, the professor got up. "Jones. May I talk to you for a moment?" He said as Jones took his backpack off of the floor. "Your essay. I need it two days ahead of time to read it before your standing ovation. You'll be speaking in front of other professors and many students. Although it says you were nominated it seems the system put you through." Jones scratched his head. "Do I

CHAPTER TWENTY-SIX – FLASH BACK

have to speak sir?" He asked, trying to dodge the responsibility. Jones hadn't practiced speaking in front of hundreds of people before. He had only practiced speaking in front of his mirror on an off day at best. "No Jones. A nominee can't turn down their position during graduation. I will help you review." Jones sighed. "Okay, sir." He said walking towards the door where Lily waited. She was leaning against the wall ready to go as she stared at the vending machine. "Ready to give me that cookie?" she said Jones rolled his eyes. "Come on, let's go," He said as the both of them started walking towards the cafeteria to order their food. "Okay, Lily, hand over the notes please," Jones said, extending his hand to hers. "No. Cookies first." She said jokingly. Jones smiled at her. "Cookies first huh?" Jones walked over to the cafeteria counter. "One giant cookie. The biggest one you have in stock please." Jones said as he ordered the cookie. "Coming right up." The student said. "Hey, I recognize you. You're that kid that researched quantum worlds or something. It was published in our school article." Jones wondered for a moment. "That doesn't seem right. I just gave my essay to the professor." The student smiled. "You didn't hear huh?" The student shook his head in dismay. "What?" Jones said completely clueless about what had happened. "When your professor read your essay, he did not only go wide-eyed but I heard he ran through the hallways as he said he hadn't seen anything like it before." Jones paid the student and walked over to Lily. "Guess who made school news," Jones said.

Lily looked at him pointing to the papers in the cafeteria with Jones' face on it. "You, dummy. Why else would I ask for your help to study?" She laughed. "Here's the notes." Extending her hand as Jones put the cookie in hers. Jones took the notes sitting down by the table as Lily split the cookie in half offering it to him. "I'm confused on question two," Lily said in her voice as she got a text from her boyfriend. "Can you help me before I go to meet up with my boyfriend?" She asked. "Sure," Jones replied as he checked over question two. "Ah, the type one loop," Jones said. "This is time differentiation. If two people are thinking of the same idea at once and trying to claim the idea without an agreement, we end up back in a time pool. This pool eventually leads to a loop where one person will be stuck and the other will be able to move forward." Lily looked at Jones in surprise. "Kind of like a time battle?" She asked out of curiosity. "Exactly like a time battle. Since it's our minds that battle for space. Only one can have that space at that point of time even if we are on the same plain." Jones continued. "I sure wish I had your smarts," Lily said.

"Well, I don't think I am," Jones said in return. "Watched a lot of YouTube and studied, I guess. This stuff interests me." Jones finished off his statement as Lily shook his hand. "Thanks for the help, Jones. I'll see you in class and at graduation!" She said excitedly while packing her suitcase. Jones walked out of the cafeteria towards the grassy field as the sunlight shone upon the school. Mira appeared right next to Jones as she sat next to him. "Are you ready to move on to the next steps soon Jones? The trip will be dangerous, you know." She said, looking at him. Her dress reflected the color of the sunlight as students walked by eating their sandwiches and racing to their next classes. "Danger is becoming my middle name," Jones said laughing at the poor situation. "Yule might even be accompanying you this time, Jones," Mira said with confidence. "You must be nicer to him. He's trying his best to get along with you." Jones looked at Mira gazing upon her dress that reflected the sunlight. "Where do you get such cool dresses anyway?" Jones asked curiously. "Well… Hestia usually makes them as I said before but this one was made by my friends back at the galactic bar. You know, the one we first met at?" Mira said, questioning Jones. "Oh yeah, I remember. You were sitting there eating ideas. Trying to feed off of them." Mira laughed, "Actually, eating those ideas had kept me from falling under Nepharius control. This has given me a chance to fight back on your side. I haven't had to worry about it since." Jones opened up his phone checking messenger as the demi-human hunter sang while walking towards his boating area. "Merry happy-with day to you good fellow!" He said filming the cracks of the sidewalk off of his phone.

CHAPTER TWENTY-SIX – FLASH BACK

Jones messaged back, "Thanks, good sir. Any trouble on your end?" He asked curiously. "None, all the best of festivities and happy days are of these docks. Nepharius has cleared out of his corners caught like a dog's tail. He is on the run with a few crystals last we saw. You'll have to chase him down the right way Jones."Jones looked at Mira curiously. "What does he mean the right way?" Jones asked as he looked around the school. "You have to capture Nepharius so he cannot leave. So, we can keep him trapped forever in his mind." Mira continued. Jones listened, he sat there thinking about the risks. "Soon I will graduate and then I will take care of this matter," Jones said. As the sun slowly set near the grass with Jones lying by the brick building, he got up. "My journey is coming to an end soon Mira, isn't it?" He asked her. "Will you disappear?" Mira sat there smiling trying to put on a poker face. "I'm not sure. I'll either be brought into reality or be separated. In these moments I will have always been here though." She grabbed Jones's hand as he got up with her. "Okay." Jones walked over to where construction was going on for the podium. He could see the football field completely cleared out as the stage was set up off to the side. "I'll be standing there huh?" He said to himself. Mira stood by. "Hope you're prepared, Jones. I'm going to head back to headquarters." Mira left in a flash before Jones could object. Jones walked back over to his car going over what Mira had told him as it rang in his head. He continuously thought of the small town of Lafayette as he drove through the highway back down towards his household. "No sleep for the inevitable," Jones said to himself as he turned up the music driving home.

Jones thought about the movie theater that had an anarchist symbol painted on it. An old movie hadn't been taken down from the place in years. Jones pulled over his car as he headed towards it where the soldier stood tall. "Here lies the town of Lafayette connected to Louisiana Lafayette." Jones sat down on the statue's bench staring out as the rounded bench connected to the other side. The old theater doors were painted an old gray as the spray paint stuck out to Jones. "I swear we will find out who did this." One voice came from around the door as Jones leaned in from the bench. "Is someone talking?" He said to himself, running his hand over the old movie poster. "Yeah; he burned down the bohemian grove! That damned council of five is always messing with us archons." Jones froze at a distance listening to the voices come out of the door as an old lady came up behind him. "Got an interest in the old theater? She said curiously as Jones looked at her. "What did they play here?" She stood at a distance from him as her black hat with a brown feather sticking out of it. "Oh, old movies. Mostly black and white." She said smiling. "You seem to like the history around this town don't you." The lady questioned Jones as he stepped away from the door. The voices subsided as Jones sat there staring out at the park. "Yeah well. I wanted to find out more about society so that I can build on it. I hope they reopen this theater one day." Jones said. A for sale sign sat above the building.

"I hope so too. You don't know what you're missing!" She smiled as the theater stood still in the dusk sunset. Jones got up to further walk towards the library as the day passed by. He blinked as the sleep deprivation took over him. A giant bear stood out in bronze made of multiple engineering tools. Jones could feel the energy forming around it as a wolf howled in the distance. "No no, I have to get home." He could hear the wolves getting closer as he thought the engineered bear started to move. A name was written on the sign below as Jones quickly read behind it. "STARS prototype one. Bear-bot." Jones looked over at the bear as he ran down the street with other people looking at him. "Sounds like Star to me. Damn them this time!" The bear attracted the wolves as Jones's scent had attracted them. The old lady in the black hat disappeared. Jones kept running down the road as the empty town didn't make a sound. Up ahead a deer sign stuck out on a building as Jones ran towards it. He had memorized all of the pathways. Jones turned down into the garage where the wolves slowly sniffed him out disappearing into the distance. Two deer stood out at the entrance of the garage. "This is what we have been protecting you from. Not only Nepharius but there are creatures of these forests that will come for you as well." The deer stomped its foot as Jones for the first time

CHAPTER TWENTY-SIX – FLASH BACK

visualized a shield over the garage. He shivered in place looking outwards towards the night sky that had befallen the town. "This way." The deer said as Jones followed it through the back of the garage out towards the veterans building where it lit up. He gulped down his Gatorade as he sat there by the cornerstone trying to read the quartz names to distract his mind off what had happened. "You still must walk the rest of the way. We will guide you towards your house." Another voice echoed in Jones's head as the squirrel appeared on the rooftop of the veterans building. "Do you understand now? The energy and the situation? You are the only free man and people want you gone for control." A squirrel continued. "I don't know what to say," Jones said as he continued to walk with the creatures making sounds in the bushes. "Thank you for saving my life," he said, talking to them as a runner gave him a weird look. The runner passed by Jones paying him no attention. Jones continued to walk into the night sky as he turned the corner towards his house. The moonlight hit the school right in the middle of the triangle as flowers with lights on them sticking out of the center of the road. Colorful lights lit up the entire pathway home through the military fence as the hillside inclined. Jones kept walking as more deer stared at him from a distance.

"Well, this is good," Jones said. "Protected by deer and squirrels instead of Mira and Yule." He said to himself. "What a joke." Mira appeared shortly after hearing that. "I thought we had a great day…these deer and squirrels are physical. I don't have the power yet to protect you." Mira kicked a rock as it moved into the gutter. Jones moved his foot kicking the same one towards the stream as it carried away. He could see his reflection off the moonlight as color went down the stream. "Oil from a car? Or cotton candy tasting water?" Jones asked himself. "Which one do I want it to be?" He said curiously as he moved in towards his home. Jones calmed down watching the moonlight move off the stream onto the cement as he slowly made his way towards his room. "What's next owl's with lasers in their eyes?" He asked Mira. "Well…" Jones threw his hand up in the air as an owl with red eyes illuminated from the moonlight's reflection. "Mira why?!" Jones said "too overkill?" Mira replied, swatting away the owl with her hand. "Okay, shoo- "she said as it flew up into a higher tree. "You're turning beauty into a destructive being. That isn't right. I'll protect myself next time." Jones said, talking to himself in his room as the door was shut. "You didn't greet your mom." Mira snapped back warning Jones that he was being too loud. "She's in her office and busy. I'm going to head to bed." Jones said as he put on his pajamas and went straight to bed. "If it weren't for me, you'd already be eaten or killed by something. From now on you're under the full watchful eye of the headquarters!" Mira said angrily. Her eyes went from calm as the room spun in Jones' mind. A galactic pattern appeared on Jones's roof as he waved his hands. "Okay, okay. Stop! I get it!" He said as Mira calmed down. The pattern disappeared. "Good. Now we've got a speech to prepare for. The CIA from your beloved hospital called. They said they wanted their specimen back." Mira said. "I've been talking to them and negotiating for you. You do realize who that specimen is right?" Jones looked back at Mira taking a deep long stare as he caught on. "I see. I'll make sure I'm not so hot on the plate. Keep them off my back. I have to graduate."Mira nodded. "Yes, you do. There's a man by the name of Bascon that understands how to code and build more than most. He's been raving about his ability to understand that gold book lately. The one with those weird inscriptions…starts with a T… I think. Anyway, to even meet Bascon you have to get into that school up in Sonoma." Mira finished her statement. "Now that you're home safe and listening to me intently. It's time for me to go again. Yule is calling me to our other tracker." Mira headed for Jones's door as Jones grabbed her hand. She stared at him for a moment. "Thanks. He said hugging Mira. She smiled back. "Right then ya troublesome man. I'll check back with you soon." She left as Jones went back to his bed to stare at the ceiling which now had a blank spot. There was no dirt showing as he stared at a small curvature from Mira's galactic point. "Reality is intermixing again," Jones said to himself. "Maybe Mira has a shot at getting onto the same plane after all…" Jones drifted off to sleep in his thoughts as they swirled around like the galaxy.

Chapter Twenty-Seven – Mira's Appearance.

The next day he sat up semi-refreshed. The rain hit the ground as his senses could hear the droplets double their normal volume. Jones recalled every piece of song in his head that he had heard during the moments he experienced. Trying not to relive how he felt in every situation he sat up looking out the window. "This place sometimes makes me feel like I wasn't born to live like this. Born for more in its own soulful way. I want to inspire many others." Jones said to himself as he tapped his foot on the key with the song playing in his head. "Each piece of this song represents each feeling of that moment in time. The universal language back in time. The only way we can truly go there." Jones recited a piece of his essay as he mimicked himself on the stands in front of the professors. "Hey, Jones, I made breakfast!" His mom shouted from the kitchen as she heard him get out of bed. "Thanks, mom!" he shouted back, quietly starting over from the beginning. Jones looked at the clock. Although he wasn't graduating it was three days until he had to speak. The pressure of standing in front of students was getting to him along with the outstanding exam he had yet to take. Lily still had not texted Jones today even though he was already late. "I wonder if the school got canceled," Jones said to himself looking at his email off of his phone. "Class is still in session." popped up on his screen along with "Buy your diploma garb." in bright blue colors. Jones clicked it looking at the price. "Hey, mom. I don't have a lot right now," he said as he scrolled through the graduation garb's pricing. "Do you think I can borrow forty bucks?" he asked her, hoping for a yes.

"You know, Jones." His mom yelled back as she flipped over an egg,
"Back when I was in college, I worked my way through with a part-time job." She scolded Jones as he came into the kitchen in his pajamas and blue tee. "Well, alright." she sighed. "Only because I heard you've been doing quite well in school lately. In three days, you are graduating it seems." She smiled, offering him a plate of eggs with bacon on the side. "Buttered toast with that?" she asked Jones as he shook his head. "I'll take the egg as is with bacon. No eggs on the buttered toast thanks." Jones said as he took the plate to sit down. "Someday, these dishes will wash themselves. Beyond even having a dishwasher," he suggested. His mom chimed in, "Yeah what? They'll grow arms and walk their little legs into the dishwasher too? While we're at it, why don't we have a robot that puts away glasses." she laughed as she ate her piece of bacon. "I swear. Robotics will be this way one day. It will be safe." Jones said happily. "Well for now it doesn't exist, even if anything is possible." his mom joked back. "So, take your little tooshie over to the sink and put them into the dishwasher for us." his mom said, trying to build a habit for Jones. "Lately you have been leaving multiple dishes. I've had to clean them in the morning. This is unacceptable behavior." She continued to scold Jones with her finger waving back and forth at him. "Mom, I'm sorry I've been busy with school," Jones said.

"In the dishwasher." His mother replied. Jones finished up his bacon and eggs with a sigh. "Trying to battle with some of humanity's worst and being reduced to a dishwasher," Jones said, annoyed by the responsibility. "I suppose I don't mind cleaning, if it's after myself I must do so anyway." he shrugged as he slowly put the dishes in the washer. "If this thing could tell me if it was run yet that'd be helpful," he said, unable to tell if they were dirty or not. "Are these dirty?" He shouted to his mom who was now by the laundry. "Yes, they are!" she shouted back. Jones put the plates

CHAPTER TWENTY-SEVEN – MIRA'S APPEARANCE.

into the dishwasher and walked towards the front door. He looked at the musical instrument hanging from the closet space as he wondered about it. "The same instrument next to the old war cane," Jones said to himself. "I will learn to play this at one point." He mentally took note of the wooden instrument that had wooden balls hanging down to each string. Picking one up he tapped it against the steel as it made noise each time the gray ball bounced. "Sounds like a mix between a violin and an erhu," Jones said, distracted by the instrument. "Are you going to school?" his mom yelled, trying to beat the sound of the dishwasher. "Oh shoot!" Jones said to himself now twenty minutes later than normal. "Yeah, mom!" He said quickly getting fully dressed and heading out the door.

Jones wandered over to his car slowly contemplating the wolf sounds that followed him to his house. "Nepharius must also have animals on his side if I have some as well. It would only make sense. The book of arbiters said nothing about this though." Jones said to himself worried about what might happen if he hadn't succeeded in slowing Nepharius down. As Jones started to drive his car towards school, he checked both sides of the road. The entire neighborhood was quiet with everyone indoors. Not a single soul walked outside. Even the wind that brushed through the trees seemed overly calm. "Today's exam day," Jones said to himself as he got on the highway. I'm going to graduate." he stated, excitedly proud of his work. As Mira and Yule suggested, Jones heeded their words of warning. He focused his main task on graduating from school. Jones parked in the back parking lot parking his car next to a tree as the show stuck out in perfect light over dark. "The perfect chi." He mentioned himself earlier. As he looked down his socks were worn in black and white. Jones walked towards his classroom where his socks showed as Lily waved. "Hey, Jones! Good to see you!" She smiled. "What's with those socks?" She questioned as he stood there at the door. "Oh…uh, trying out a new fashion. I got kind of bored at home." Jones lied as he tried to stay in tune with himself. "Thanks for helping me study. We've been doing so well you could practically bomb this final exam and pass the course. It's to be an open book so we can take it in the study room." Lily said as the professor walked up towards the classroom door.

"Good morning Lily," he said. And turning to Jones, "Good morning to you as well Mr. Harver." as he unlocked the classroom door. "You two always seem to be first to school these days. Makes me proud to have students like yourselves." The rest of the students slowly poured in chattering, as the topics of graduation sparked conversations throughout the room. Even Tom, who was generally quiet, seemed chipper about being done. "Today's final will be an open book as most of you know. However, for those who have been in our school newspaper, we expect more. You will be receiving a different exam." the professor said. The entire class looked over at Jones as he raised his hand, "I object to this sir. You can't change the whole curriculum at my expense!" Jones complained as the two of them glared at one another. "The teachers would like to invite you into our lab research depending on how well you do. You have already passed the course." Jones sat back down. Was the school allowed to do this or was it of special request? Jones' head spun as he was now not only giving a speech but writing a lab research report for his last few days at school. Lily patted Jones on the back. "Isn't that great Jones? You've got everything you've wanted." she smiled. Jones frowned, "What if I don't want to be inducted in the school lab?" Jones asked the professor. "I don't see why not. Don't you love this type of work?" the professor said as the rest of the class sat there watching their conversation. "Well. No, I have other plans." Jones said. "Suit yourself. The lab will be open to you if you're interested in the future. In that case, I want you to practice your speech. You're dismissed for the day." said the professor. Jones got up taking his backpack as the rest of the class discussed curiously. "Well alright then," Jones said in return. He walked outside of the classroom taking the few papers in his hand as he went out to the field practicing what he was going to say. Mira walked up from behind the red-bricked wall. "Hey crazy!" she said. "I saw what happened." she happily continued. Jones looked back

CHAPTER TWENTY-SEVEN – MIRA'S APPEARANCE.

at Mira in wonderment. She was wearing black and green again, ready to go out. "You know. I might have a way to get you here." She laughed. "I am already here!" Jones shook his head. "I mean actually here." As he read over his research paper Jones realized the connectivity. "You see if I can build you in others' minds collectively before graduation. During the graduation, I might be able to help you." Jones said as he read over the paper.

Jones pointed to the paragraph that stated about minds working together to formulate ideas. "Right here. I have a plan. First I will draw you into existence." Mira laughed questioning Jones, "So I get to pose? She took one arm and put it over her head moving back and forth as she spun out on the grassy field. "This wouldn't be a bad break from worrying about Nepharius." Jones took out a sheet of paper. He began drawing what he saw in his mind. Mira's long hair and yellow eyes started to come together on the piece of paper as Kali walked by. "Jones! That application idea — it's not bad. I started to build it with my team." Kali said excitedly looking back at Jones. Jones looked up at Kali as he spoke. The wind blew as Jones followed the direction through the trees looking around him. Lily also saw Jones from a distance and approached him. "Hey, Jones!" The both of them now stood there looking at the piece of paper. "I didn't know you drew. What character's that supposed to be?" Kali asked Jones curiously. "It's someone called Mira. She's been really helpful lately." Jones said. Lily and Kali looked at one another confused. "Okay…?" Kali said. "I assume that what she's wearing here isn't actually what she wears around you?" he said with his eyebrows raised. Jones thought about it for a moment. "Uh, no, she usually wears a yellow dress. Like the sun," he said smiling as Mira stood off to the side pouting that she got interrupted. "Did you pass your exam?" Jones asked Lily as the two of them looked at the piece of paper, curious about Mira. "Oh, yeah! I think I did quite well thanks to you. I was headed home and saw you up here so I decided to say thanks and see you at graduation" Lily said. "Well, you can say it now." Jones laughed, making his first joke. The tension slowly released as Mira stood there.

"How much longer do I have to stand here? Yule is calling me." Mira inquired. Jones looked at Mira and moved his head signaling her to go. "Go on, go," Jones mumbled as Kali and Lily talked to one another. "Hey, I have to go as well," Lily said as she started walking away. "As well? Jones called out after Lily. What do you mean as well?" Jones stopped for a second waiting for a response. "Didn't Kali say he was leaving?" Lily looked at Jones confused. Kali shook his head. "I was about to, but I've said nothing. I was here simply to thank Jones and tell him if he needed an app, I'd make one for him." Jones smiled. "There may be hope after all," he said softly to himself as the two of them looked at Jones. "Right man. Well, we're going to go now. We'll see you at graduation." Kali and Lily walked down the hillside towards the front of the school as Jones finished his sketch of Mira. "This better have been a good use of our time Jones," Mira said as she slowly disappeared towards the other side. Jones stood up staring at the sheet of paper he had done feeling proud of his mediocre art skills. He was going to show it at graduation and make it into a joke about the mind. "My plan is foolproof. No one will suspect a thing." He said smiling to himself. Jones continued to practice his speech as the sunset slowly came upon the school. He meandered slowly towards his car ready to go home. Jones saw a flower popping up out of the grass. He stopped to stare at it trying to give himself a piece of mind. He hadn't forgotten that humanity's imagination was still at risk. That the watchers had their own problems. He wondered what would happen when their newer technology was freed. When each watcher was no longer suppressed by the confinement of societal hierarchy. Jones bent down to run his hand over the flower, trying to give himself a sense of his little humanity. He felt desensitized to people around him after all that had happened. He started to wonder if there were others out there like Axel and Bey who saw the world the way he did. Others with more control over their mindset collectively coming together to secretly improve upon the world humanity lived in. Jones picked the flower giving it a smell before tossing it aside to the ground where it would be forgotten. That is until his action would later lead to that flower growing into a tree. A net

CHAPTER TWENTY-SEVEN – MIRA'S APPEARANCE.

cast upon itself the same as Jones had unknowingly done by all the people he had talked to. Time ripples were different from Jones's conversations now. Since Jones had made those conversations without realizing it, he thought he had changed the world around him through the missions given while living inside of his own head. However, Jones had inspired some of the smartest people in the world to create his ideas into existence. Ideas where he could not build, others did not. Jones walked towards his car as he looked out over the horizon watching the sunset go down.

Soon his graduation would prove the end of a new beginning and a call he didn't ask for. "Expect the unexpected. Isn't that what I have always told you?" Yule's voice rang in his head. "No Yule. We have only met this year." Yule stopped for a moment. "You're right. I have been telling you in other ways with signs by leaves and wind. This is the first time I've used my words with you." Jones sat back in his chair driving his car. "Oh. So, it's been you leading me in these directions this whole time, has it?" Jones asked. "Yes. I am the one guiding you. Nepharius had been watching you directly. I have been secretly pulling these signs behind him so he would not recognize me." Yule moved his finger as a leaf went in front of Jones' car. Jones continued to watch the leaf as a red light initiated at the same time. "You understand now? All of the pieces of time make sense to you again don't they arbiter? He said in a low tone. "I suppose I can connect the dots that aren't there more easily," Jones said in retort. He continued to drive forward, irritated that Yule was showing him the opposite of what Jones thought was to be his fate. "You're lucky you were only baited to that hospital. It will be shut down soon for further renovations." Yule said. "I'm sorry to have put your life in danger. You have been a great help thus far." Jones didn't know if he was to feel angry or happy. Yule's voice disappeared as Jones made his turn. He arrived back at his house where the door was open. His mother was gardening out front. "Mira will become real, won't she?" Yule asked Jones. "A helpful agent would be nice," Jones said in return, trying to be kind to Yule. "I have an idea and it seems to work." Yule nodded. "Right then. You've got work to do." Jones smiled at Yule. "Thanks, without you I don't know where I'd be."

His mother walked up to his car window as Jones waved. "Hey, mom!" Jones said as he got out of the car hugging her. His mom ran up to him "Congrats on finishing your associate's degree!" she said beaming. Jones turned to her, "I'm going to go get my bachelor's degree now mom. I think it's time." She smiled, "I didn't think you'd ever go back to school. I'm proud of you son. We will work out the finances to get you in." She smiled. "I've already discussed it with your father. We didn't expect you to get your transfer credits, but you did it." Jones cheered his mom as he looked inside of the house. "I guess we're celebrating tonight?" he asked his mom. "Yes, I have champagne on the table for your accomplishment!" she said, encouraging him. "Well, I still have a speech to say on graduation day," Jones said in return. "A speech?" she asked. "Yeah, I'm supposed to speak in front of everyone," Jones said as his mom looked at him confused but surprised. "Well, okay sir." She scoffed as she stopped hugging him. "I find that odd. Are you well prepared?" she asked. Jones poured himself a glass. "Yeah, mom. I've been studying it all day. Everything I wrote is in that essay format." Jones said. "I'm feeling pretty good that I'll be able to deliver it." She looked at him. "We are proud of you. Your father and I are both still surprised. We are happy that you've decided to continue higher education." She continued. "As I mentioned before we still have to work out the finances, but your father will cover half of your housing for the state school system." Jones smiled. "Thanks, mom. That will be a great help. What do you think of this character I drew?" He said holding it up to his mother. "That's interesting. What does she represent?" Jones said to his mom. "Her name is Mira. She's sort of an idea I have going. She's an agent." His mom played along with Jones's idea. "An agent? That sounds interesting. Tell me more." She said as he sat down at the table. "Well, she is sort of this agent of humanity. She's meant to protect our imaginations and watch over us from close by while still being far away." His mom replied, "Like a deity or god?" Jones shook his head. "No, a human-like us hidden within the confinements of our own thoughts." He replied.

CHAPTER TWENTY-SEVEN – MIRA'S APPEARANCE.

His mom nodded her head. "Okay…that's a cool idea." She said, trying to follow Jones' thoughts. "What does this agent do?" Jones shook his head. "Protect our thoughts." His mom looked at him. "Well, it sounds like a fun story." She dismissed Jones's admittance of Mira as she put dinner on the table. "We have spaghetti and meatballs tonight. We can make a special dinner after your speech day." Jones nodded as he headed towards his room. "Call me when dinner is ready." He said smiling as he got up to sit on the computer and closed his door. Jones sat on his chair thinking about the galaxy and his experiences. Had it all really been for nothing? What else had he done in his state of mind? He loaded up the app messenger looking through it as he noticed he had added the people he ran into along the way. "Who is this?" He questioned. "Hey, we need your help." It read, "Hiynkly here, we have a big problem." Jones read it again. "A big problem." He thought to himself. Should he reply? He blinked his eyes again as the message disappeared. Right, I doubt this is real after all… Right? He blinked again, "We have a big problem. The council of five needs you. Our bus has broken down and we're unable to inspire the watchers. It's out of control up here in Los Angeles. We'll call it crazy-villa." Jones sighed. "Give me a night to think it over." He said hanging up. The man replied, "okay, get us that yellow bus." Jones rolled over and fell asleep as tomorrow's graduation went through his mind. The next day Jones woke up heading to school as he got ready. Fossils in the ground that represented dinosaurs in different poses were seen as Jones got into his silver Jetta. As the car flickered off of the sun. Emotional tears rolled down Jones' cheek as he continued towards school. The way the football field extended across the field stuck out for Jones as he stood on the wooden stage. "Today we have many great students who have contributed a good amount to society." Jones got in the line that extended across the bleachers. "Was I late?" He whispered to Lily as she stood right next to the line "Yeah!" She waved as Jones now stood in line with the rest of them. "Our first guest speaker is a lady who knows no bounds. With three of her children she graduated. Please welcome the student to the stage!" "Thank you! Oh, thank you for letting me speak to the professor. When I first came to the stage, I thought I would never make it. By stage I mean school. I was front and center fighting through life with three hard-to-feed children and a nanny at a hire. I never once gave up and you students shouldn't either. Now I'm standing here speaking to all of you going to a top school on transfer. A top school in America. She took a step down as she waved to everyone. The bleachers slowly filled up as people sat down in their respective places.

"Oh! That's Jones up there!" Jones's mom said to his own two family members. Jones stood behind the woman giving the speech as he prepared to speak next about his essay. The woman continued her speech. "I'm going to hand over the microphone. I want you all to remember. If you feel like giving up. Don't! Keep going strong." The lady stepped down from the podium feeling everything out of control. "This has everything. Everything is worthwhile." She continued privately speaking to Jones. "Even if you freeze up there. Remember that you're not alone."Jones stepped on the stairs looking out among the crowd. "Yeah, man. Yeah!" Jones yelled at the crowd. "Hold on. I'm not here to speak on these matters. I'm just a kid who did some research. I'm not here to stay in the same problems over and over. So, I want you to know that this is all based on a character I called Mira." Jones continued as the crowd tried to follow what he was talking about. "Then so be it"! Jones said. "See this paper? This is how you travel!" Jones showed the paper as no reaction happened. The crowd laughed as Jones held up the paper. "Oops. I meant it as a joke." Jones said laughing and scratching his head. He continued his speech as Mira was posing right beside Jones unseen by the crowd. "I'm waiting for my big debut," Mira said, rolling her eyes. "Come on Jones!" "Ahem," Jones said, starting his speech. "Time is a construct ripped from the hole of one's own emotion. In each plane, characters formed in our minds to create what we love and want. If we imagine ourselves in the world on the same plane new people come to light by the massive force of energy through our creation of ideas. In time we get thirty seconds to think, differentiate and feel. Within those thirty seconds, we think of these ideas.

CHAPTER TWENTY-SEVEN – MIRA'S APPEARANCE.

These things then become real as our ideas now exist within many people now generating that energy. By pushing all of our energy forward in time to that singular point of thrown energy particles from our minds we can open portals to other planes, much like a black hole that sucks inconsistent energy until you reach the other end coming out in pure light. Take Mira for example. If shared with you, she becomes real in your mind. Now that idea is twice as strong." Jones continued his theory.

"See, Mira will appear if all of us think of her." The professors scratched their heads as one person waved for Jones to get off of the stage and finish his speech. "Jones, it's time to go." Jones fought for a moment, "Wait, it's true." He said as a person now grabbed his shoulder lightly and tugged at it. Mira started to be seen by multiple people as they looked at the piece of paper on the stage. Mira appeared by the stairs as the crowd gasped. "This is my research! The research I've been trying to tell you." Jones further proved his case as Mira stood there waving. "You did it, Jones! You gave me reality." Mira smiled as the crowd sat there for a moment before the crowd forgot that it happened. Jones started to walk down the stairs as the professor who grabbed Jones' shoulder paused for a moment. The reaction briefly altered the crowd's memory as people looked at one another as talks of Deja vu echoed through the crowd. Mira stood there in happiness. She stared out over the crowd as each person had questioned why a random lady sat up top of the graduation stage. "Alright then. I'm going to head home." She said towards Jones. Mira went down the stairs excitedly before the crowd realized something. "Is this a trick?" The crowd looked. "Who's that girl?" They asked as each one looked at Jones. "That's my girlfriend congratulating me." Jones lied. Mira had already started walking. "So, to continue my speech I will continue talking about different times. This is time fused together. From the energy we create we temporarily lose our memory if it is too strong which is why many people can't keep up with their ideas. Not remembering moments created collectively or writing them down." Mira joined society happily moving around. "Since then, time has always thrown you for a loop.

However, I will never be stuck in this loop of time forever. Neither will you. The words we have forgotten by society's mediations, hiding them away from our dictionaries and scriptures will continue to dictate this planet's underdevelopment." The crowd slowly sat there confused and then clapped as Jones finished his speech "Thank you," Jones said, stepping down into the new type of life. Other students started to be called out for their diplomas.

"This would be a good time to go back to normal Jones," Mira said anxiously, taking his hand as she walked further escorting him fully away from the stage. She pulled him down towards the front of the place as people looked around for Jones. Jones headed towards his car with Mira as she could be seen. "Nice girl Jones!" A voice yelled as Lily and Kali cheered from a distance. "Best graduation speech I've ever heard. Made zero sense yet so much!" The professors scratched their heads. "That wasn't the original speech we saw in the paper. The professors said to one another trying to read their notes. It was pointless for the professors. None of them were understanding what Jones had said. Jones walked away towards his car as he snuck away while graduation was finishing up. He heard people starting to disperse from the football field where their kids would go on to higher education. Jones drove slowly away towards his home. As he arrived close by, Mira stopped Jones. "Stop, I have to go somewhere. I don't think your mother is ready to see my existence. You did it. I'm here. You can come back to normal for a moment now." Mira put her hand on Jones's shoulder as he woke up out of his own mind. "Where am I?" Jones said Mira laughed. "Home. You really zoned out there." Jones looked at Mira free from his hypnotism as he looked at his cap and gown. "I did it! I really graduated!" He smiled getting out of the car. Jones and Mira smiled as his mom saw them through the window.

"Bye Jones!" Mira waved as she headed down the road towards where the headquarters were. Jones assumed Mira already had a place to stay as he waved her off. His mom walked up to him. "Who was that? She looked

CHAPTER TWENTY-SEVEN – MIRA'S APPEARANCE.

familiar." Jones had connected both of the plains in this instance. He brought Mira into the real world as he had also proven his essay. Although the entire school had forgotten the incident Jones remembered. "No one mom. A friend who lives close by. Her name is Misa. You probably won't see her again" Jones lied. His mother accepted it. "Okay. Welcome home." "As I said I would. I have Mira now on my side." His voice echoed across the galactic space as the watchers cheered in his mind. Jones mumbled under his breath. "It's time to chase Nepharius to where he belongs! Locked up!" Jones said. He went back into his room where he closed the book of arbiters. "I better return this," Jones said as he put it off to the side to return it to the library. His cellphone rang again. Jones reached over to his phone. "I'm in. I have to go to school up in Sonoma though," He looked up at his family and his mom celebrating.Jones realized a new journey awaited him. Sometimes when you're looking for that solution, that item, that big break. You become self-absorbed and start to miss other opportunities. Instead of searching for your solution, if you stop looking it might just appear in front of you, quite like love. "So, what are you going to do now Jones?" An inaudible voice echoed in his head as Jones looked up at the sky. "Finish saving our imaginations." The phone clicked as Jones walked out the door back into the small earth that waited for him. Jones reached into his pocket to look at the compass.

"Time to head west." He said to himself as a squirrel looked at him following Jones from behind. The sun shined down as Jones looked at the sky following the wind that pushed him forward. "You are no match for us, Nepharius!" He said putting the compass back in his pocket. Silence ensued as he smiled to himself while walking down the open road. Jones's roommate stared at him blankly for a moment. "That's why we're in this high-end security place with no way out?" Jones scoffed, he wrote in his journal further documenting the ward. "I have a plan, now that you understand who you are." "Jones! It's time for dinner!" The psychiatrist came by again offering him a plate of food with a packet of salt. Jones sat silently to himself, "Iodine. Follow me Mars 42 we have a chip to find."

Jones's roommate laughed, "Lead the way."

CHAPTER FINALE - THE LETTER

So how does one wake up from reality if that's their own reality? Remember the letter I wrote to you in the beginning about the promise of a tale, my grandfather's woven book? Good old grandfather Niles. He knew something I didn't and when I read that, I dipped into his world! So here I am! A tale full of worthwhile experiences that I, Jones, have taken. To wake up from a reality you've created, you must first understand the reality you've built around you and reverse engineer that to nothing. This is something I should have done sooner. I'm now stuck here at these damned CIA agent hospitals looking for someone. I'm sitting next to another man who gets angry over the fact that we're made of golden stardust. As I mentioned in the beginning, I would be exposing the man of Mars 42, among other things... I'm still sitting in this ward for the second time and the computer nanochip is somewhere around here. I'll find it...

Endorsements

Kufanya Gentry – Captivates the reader from the introduction, this book brings a new perspective on electronic dance music and life taking relatable experiences which turns this into a fun read.

Eric Diaz (Wolf Beats) – As a passionate leader in the music industry and a heartfelt person towards people who need help with mental health this book is entertaining and hits home. Humorous and relatable, who knew space pirates could be so intense?

Bobby K (Treasure Team) – Loved this book, filled with intensity and it's different. You don't really know what's going to happen next. It really takes you through a galactic musical journey.

www.ingramcontent.com/pod-product-compliance
Lightning Source LLC
Chambersburg PA
CBHW031602210526
45464CB00004B/1397